# The Inflammatory Myopathies

Lawrence J. Kagen
Editor

# The Inflammatory Myopathies

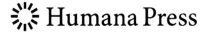 Humana Press

*Editor*
Lawrence J. Kagen
Department of Rheumatology
Weill Medical College of Cornell University
Hospital for Special Surgery
New York Presbyterian Hospital
New York, NY
USA
kagenl@verizon.net

ISBN 978-1-60327-828-7     e-ISBN 978-1-60327-827-0
DOI 10.1007/978-1-60327-827-0
Springer Dordrecht Heidelberg London New York

Library of Congress Control Number: 2009926029

Printed on acid-free paper

Springer is part of Springer Science+Business Media (www.springer.com)

# Preface

This book is dedicated to our readers with the intention of providing an informative exposition of the myositis syndromes. It is also presented in the hope that perhaps it may serve to inspire and stimulate discussion and research into these disabling disorders. Included are descriptions of clinical features, differential diagnosis, pathogenetic mechanisms, and approaches to therapy. Current concepts of classification and diagnostic techniques are also presented.

The production staff at Humana Springer, especially Ms. F. Louie and Ms. C. Walsh, have been instrumental and invaluable in allowing this work to see the light of day.

Above all, the scholarly essays of the contributing authors are acknowledged with gratitude. They have given this volume its character and existence.

New York, NY                                                            Lawrence J. Kagen

# Contents

# Contributors

**Ronald S. Adler, MD, PhD**
Division of Ultrasound and Body Imaging,
Hospital for Special Surgery, Weill Medical College of Cornell University,
New York, NY, USA

**Helene Alexanderson, PhD, RPT**
Department of Physical Therapy,
Orthopedic and Rheumatology Unit, Karolinska University Hospital,
Rheumatology Unit, Department of Medicine, Karolinska Institutet Solna,
Stockholm, Sweden

**Alan N. Baer, MD**
Division of Rheumatology, Johns Hopkins University
School of Medicine, Baltimore, MD, USA

**Hans L. Carlson, MD**
Department of Orthopaedics and Rehabilitation,
Oregon Health and Science University, Portland, OR, USA

**Stephen J. DiMartino, MD, PhD**
Division of Rheumatology, Hospital for Special Surgery,
Weill Medical College of Cornell University, New York,
NY, USA

**Giovanna Garofalo, MD**
Unità Operativa di Immunologia e Allergologia, Ospedale A. Murri,
Fermo, Italy

**Robert A. Greenwald, MD**
Medicine Department, Long Island Jewish
Medical Center, Lake Success, NY, USA

**Thomas A. Griffin, MD, PhD**
William S. Rowe Division of Pediatric Rheumatology, Cincinnati Children's
Hospital Medical Center and University of Cincinnati College of Medicine,
Cincinnati, OH, USA

**Sakir Humayun Gultekin, MD**
Department of Pathology, Division of Neuropathology,
Oregon Health and Science University, Portland, OR, USA

**Lawrence J. Kagen, MD**
Department of Rheumatology, Weill Medical College of Cornell University,
Hospital for Special Surgery, New York Presbyterian Hospital,
New York, NY, USA

**Mark Kagen, MD**
Riverchase Dermatology, Naples, FL, USA

**Eun Ha Kang, MD, PhD**
Division of Rheumatology, Department of Internal Medicine,
Seoul National University Hospital, Seoul, Korea

**Asaf Klein, BSc**
State University of New York, Downstate College of Medicine,
Brooklyn, NY, USA

**Ingrid E. Lundberg, MD, PhD**
Rheumatology Unit, Department of Medicine,
Karolinska University Hospital, Karolinska Institutet Solna,
Stockholm, Sweden

**Galina S. Marder, MD**
The Myositis and Vasculitis Center, North Shore Long Island Jewish Health
System, Albert Einstein College of Medicine, Lake Success, NY, USA

**Frederick W. Miller, MD, PhD**
Environmental Autoimmunity Group,
National Institute of Environmental Health Sciences, National Institutes
of Health, Bethesda, MD, USA

**Lauren M. Pachman, MD**
Division of Rheumatology, Children's Memorial Hospital,
Northwestern University's Feinberg School of Medicine,
FOCIS/CMRC Center of Excellence in Clinical Immunology,
Cure JM Program of Excellence in Juvenile Myositis, Chicago, IL, USA

**Ann M. Reed, MD**
Departments of Pediatrics and Medicine, Division of Rheumatology,
Mayo Clinic College of Medicine, Rochester, MN, USA

**Lisa G. Rider, MD**
Environmental Autoimmunity Group, National Institute
of Environmental Health Sciences, National Institutes of Health,
Bethesda, MD, USA

**Michael Rubin, MD, FRCP(C)**
Department of Neurology, Division of Neuromuscular Disease,
Weill Medical College of Cornell University,
New York, NY, USA

**Carolyn M. Sofka, MD**
Department of Radiology and Imaging, Hospital for Special Surgery,
Weill Medical College of Cornell University, New York, NY, USA

**Yeong Wook Song, MD, PhD**
Division of Rheumatology, Department of Internal Medicine,
Seoul National University Hospital, Seoul, Korea

**Ira N. Targoff, MD**
Department of Medicine, University of Oklahoma Health Sciences Center,
Department of Veterans Affairs Medical Center Oklahoma City, Oklahoma
Medical Research Foundation, Oklahoma City, OK, USA

**Robert L. Wortmann, MD**
Department of Rheumatology, Dartmouth Hitchcock Medical Center,
Lebanon, NH, USA

# Chapter 1
# Evaluation of the Patient

Lawrence J. Kagen

**Abstract** The evaluation of the patient with inflammatory myopathy takes into account the history, physical findings, and ancillary examinations, including laboratory assessment, electromyography, imaging studies, and muscle biopsy. Weakness and its pattern of presentation are the cardinal features. Rash should also be evaluated, if present. Beyond these systems, the possibility of pulmonary, gastrointestinal, or cardiac involvement should be considered and vascular abnormalities, as well as calcification, noted. In active disease, elevation of the activities of certain enzymes in the serum (e.g., creatine kinase) and of serum myoglobin will reflect their loss from muscle tissue and may serve as guides to disease severity or course. Clinical evaluation of these elements, carried out in an ongoing manner, can be used to assess progress and response to therapy.

**Keywords** Weakness • Myalgia • Enzymes • Myoglobin • Creatine kinase

## Introduction

Skeletal or voluntary muscles represent, in the aggregate, approximately 40–45% of our body's weight. The contractile proteins, the molecular mechanisms inherent in muscle structure, account for its ability to contract, relax, and develop force. As a consequence of this property, movement is made possible. Locomotion, skill of performance of tasks, and even the quality of voice depend on the integrity and function of our muscles. The image we present to the world and to ourselves therefore relates in large measure to this tissue system. In this

L.J. Kagen
Department of Rheumatology, Weill Medical College of Cornell University,
Hospital for Special Surgery, New York Presbyterian Hospital, New York, NY, USA
e-mail: kagenl@verizon.net

L.J. Kagen (ed.), *The Inflammatory Myopathies*,
DOI 10.1007/978-1-60327-827-0_1,
© Humana Press. a part of Springer Science + Business Media, LLC 2009

regard, it might be imagined that because of the prominence and visibility of muscle function, disorders of the voluntary muscles would be immediately apparent. However, disorders of the muscular system, the myopathies, in some cases may go undiagnosed for long periods of time.

There are in general two reasons for this seeming paradox. First, muscular dysfunction can arise insidiously and slowly and cause subtle changes that may not be immediately evident. Second, it may be difficult to assign symptoms of muscle disease to the skeletal muscles even when abnormalities in their function are recognized. Symptoms such as weakness or fatigue may be ascribed to other causes or to other organ systems. Even when myopathy is considered and a diagnosis is made, the assessment of its course and the clinical state of the affected individual may at times be difficult to delineate with precision *(1)*.

The recognition of myopathy generally begins with symptoms of weakness, fatigue, or muscle pain. As mentioned, the relation of these symptoms to muscle dysfunction may initially be difficult to ascribe. This is particularly true early in the course of inflammatory myopathy. For example, in inclusion body myositis, which usually affects older individuals, symptoms may be thought to be due to the natural course of aging or to poor conditioning rather than to a pathological process of muscle. If present, cardiovascular, pulmonary, or metabolic comorbidities can confound the diagnosis. Further, techniques of physical examination may lack the sensitivity needed to detect small changes in strength from normal or from what was earlier present.

All of this presents the paradox of a large and evident tissue system whose dysfunction may yet remain enigmatic and elude diagnosis. For these reasons, in appropriate situations, the presence of myopathy should be considered and the history taken and physical examination performed with this possibility in mind.

## Clinical Findings

### *Weakness*

Weakness is a prominent feature of myopathic states. It is important to ascertain which muscle groups are involved and the degree to which they are affected. Most symptoms in patients with inflammatory myopathies are prominent in proximal musculature.

With involvement of these muscles in the upper extremity, patients will experience difficulty in lifting objects, particularly overhead; brushing the hair; using a hair dryer; hanging up clothing; or putting objects into cabinets or the refrigerator. In acquiring the history, it is good to make note of specifics, such as the weights or types of objects, that cause difficulty. This will prove useful for comparison over time in assessing progress or response to therapy.

Weakness of the proximal musculature in the lower extremity is manifested by difficulty in arising from a chair or toilet seat, going up or down stairs, getting out of an automobile, or lifting the legs to put on pants or other garments. Again, to the degree possible, specifics should be noted.

Symptoms arising in distal musculature usually suggest more severe or more chronic forms of myositis. Difficulty in writing or opening jars is noted with upper extremity distal involvement; tripping on curbs or uneven surfaces occurs with muscle dysfunction of the lower extremities. In inclusion body myositis, however, distal weakness can be present initially. A peculiarly weak handshake with fingers not capable of full firm flexion may be a clue to this illness when the physician first meets the patient. Myotonic dystrophy and the myopathy associated with anti-signal recognition particle (anti-SRP) antibodies are two other examples of myopathies with distal weakness occurring early in the course of illness.

Proximal lower extremity and pelvic girdle weakness make it difficult to arise from the floor after a fall. This can be frightening, and patients affected in this manner can be forced to creep to an article of furniture, or to a means of communication, to secure help in standing. Weakness of the trunk and abdominal muscles may prevent arising from the supine position when in bed. In this case, affected individuals will try to arise by rolling laterally, swinging the legs downward while pushing against the bed with the arms.

The etiology of muscle weakness in patients with myositis likely is multifactorial. Cellular, immune damage, and destruction with resulting loss of myofibers as well as inefficiency of the contractile process in the inflammatory milieu are important elements. In addition, nonimmunological processes resulting from class 1 major histocompatibility complex (MHC) molecule overexpression may initiate endoplasmic reticulum (ER) stress responses. These may arise from overload of the ER with newly synthesized, unfolded peptides, which can then lead to the upregulation of proteolytic, destructive pathways *(2)*. Table 1.1 lists the areas of weakness seen in several of the musculoskeletal disorders.

## *Pain*

Severe muscle pain is not common in the myositis syndromes. Soreness or aching is frequently described by patients with inflammatory myopathy, especially in virally induced syndromes.

Many disorders other than primary myopathies, however, do present with severe muscle pain as the prominent or initial symptom. Polymyalgia rheumatica, for example, is characterized by severe pain and morning stiffness. Fibromyalgia also typically presents with diffuse myalgia. Patients with rheumatoid arthritis complain of stiffness and, on occasion, of muscle pain.

Cramping (painful, sustained involuntary contractions) is a feature of lower motor neuron disorders. Pain with exercise is noted in patients with myopathy

**Table 1.1** Weakness in musculoskeletal disorders

| |
| --- |
| Proximal musculature |
|   Most myopathies, including myositis syndromes and muscular dystrophy |
| Distal musculature |
|   Inclusion body myositis |
|   Myotonic dystrophy |
|   Distal myopathies |
|   Neurogenic disorders (e.g., neuropathy, radiculopathy, myelopathy) |
| Facial musculature |
|   Facioscapular humeral dystrophy |
|   Myasthenia gravis |
|   Myotonic dystrophy |
|   Mitochondrial myopathy (e.g., Kearns Sayres syndrome) |
| Cranial nerve disorders and central nervous system conditions (e.g., Bell's palsy, myasthenia gravis, cerebrovascular accident) |
| Palatal musculature |
|   Inflammatory myopathy (rarely) |
|   Central nervous system disorders |
|   Myasthenia gravis |

Adapted from **Ref. 1**

**Table 1.2** Myalgia

| |
| --- |
| Myositis (e.g., dermatomyositis, polymyositis, infectious, parasitic) |
| Rheumatoid arthritis |
| Polymyalgia rheumatica |
| Metabolic myopathies (disorders of glycogen and lipid metabolism, e.g., McArdle syndrome) |
| Hypothyroidism |
| Drugs (e.g., statin myopathy) |
| Fibromyalgia |
| Lower motor nervous disorders (cramps and fasciculations) |
| Ischemic claudication (arterial insufficiency) |
| Neurogenic claudication (e.g., spinal stenosis) |

Adapted from **Ref. 1**

related to abnormalities in carbohydrate or lipid metabolism as well as in those with mitochondrial myopathies. The myopathy associated with lipid-lowering agents (statin myopathy) is another disorder characterized by pain and spasm of muscles with exertion. Hypothyroidism can be manifested by pain as well as weakness of muscles. Table 1.2 lists a number of disorders that present with muscle pain.

## *Atrophy*

In the early course of most patients with myopathies, muscle volume appears preserved, so that weakness is out of proportion to atrophy. This is in contrast to lower motor neuron disorders in which weakness and atrophy are generally concomitant findings. Later in the course of myopathies, however, atrophy does occur and may become prominent.

## Dermal Manifestations

### *Rash*

Dermatomyositis is characterized by rash over the face, torso, and boney prominences. See Chap. 13 for full discussion.

### *Calcification*

Deposition of calcium, usually in the form of hydroxyapatite, may be a disabling complication in patients with myositis. It is most common in juvenile dermatomyositis but may be seen in adults as well. Calcinosis can occur in the connective tissue investing muscle, resulting in disabling woody induration, or it may be present superficially under the skin. Deposits of calcium can erupt from the latter location as small pebbly masses, as a semisolid cheesy paste, or in semiliquid form. In addition to the hydroxyapatite mineral, these deposits also contain bone matrix proteins such as osteopontin, osteonectin, and bone sialoprotein *(3, 4)*.

## Pulmonary Disorders

Disorders of respiratory function occur frequently in patients with myositis. These may be due to weakness of muscles of respiration or to interstitial pulmonary disease. Interstitial lung disease is not only a concomitant finding in myositis but may even appear prior to the recognition of muscle involvement. In addition, interstitial pulmonary disease may occur as the result of muscle disease with hypoventilation and poor pulmonary mechanics. It can also be due to aspiration in patients with pharyngeal or esophageal dysmotility. Infection or, rarely, drug sensitivity or toxicity (e.g., to methotrexate, cyclophosphamide) may also give rise to pulmonary disorders. See Chap. 12 for a full discussion of this entity.

## Cardiac Manifestations

Electrocardiographic abnormalities, including heart block and dysrhythmias, have been noted in patients with myositis. Even though clinical features of heart disease are rarely marked, congestive heart failure has occurred as the result of myocardial involvement, and postmortem evaluation has demonstrated inflammation and fibrosis of the cardiac muscle in patients with myositis *(5–9)*.

## Vascular Findings

Vascular involvement can be prominent in inflammatory myopathy, particularly in children with dermatomyositis. In these patients, the terminal components of the complement system, C5–C9, are found on the endothelium of affected vessels. These vessels may appear histologically normal or may exhibit endothelial swelling, inflammation, and obliteration. Other tissues can be affected in this way as well and consequently may undergo loss of vasculature. Capillaries, venules, and arterioles in many areas, including the skin, gastrointestinal tract, nerves, fat, nail beds, and even the retina, may be affected. These vascular changes, if severe, may lead to thrombosis, causing infarction and ischemia of involved tissues. Ischemic vasculopathy of the bowel can result in perforation, a grave complication of childhood dermatomyositis. Ischemia of the skin may be the cause of ulcerative lesions. Raynaud's phenomenon, representing transient digital ischemia, is common in patients with myositis *(10–14)*.

## Gastrointestinal Involvement

Although dysmotility of the stomach and small and large bowel may occur, dysphagia secondary to esophageal dysfunction is the most prominent gastrointestinal symptom in patients with myositis syndromes. It represents a serious manifestation that may be complicated by aspiration, either acutely or chronically. Dysphagia can be caused by abnormalities of muscle function of the oropharynx; however, it is esophageal dysfunction due to dysmotility or cricopharyngeal achalasia that is most prominent.

   In addition to dysphagia and dysmotility, vascular involvement of the bowel may rarely lead to ischemic ulceration, necrosis, perforation, and catastrophic complications, most notably in juvenile dermatomyositis, but even in adults *(15–19)*.

## Laboratory Assays

### *Serum Enzymes*

During the course of muscle disease or following injury, muscle tissue cytoplasmic enzymes may appear in the circulation in increased amounts. Assay of these enzymes has become the most commonly used laboratory approach for the evaluation of patients with a myopathy. Indeed, the presence of elevated levels of these enzymes on routine examination, especially those of creatine kinase (CK), has often led to the discovery of subclinical or otherwise unsuspected myopathic disorders.

It should be kept in mind, however, that these enzymes are present in many tissues of the body, so that none is absolutely specific for the detection of skeletal muscle disease. Lactate dehydrogenase (LDH), aldolase, and the transaminases are widely distributed in many cell types. CK, however, is present mainly in muscle and nervous tissue, and on this account its assay has a greater degree of tissue specificity than that of the other enzymes mentioned. Only rarely will disease of skeletal muscle cause elevation in the serum activity of the other enzymes in the absence of an elevation of that of CK.

In an attempt to increase the specificity of the total enzyme assay, detection of isoenzymes has been employed. Many of the enzymes (e.g., CK and LDH) occur in isoenzymic forms that differ in concentration in different tissues. The determination of the isoenzyme type of enzyme protein giving rise to the serum activity assayed can therefore be used as a guide to the tissue from which the enzyme was released. Although isoenzyme analysis of serum (commonly by electrophoresis) was frequently used in the past, this approach is currently employed less often, and total enzyme activity alone is most commonly assayed.

The clinician should also keep in mind that not only may enzymes arise from different tissues or organs, but most clinically employed assays reflect enzyme activity rather than molecular content. Artifacts resulting from specimen handling or the presence of inhibitors or interfering substances may affect the final reported values. In this connection, effects on enzyme assay due to interfering factors have been noted for CK, aldolase, LDH, and transaminases (1). Fortunately, these effects will only rarely cause major variations but nonetheless on occasion may be of importance. In addition, hyperlipoproteinemia and hemolysis of the serum sample may also cause interference with assay results (20, 21).

## Creatine Kinase

Creatine kinase catalyzes the interconversion of adenosine triphosphate (ATP) and creatine phosphate and controls the flow of energy, in the form of high-energy phosphate, within the muscle cell.

### Action of Creatine Kinase

$$\text{Creatine} + \text{ATP} \leftrightarrow \text{creatine phosphate} + \text{ADP}$$

In clinical practice, estimation of serum levels of the CK enzyme is one of the most useful and practical guides to the presence, severity, and course of muscle disorders. CK is present in greatest concentration in muscle and nervous tissue. It exists as a dimer composed of two subunits, M and B, therefore giving rise to three isoenzymic forms: CK MM, CK MB, and CK BB.

### Isoenzymes of Creatine Kinase

Within skeletal muscle, 90–95% of the enzyme is in the MM isoenzyme form. Small amounts of MB are also present. In cardiac muscle, 20–30% of the enzyme is in the MB isoenzyme form. The BB form is predominant in nervous tissue and smooth muscle. The MB form of CK is present in embryonic muscle, and elevated levels of this isoenzymic form have been found in skeletal muscle of infants.

With inflammation or injury of skeletal muscle, rapid and dramatic increases in serum levels of CK MM occur. The MB form, however, can also be found in increased amounts in serum not only after cardiac injury but also in chronic disorders of skeletal muscle such as dystrophies and inflammatory muscle disease. In the last cases, these increases have been postulated to be the result of release from regenerating myofibers or from chronically damaged myofibers, which may synthesize increased amounts of the B subunit, as was the case in their earlier development.

On rare occasions, a patient with active myositis may present with CK values in the normal range. The reason for this remains obscure, although the presence of an inhibitor to the assay in serum may play a role *(22–25)*.

## *Aldolase*

Aldolase is widely found in tissues of the body. It catalyzes the aldol cleavage of fructose-phosphate, a 6-carbon moiety, to the two 3-carbon moieties dihydroxyacetone phosphate and glyceraldehyde-phosphate.

### Action of Aldolase

Fructose-1, 6-diphosphate $\leftrightarrow$ glyceraldehyde-3-phosphate + dihydroxyacetone phosphate

Human aldolase exists in enzyme subtypes denoted A, B, and C (Table 1.3). Aldolase A is expressed primarily in muscle and erythrocytes; B in liver, kidney, and small intestine; and C in brain and smooth muscle. In addition to its dominant

**Table 1.3** Tissues rich in aldolase

| Aldolase type | Tissue |
| --- | --- |
| A | Muscle |
| B | Liver, kidney, small intestine |
| C | Brain, smooth muscle |

role in the glycolytic pathway, aldolase may also have other intracellular functions, binding to macromolecules such as F-actin and vacuolar $H^+$-ATPase (adenosine triphosphatase).

Aldolase is composed of four subunits. During embryogenesis, both types A and C are present in skeletal muscle. After birth, aldolase A is the predominant form present in muscle. Aldolase A therefore is the form released into the circulation in patients with myositis and other myopathies. In chronic myopathic states, however, the C form may be produced and released from muscle, resulting in the presence of A C hybrid forms of the enzyme in the serum.

Increases in total serum aldolase activity are noted in skeletal and cardiac muscle disorders as well as disorders of many other tissues, such as liver and the blood-forming organs *(26, 27)*.

## Lactate Dehydrogenase

Lactate dehydrogenase is widely distributed in body tissue. It catalyzes the interconversion of lactate and pyruvate.

### Action of Lactate Dehydrogenase

$$Pyruvate + NADH \leftrightarrow lactate + NAD$$

The enzyme is a tetramer, consisting of four subunits, of two types, M and H. There are therefore five isomeric forms that exist in serum: LDH-1, $H_4$; LDH-2, $H_3M$; LDH-3, $H_2M_2$; LDH-4, $HM_3$; and LDH-5, $M_4$.

### Isoenzymes of LDH

Skeletal muscle contains each of the LDH isoenzyme species, with the M subunit in greatest concentration in fast-twitch fibers and the H subunit greatest in the slow-twitch fibers. The proportions of these isoenzymes in individual muscles vary between different individuals; however, certain muscles, such as the gluteus medius and soleus, are richest in LDH-1 and LDH-2, whereas the gastrocnemius and triceps brochii generally contain greater amounts of LDH-3 and LDH-4. In skeletal muscle disease, LDH levels in serum increase, with the isoenzyme pattern reflecting which muscles are involved. Cardiac muscle damage results in greatest increases in LDH-1 and LDH-2. In cases of muscle trauma, the rise in LDH may occur after that of CK and be more prolonged. In some patients with myositis in remission, levels of LDH may remain elevated after CK levels have diminished. Marked increases in LDH activity in the circulation also are seen in hepatic disorders, renal disease, and hemolytic anemia *(28–31)*.

## *Transaminases*

### Aspartate Aminotransferase

Aspartate aminotransferase (AST) is present in greatest activity in skeletal and cardiac muscle and liver. It is also widely distributed in other tissues. This enzyme catalyzes the reversible reaction, converting aspartate to glutamate.

### Action of Aspartate Aminotransferase

Aspartate + alpha ketoglutarate $\leftrightarrow$ oxalacetate + glutamate

Elevated levels in the serum are found in myopathy, cardiac disorders (e.g., myocardial infarction), as well as liver disease and in patients with pulmonary emboli.

### Alanine Aminotransferase

Alanine aminotransferase (ALT) *(32, 33)* is present in greatest activity in liver, kidney, and cardiac and skeletal muscle. It is also widely distributed in other tissues. Elevated serum levels occur not only in liver diseases such as hepatitis and biliary obstruction but also in cardiac disorders and myopathies.

The enzyme catalyzes the interconversion of alanine to glutamate.

### Action of Alanine Aminotransferase

Alanine + alpha ketoglutarate $\leftrightarrow$ pyruvate + glutamate

Interference in the assay for ALT, caused by elevated levels of immunoglobulins in sera of patients with multiple myeloma, can artifactually cause results that are higher than expected.

## *Myoglobin*

Myoglobin is the oxygen-binding respiratory protein of skeletal and cardiac muscle. Each molecule is made up of a heme group linked to a single polypeptide globin chain. An iron atom coordinated with a porphyrin group makes up the heme moiety, where molecular oxygen is reversibly bound. For comparison, molecules of hemoglobin, the respiratory protein of the red blood cell, are roughly four times the size of myoglobin molecules. They each contain four globin chains and

**Table 1.4**   Characteristics of myoglobin and hemoglobin

|  | Myoglobin molecule | Hemoglobin molecule |
|---|---|---|
| Size | One iron atom | Four iron atoms |
|  | One heme group | Four heme groups |
|  | One globin chain | Four globin chains |
| Function | Oxygen binding | Oxygen binding |
| Site | Muscle cell | Red blood cell |

four heme groups, in contrast to the single heme group and globin chain of the myoglobin molecule (Table 1.4). Myoglobin binds oxygen at lower oxygen tensions than does hemoglobin, favoring the ability of myoglobin to upload oxygen into muscle tissue under conditions in which hemoglobin would release it. Myoglobin therefore may function to facilitate oxygen transport into muscle as well as an oxygen storage protein for muscle.

As in the case of the cytoplasmic enzymes, muscle injury (whether to cardiac or skeletal muscle) results in the efflux of myoglobin into the circulation. Its levels there reflect the severity of muscle damage and disease. Unlike the enzymes, however, myoglobin occurs only in muscle, so that assay of its content in serum has specificity for skeletal or cardiac muscle. Its serum levels can be used not only to indicate the severity of myopathy but also to guide assessments of its course and response to therapy.

In severe states of muscle injury, such as those that occur with massive trauma, burns, or chemically induced rhabdomyolysis, large amounts of myoglobin can be released into the circulation and from there appear in the urine. Severe or persistent myoglobinuria may be associated with renal failure. In inflammatory muscle disease, levels of myoglobin in the circulation generally do not reach these amounts, so myoglobinuric renal failure usually does not occur and is rarely reported *(34–36)*.

# References

1. Kagen LJ. History, physical examination and laboratory tests in the evaluation of myopathy. In: Wortmann RL, ed. Diseases of skeletal muscle. Philadelphia, PA: Lippincott Williams and Wilkins, 2000:255–66.
2. Nagaraju K, Casciola-Rosen L, Lundberg I, et al. Activation of the endoplasmic reticulum stress response in autoimmune myositis. Arthritis Rheum 2005;52:1824–35.
3. Stock S, Ignatiev K, Lee P, et al. Pathological calcification in juvenile dermatomyositis (JDM): micro CT and synchotron X-ray diffraction reveal hydroxyapatite with varied micro structures. Connect Tissue Res, 2004;45:248–56.
4. Pachman LM, Veis A, Stock S, et al. Composition of calcifications in children with juvenile dermatomyositis: association with chronic cutaneous inflammation. Arthritis Rheum 2006; 54:3345–50.
5. Denbow CE, Lie JT, Tancredi R, Bunch TW. Cardiac involvement in polymyositis. Arthritis Rheum 1979;22:1088–92.
6. Haupt HM, Hutchins GM. The heart and cardiac conducting system in polymyositis-dermatomyositis. Am J Cardiol 1982;50:998–1006.

7. Lundberg IE. The heart in dermatomyositis and polymyositis. Rheumatology 2006;45(Suppl 4): 18–21.
8. Senechal M, Crête M, Couture C, Poirier P. Myocardial dysfunction in polymyositis. Can J Cardiol 2006;22:869–71.
9. Finsterer J, Stöllberger C, Avanzini M, Rauschka H. Restrictive cardiomyopathy in dermatomyositis. Scand J Rheumatol 2006;35:229–32.
10. Kissel JT, Mendell JR, Rammohan KW. Micro-vascular deposition of complement membrane attack complex in dermatomyositis. N Engl J Med 1986;314:329–34.
11. Crowe WE, Bove KE, Levinson JE, Hilton PK. Clinical and pathogenetic implications of histopathology in childhood polydermatomyositis. Arthritis Rheum 1982;25:126–39.
12. Bowyer SL, Clark RAF, Ragsdale CG, et al. Juvenile dermatomyositis: histological findings and pathogenetic hypothesis for the associated skin changes. J Rheumatol 1986;13:753–9.
13. Gunawadena H, Harris ND, Carmichael C, McHugh NJ. Microvascular responses following digital thermal hyperaemia and iontophoresis measured by laser Doppler imaging in idiopathic inflammatory myopathy. Rheumatology 2007;46:1483–6.
14. Venkatesh P, Bhaskar VM, Keshavamurthy R, Garg S. Proliferative vascular retinopathy in polymyositis and dermatomyositis with scleroderma (overlap syndrome). Ocul Immunol Inflamm 2007;15:45–9.
15. Kagen LJ, Hochman RB, Strong EW. Cricopharyngeal obstruction in inflammatory myopathy. Arthritis Rheum 1985;6:630–6.
16. Oh TH, Brumfield KA, Hoskin TL, et al. Dysphagia in inflammatory myopathy: clinical characteristics, treatment strategies and outcome in 62 patients. Mayo Clin Proc 2007; 82:441–7.
17. McCann LJ, Garay SM, Ryan MM, et al. Oropharyngeal dysphagia in juvenile dermatomyositis (JDM): an evaluation of videofluoroscopy swallow study (VFSS) changes in relation to clinical symptoms and objective muscle scores. Rheumatology 2007;46:1363–6.
18. Tweezer-Zaks N, Ben-Horin S, Schilby G, et al. Severe gastrointestinal inflammation in adult dermatomyositis: characterization of a novel clinical association. Am J Med Sci 2006; 332:308–13.
19. Mamyrova G, Kleiner DE, James-Newton L, et al. Late onset gastrointestinal pain in juvenile dermatomyositis as a manifestation of ischemic ulceration from chronic end arteropathy. Arthritis Rheum (Arthritis Care Res) 2007;57:881–4.
20. Kagen LJ. Laboratory assays useful in assessment of patients with disorders of muscle. In: Cohen AS, ed. Laboratory diagnostic procedures in the rheumatic diseases. Orlando, FL: Grune and Stratton, 1985:315–27.
21. Wu AHB, Perryman MB. Clinical applications of muscle enzymes and proteins. Curr Opin Rheumatol 1992;4:815–20.
22. Dawson DM, Fine IH. Creatine kinase in human tissues. Arch Neurol 1975;16:175–80.
23. Eppenberger HM. A brief summary of the detection of creatine kinase isoenzymes. Mol Cell Biochem 1994;133-134:9–11.
24. Wallimann T, Wyss M, Brdiczka D, et al. Intracellular compartmentation, structure and function of creatine kinase isoenzymes in tissues with high and fluctuating energy demands: the phosphocreatine circuit for cellular energy homeostasis. Biochem J 1992;28:21–40.
25. Kagen LJ, Aram S. Creatine kinase activity inhibitor in sera from patients with muscle disease. Arthritis Rheum 1987;30:213–7.
26. Arakaki TL, Pezza JA, Cronin MA, et al. Structure of human brain fructose 1,6-(bis) phosphate aldolase: linking isozyme structure with function. Protein Sci 2004;13:3077–84.
27. Tzvetanova E. Aldolase isoenzymes in patients with progressive muscular dystrophy and in human fetuses. Clin Chem 1971;17:926–30.
28. Emery AEH. The determination of lactate dehydrogenase isoenzymes in normal human muscle and other tissues. Biochem J 1967;105:599–604.
29. Markert CL. Lactate dehydrogenase isoenzymes. Cell Biochem Funct 1984;2:131–4.
30. Gollnick PD, Armstrong RB. Histochemical localization of lactate dehydrogenase isoenzymes in human skeletal muscle fibers. Life Sci 1975;18:27–31.

31. Bruns DE, Emerson JC, Intemann S, et al. Lactate dehydrogenase isoenzyme-1. Changes during the first day after myocardial infraction. Clin Chem 1981;27:1821–3.
32. Edge K, Chinoy H, Cooper RG. Serum alanine aminotransferase elevations correlated with serum creatine kinase levels in myositis. Rheumatology 2006;45:487–8.
33. Nathwani RA, Pais S, Reynolds TB, Kaplowitz N. Serum alanine aminotransferase in skeletal muscle diseases. Hepatology 2005;41:380–2.
34. Kagen LJ. Myoglobin. New York: Columbia University Press, 1973.
35. Lovece S, Kagen LJ. Sensitive rapid detection of myoglobin in serum of patients with myopathy by immunoturbidometric assay. J Rheumatol 1993;20:1331–4.
36. Targoff IN. Laboratory testing in the diagnosis and management of idiopathic inflammatory myopathies. Rheum Dis Clin North Am 2002;28:859–90.

# Chapter 2
# Classification of Idiopathic Inflammatory Myopathies

**Frederick W. Miller**

**Abstract**  Although it has been long recognized that inflammatory muscle disease of unknown etiology may present clinically and respond to therapy in a variety of ways, our approaches regarding how to best classify or divide these entities into more understandable groups of patients has evolved as larger series have been studied using advanced laboratory, immunopathologic, and genetic technologies. In addition to the traditional clinicopathologic classifications of these entities, there is increasing interest in using newer methods, including serology, environmental exposures, and molecular genetics, to divide these syndromes into more homogeneous subsets. While our understanding of these disorders is far from complete, it is clear that the inflammatory myopathies are composed of many separate and distinct disorders with widely divergent clinical signs, symptoms, pathology, laboratory abnormalities, immune responses, genetic and environmental risk factors, and prognoses. Classification of the inflammatory myopathies remains unsatisfactory and controversial, with a number of competing approaches currently in use. Nonetheless, while many different schemes have been proposed, this chapter focuses on the classifications based on clinical signs, pathology, and autoantibodies that today are useful in assessing subjects, as well as possible new approaches that take into account environmental exposures and immunogenetics. Our understanding of the pathogenesis, classification, and prognosis of the inflammatory myopathies will become more complete as we decipher the interrelationships among all the critical features of disease—including the genetic and environmental risk factors necessary and sufficient for the induction of myositis—and develop more rational ways of dividing and treating these increasingly recognized syndromes.

F.W. Miller

Environmental Autoimmunity Group, Office of Clinical Research, National Institute of Environmental Health Sciences, NIH, HHS, National Institutes of Health Clinical Research Center, Bethesda, MD 20892-1301, USA

e-mail: millerf@mail.nih.gov

L.J. Kagen (ed.), *The Inflammatory Myopathies*,
DOI 10/1007/978-1-60327-827-0_2,
© Humana Press. a part of Springer Science + Business Media, LLC 2009

**Keywords** Clinicopathologic • Serologic • Myositis-specific autoantibodies • Environmental • Genetic • Phenotypes

## Defining the Idiopathic Inflammatory Myopathies

It is often difficult to define rare forms of disease whose pathogeneses remain obscure, and the idiopathic inflammatory myopathies (IIMs) are no exception. A primary problem is that sharp boundaries do not exist among many of the syndromes that result in muscle weakness, and none of the multiple competing current diagnostic criteria is able to divide reliably all IIM cases from the many dystrophic, metabolic, infectious, and other causes of myopathy *(1)*. Whatever classification criteria are used, a significant number of patients seen in referral centers still defy diagnosis, and empiric therapies are often required. Also, because different specialists tend to use different ways to identify and evaluate myositis patients, it remains difficult to integrate the literature in the field regarding the clinical utility of different classification schemes. Furthermore, the systemic nature of many of these disorders and the resulting cutaneous, cardiac, pulmonary, and gastrointestinal manifestations can confuse the presentation and result in misdiagnosis and delayed therapy.

While imperfect, the criteria for the diagnosis of polymyositis (PM) and dermatomyositis (DM) proposed by Bohan and Peter *(2)* over 30 years ago remain useful today with certain modifications. Due to the limitations inherent in the Bohan and Peter criteria, a group of specialists interested in standardizing the assessment and study of IIMs, the International Myositis Assessment and Clinical Studies Group, or IMACS, has revised these criteria to include the need for a muscle biopsy consistent with the diagnosis of PM and the need for the presence of specific rashes to define DM *(3)*. Thus, after rigorously excluding the many other causes of myopathy, the presence of the following criteria usually establishes a diagnosis: for PM, the finding of proximal muscle weakness, elevated serum levels of sarcoplasmic enzymes, myopathic changes on electromyography, and a muscle biopsy showing myofiber degeneration and regeneration with chronic inflammatory infiltrates; in the case of DM, the presence of the heliotrope rash or Gottron's papules. The diagnosis of inclusion body myositis (IBM) was accepted by IMACS as that defined by Greggs et al. *(4)*.

Some groups have proposed that using the Bohan and Peter criteria *(2)* will over- or misdiagnose these conditions and proposed alternative pathologic approaches *(5)*. However, given the limited data available today, it remains unclear if use of these alternative approaches will actually improve patient therapies or outcomes *(6)*. Nonetheless, it is clear that even the IMACS-modified Bohan and Peter criteria have limitations, and it is useful to consider additional clues that can lead to the diagnosis of IIM in unclear cases. These include the presence of certain autoantibodies, a family history of autoimmunity, other signs of connective tissue disease in the patient, symmetric inflammatory changes on magnetic resonance imaging of muscle, and a clinical response to immunosuppressive therapy *(7)*. In fact, it has been clear for some time that new criteria are needed to define the IIMs and to subclassify them; a large international study is now ongoing to accomplish these tasks (see http://www.niehs. nih.gov/research/resources/collab/imacs/classificationcriteria.cfm). Until the patho- genetic mechanisms of these disorders are defined and the distinctions among the types of IIMs substantiated, these syndromes will remain diagnoses of exclusion and heterogeneous complexes of clinical signs, symptoms, and laboratory findings that fulfill the criteria discussed rather than unique disorders. It is hoped that the deficiencies in the current classifications will become clearer as we understand the interrelationships of the many features of the different forms of myositis. Many new biomarker technologies, including advances in genetics, proteomics, and gene expression arrays, will also surely have an impact in assisting in the future diagnosis and classification of myositis.

## Clinicopathologic Classifications

Since clinical and histopathologic features are what physicians focus on in the evaluation of patients with muscle weakness or elevated creatine kinase (CK) activity and because these features have been useful in defining different groups of myositis patients in terms of severity of disease, responses to therapy, and prognoses, the major classification schemes are based on these elements. As is the case with all forms of classification, however, there remains disagreement in the field regarding the appropriate ways of applying clinicopathologic features to divide the myositis syndromes. A modification of several previously proposed clinicopathologic clas- sifications is listed in Table 2.1. Unfortunately, these categories are not all mutually exclusive. For example, juvenile myositis patients may also be categorized as having PM, DM, myositis in association with another connective tissue disease (overlap myositis), or even rarely cancer-associated myositis (CAM), or IBM. It remains unclear which of these diagnostic divisions is more important because no study has had adequate numbers of patients within these many categories to address this question appropriately in a multivariate analysis. Certain entities (e.g., focal or nodular myositis, myositis ossificans, and macrophagic myofasciitis) have been included in this discussion because they may develop as a result of distinct etiologic mecha- nisms; however, definite clinicopathologic differences have yet to be documented among all these disorders.

Many lines of evidence suggest that primary idiopathic PM differs from primary idiopathic DM. Support includes differences in clinical presentation, histopathol- ogy, the number and distribution of both circulating and muscle-infiltrating CD4+ and CD8+ T cells and B cells, responses to therapy, different environmental exposures, and genetics (reviewed in *(7)*. Controversy continues regarding whether a distinct entity known as DM without myositis (*dermatomyositis sine myositis*) exists or if this is simply one end of a spectrum of disease severity *(8)*.

**Table 2.1** A clinicopathologic classification of the idiopathic inflammatory myopathies[a]

| Clinicopathologic category | Associations and comments |
|---|---|
| Polymyositis | A diagnosis of exclusion: defined by the absence of all the features below in a patient meeting IIM criteria; muscle biopsy often shows endomysial infiltration of myocytes, primarily by CD8[+] T cells |
| Dermatomyositis | Heliotrope rash or Gottron's papules are pathognomonic, but other rashes may be present; myositis may be clinically absent but can be seen by biopsy or magnetic resonance imaging (MRI); muscle biopsy often shows perifascicular atrophy, microvascular changes, and deposits of the membrane attack complex and prominent perivascular CD4[+] T cells and B cells |
| Myositis associated with another connective tissue disease | Mild myositis, good response to therapy; rheumatoid arthritis, systemic sclerosis, and lupus are most common as overlaps |
| Juvenile myositis | Age of onset <18 years, frequent calcifications, occasional gastrointestinal vasculitis; better responses to therapy and outcomes than adult forms |
| Cancer-associated myositis | Myositis onset often within 2 years of the diagnosis of cancer; different cancers may be overrepresented in polymyositis (PM) and dermatomyositis (DM) |
| Inclusion body myositis | Occurs mainly in older white men with insidious onset and progression and poor response to therapy; asymmetric distal weakness with wrist and index finger flexors weaker than extensors; rimmed vacuoles and amyloid found in myofibers with characteristic tubulofilaments on ultrastructural analysis |
| Granulomatous myositis | Granulomas prominent in muscle biopsy; can be seen in sarcoidosis |
| Eosinophilic myositis | Eosinophils prominent in muscle; can be a part of hypereosinophilic syndrome or eosinophilic fasciitis |
| Vasculitic myositis | Vasculitis prominent in muscle; can be part of other vasculitides, including polyarteritis nodosa |
| Orbital or ocular myositis | Involvement of extraocular muscles only; periorbital pain, proptosis, and diplopia; diagnosis confirmed by ultrasound, computed tomography (CT), or MRI |
| Focal or nodular myositis | Focal involvement of one or more limbs; can progress to polymyositis, remain isolated, or resolve |
| Myositis ossificans | Occurs as a local limited phenomenon or more generalized excessive proliferation of connective tissue and replacement by bone |
| Macrophagic myofasciitis | Persistent fatigue, localized then diffuse myalgia mostly in lower limbs with little or no loss of muscle strength and no muscle wasting; biopsy shows perifascicular cellular infiltrate of clusters of macrophages with occasional CD8[+] lymphocytes and intact muscle fibers; in most cases develops after immunization with aluminum hydroxide-containing vaccines |

[a]Modified from *(53)*; information derived from *(3,4,7,11,18,22,54,55)*; categories are not mutually exclusive

Difficulties in assessing whether a classification scheme should include this as a separate category relate to the frequent delay between the development of the rash and muscle involvement in DM, the relatively mild muscle weakness and lower serum CK levels in DM, and the understandable reluctance of physicians to perform muscle biopsy or electromyography to confirm muscle disease in a patient without clinical evidence of weakness. Magnetic resonance imaging and histopathologic studies suggest that there are alterations in the muscles of at least some patients who have Gottron's papules or heliotrope rash but do not have clinical evidence of muscle weakness.

The category known as overlap myositis has been proposed to occur when a subject meets PM/DM or IBM criteria and criteria for another connective tissue disease, such as systemic sclerosis, rheumatoid arthritis, systemic lupus erythematosus, or Sjogren's syndrome *(9)*. Other researchers, however, have more recently defined this group in other ways on the basis of the presence of certain autoantibodies *(10)*. Using the original definition, connective tissue disease overlap myositis (CTM) appears to differ from primary PM or DM in several ways. CTM tends to be characterized by different frequencies of certain clinical signs and symptoms, different frequencies and types of autoantibodies, possible histopathologic differences, and a less-severe myositis with a better response to therapy *(9)*.

As mentioned, our recognition of the diversity of clinical, serologic, and pathologic presentations of juvenile myositis is increasing, and there may be fewer differences from the adult forms of myositis than previously believed. Nonetheless, juvenile myositis patients tend to have a higher frequency of vasculitic complications and soft tissue calcifications and a better response to therapy than that seen in most adult myositis patients *(11–13)*.

Cancer-associated myositis has been controversial, although early anecdotes and later epidemiologic data suggested that PM, DM, and IBM patients have an increased risk of a variety of cancers, with most, but not all, cancers diagnosed within 2 years of the onset of myositis *(14,15)*. Since DM appears to respond in some cases to simple resection of the associated cancer and because a return of the rash can herald the reappearance of the cancer, it seems likely that the development of the myositis is closely linked either to factors generated by the neoplastic cells or to immune responses to the malignant cells. Although any cancer can occur in myositis patients, certain ones may be more common. In DM, ovarian, lung, pancreatic, stomach, and colorectal cancers, and non-Hodgkin lymphoma were significantly increased in a study in Scandinavia *(15)*. In contrast, PM was associated with a raised risk of non-Hodgkin lymphoma and lung and bladder cancers. CAM patients have a poorer prognosis as a result of their cancer compared to other myositis patients. Features that are statistically less likely to be associated with CAM include myositis-specific and -associated autoantibodies and interstitial lung disease *(9,16)*.

The different clinical, serologic, prognostic, and pathologic features of IBM certainly justify a separate category for this entity, but recent information suggests the line between PM and IBM may not be so clear, and intermediate forms may be more common than generally appreciated *(17)*. The variants of eosinophilic, granulomatous, and vasculitic myositis have distinctive muscle pathology features as well *(18)*, and they are also likely to have different pathogenetic mechanisms; their rarity, however, has not allowed a careful documentation of clinical differences from the other forms of IIMs.

A number of rare and unusual IIMs have also been described that are focal in nature and are not systemic disorders and thus are not typically considered IIMs *(19)*. One form, called ocular or orbital myositis, involves chronic inflammation of structures within the orbit. Ocular or orbital myositis often begins with unilateral periorbital pain usually made worse with eye movement, proptosis, diplopia, and swelling of the eyelid. The diagnosis is often made by orbital ultrasonography, high-resolution computerized tomography, or magnetic resonance imaging. Another group of exceedingly rare syndromes is defined by local areas of pain, swelling, or weakness and on biopsy shows the typical features of inflammatory myopathy. These cases have been called variously focal, nodular, or focal nodular myositis *(20)*. Although trauma has been implicated in some of these cases, in other cases no evidence of trauma occurred. The fact that patients with these disorders can progress to systemic PM, remain chronically focal, or spontaneously resolve suggests that this syndrome may represent a variety of disorders with heterogeneous etiologies and pathogeneses. Similarly, myositis ossificans, in which either local or more generalized areas of soft tissue, including muscle, undergo proliferation, inflammation, and finally replacement by bone, probably represents a variety of disorders and needs additional study for definite categorization *(21)*. A more recently identified type, macrophagic myofasciitis, is a focal form of myositis that was originally described as developing in association with aluminum hydroxide-containing vaccines but has also been reported occurring without vaccinations *(22)*.

## Serologic Classifications

Another approach to classifying the IIMs utilizes the immune responses in these patients. The myositis autoantibodies have an important role in identifying additional groups of patients who share common features and may eventually assist in defining their pathogeneses. Table 2.2 lists a serologic classification of the IIMs using these autoantibodies and their major associations as understood today.

The more studied autoantibodies—such as the antisynthetase, anti-p155/p140, anti-MJ (autoantibody directed against nuclear matrix protein NXP-2), anti-signal recognition particle (SRP), and anti-Mi-2 autoantibodies (directed against chromodomain helicase DNA binding protein 4) —are particularly useful in that each appears to define a syndrome different enough from the others in epidemiology, clinical features, severity of myositis, immunogenetics, responses to therapy, and prognosis to be considered a distinct disorder *(9,23,24)*. Yet additional studies of the newer myositis autoantibodies are needed to determine fully their usefulness in this regard. Overall, these myositis autoantibodies have been helpful in assisting in the diagnosis of certain patients with confusing presentations and in predicting clinical courses and responses to therapy.

Most of the studies of myositis autoantibodies have defined them by protein and RNA immunoprecipitation methods, which remain the gold standard for their

**Table 2.2**  A serologic classification of the idiopathic inflammatory myopathies

| Serologic category | Associations and comments |
| --- | --- |
| Antisynthetase[b] | Frequent symmetric nonerosive arthritis, interstitial lung disease, low-level fevers, mechanic's hands, Raynaud's phenomenon and often occurs as an acute, severe myositis with onset in the spring, moderate response to therapy, myositis flare with tapering of therapy; seen in 20–25% of all myositis cases |
| Anti-signal recognition particle | Frequent palpitations and myalgias; very acute onset of severe polymyositis; most often in black women; poor response to therapy; seen in <5% of myositis patients |
| Anti-Mi-2[c] | Classic dermatomyositis with V sign, shawl sign, and cuticular overgrowth; good response to therapy; seen in 5–10% of myositis patients |
| Anti-p155/p140 | Associated with dermatomyositis in children and adults and cancer in adults |
| Anti-MJ | Associated with dermatomyositis in children and adults |
| Anti-CADM-140 | Japanese patients with amyopathic dermatomyositis and interstitial lung disease |
| Anti-PM-Scl | High incidence of scleroderma/myositis overlap syndromes |
| Anti-Ku70/80 | Seen primarily in scleroderma/myositis overlap syndromes |
| Anti-U1RNP | Seen primarily in myositis overlap syndromes |
| Anti-U2RNP | Associated with scleroderma/myositis overlap syndromes |
| Anti-Ro52 | Seen primarily in myositis overlap syndromes |
| Anti-La | Seen primarily in myositis overlap syndromes |

[a] Modified from *(53)*; information derived from *(7,9,23,24,56–58)*
[b] Includes patients with anti-Jo-1 autoantibodies (directed against histidyl-transfer RNA synthetase) and those with autoantibodies to threonyl-, alanyl-, isoleucyl-, glycyl-, tyrosyl-, asparaginyl- and phenylalanyl-transfer RNA synthetases
[c] Abbreviations: *anti-Mi-2* autoantibody directed against chromodomain helicase DNA binding protein 4; *anti-p155/p140* antibody directed against transcriptional intermediary factor 1gamma; *anti-MJ* autoantibody directed against nuclear matrix protein NXP-2; *anti-CADM-140* autoantibodies directed against a 140 KD protein seen initially in clinically amyopathic dermatomyositis patients

determination but are only performed by a few laboratories. The more common tests for these autoantibodies in clinical practice, using solid-phase assays, have not been as fully validated and can result in false-positive and false-negative results (*(25)* and Miller, personal observations). Thus, more study is needed to assess the most cost-effective and accurate ways to identify these autoantibodies.

## Environmentally Associated Myositis

Myositis in association with environmental exposures—to drugs, toxins, or other agents—has been traditionally considered in a different category from the IIMs. Nonetheless, the lines demarcating these disorders are not clear, and environmentally associated myositis can be indistinguishable in clinical presentation, pathology, and response to immunosuppressive therapy from IIMs. Defining these forms is difficult because, although there may be a temporal association between the exposure and the development of myositis, a cause-effect relationship with the exposure and the pathophysiologic mechanisms involved in the evolution of the inflammation are often not clear. Attempting to define an appropriate temporal association (challenge), assessing if the myositis ameliorates after removal of the suspect agent (dechallenge), determining if the myositis recurs after reexposure to the suspect agent if appropriate (rechallenge), eliminating all other possible causes for the myositis, assessing if any prior similar or identical cases have been reported, and determining if there is any biologic rationale for the association are all useful approaches to help define if there is a true association with the suspect agent *(26)*. Given the increasing evidence that many immune-mediated disorders are the result of gene-environment interactions *(27)*, a classification based on environmental exposure history is useful for the purpose of differential diagnosis and to increase awareness and research of these entities (Table 2.3).

**Table 2.3**  An environmental classification of the inflammatory myopathies[a]

| Environmental exposure category | Associations and comments |
| --- | --- |
| Penicillamine | Can mimic classic polymyositis; different genetic risk factors from primary polymyositis |
| Lipid-lowering agents | Most commonly associated with noninflammatory myopathies, but some polymyositis (PM), dermatomyositis (DM), and inclusion body myositis (IBM) cases have been reported |
| Hydroxyurea | A dermatomyositis-like eruption is most often seen |
| Other drugs | Rarer reports of myositis after antithyroid agents (carbimazole, propylthiouricil); omeprazole; cimetidine; leuprolide acetate; procainamide; hydralazine; penicillin; minocycline; cytokines (interferon $\alpha$ and interleukin 2); growth hormone; and others |
| L-Tryptophan | A polymyositis-like syndrome was sometimes seen in the eosinophilia myalgia syndrome |
| Adulterated rapeseed oil | Myositis occasionally was seen in the toxic oil syndrome |
| Transplants (graft-versus-host myositis) | Rare reports of a polymyositis-like syndrome after bone marrow transplants and in mice |
| Ciguatera toxin | Three cases of polymyositis following classic ciguatera poisoning have been described |
| Silica | Rare cases of myositis reported in stonemasons and house cleaners |
| Collagen implants | Frequent dermatomyositis; onset often within 6 months of implant |
| Silicone implants | Frequent dermatomyositis; late onset after implants, possible different genetic predisposition from other forms of myositis |
| Ultraviolet radiation | Associated with DM in the first worldwide study of myositis |
| Physical exertion | A sixfold increase in PM/DM was seen in a case in a sibling control study |
| Aluminum hydroxide vaccines | Focal macrophagic myofasciitis and diffuse inflammatory myopathy with abundant macrophages are described occurring after receiving vaccines containing aluminum hydroxide |

[a]Modified from *(53)*; information derived from *(27,31–33,59–63)*; categories are not mutually exclusive

While a wide array of infectious agents, including bacteria, viruses, and parasites, has also been associated with myositis, these agents are considered infectious myopathies responsive to anti-infective therapy and are not covered in this review.

Drug-associated myositis has been increasingly identified as the number of agents in use multiplies and associations have become better known. The prototypic example of penicillamine-induced myositis is well documented as an entity that usually responds to dechallenge but can cause fatal complete heart block *(28)*. Although the dose of the drug does not appear to be a factor in development of myositis, the immunogenetic risk factors for the development of myositis after penicillamine exposure appear to differ from those of idiopathic myositis *(29)*.

Most classes of lipid-lowering agents have been associated with myopathies, but smaller numbers of cases of PM, DM, and IBM have also developed in subjects taking these agents *(30)*. The role of other drugs in inducing myositis, such as antithyroid agents (carbimazole, propylthiouricil); omeprazole; cimetidine; leuprolide acetate; procainamide; hydralazine; penicillin; minocycline; cytokines (interferon-alpha and interleukin [IL] 2); and growth hormone are only based on case reports and remains less clear *(31–33)*.

Other relatively rare environmentally associated IIMs listed in Table 2.3, which may be distinct entities but need additional study to clarify their nature, include myositis occurring after transplantation (graft-versus-host myositis); the myositis associated with the L-tryptophan-related eosinophilia myalgia syndrome and the toxic oil syndrome; other toxin-associated myositis; myositis developing after silica exposure in stonemasons and house cleaners; and the myositis, especially DM, that occurs after collagen and silicone implants. Of interest, the myositis that develops after silicone implants appears to be associated with a different genetic risk factor, human leukocyte antigen (HLA) DQA1*0102, compared to the genetic risk factors seen in other forms of IIMs *(34)*.

# Genetic Classifications

A genetic role for the development of myositis has been suspected for some time based on early immunogenetic associations and familial forms *(35,36)*. Yet, although these immunogenetic associations have been known for several decades, the specific major histocompatibility complex (MHC) loci associated with the many different IIM phenotypes have only recently been elucidated. While the ancestral MHC 8.1 haplotype defined by HLA A*0101-B*0801-Cw*0701-DRB1*0301-DQA1*0501 has been confirmed to be a risk factor for all forms of myositis in Caucasians, the major clinical and serologic subgroups in different ethnic groups have different immunogenetic associations *(37–46)*. There is also increasing evidence that polymorphic genes beyond those regulating the immune system in the MHC are likely important in the development of one or more forms of myositis. These other genes, which play important regulatory roles in immune activation and regulation, include those for tumor necrosis factor $\alpha$ (TNF$\alpha$), IL-1$\alpha$, IL-1$\beta$, IL-1RN, interferon gamma (IFNγ), protein tyrosine phosphatase N22, and immunoglobulin (Ig) G and IgK constant gene polymorphisms *(35,47–50)*; however, this review focuses on how MHC and immunoglobulin gene associations can help classify the IIMs given their more extensive evaluation in the clinical and serologic groups. Studies of a number of autoimmune diseases suggested that gene-environment interactions are likely critical for the development of subgroups of disease *(27)*; therefore, a focus on only the environment or genetics alone may be limiting. Nonetheless, given our inability to detail these interactions now, it is useful to consider how genetics alone can help in dividing and understanding the myositis syndromes.

The best-studied genetic markers for myositis are HLA alleles, and a division of IIM phenotypes based on currently identified major HLA genetic factors is summarized in Table 2.4. It is clear that the risk factors differ in many of the different clinical and serologic groups, and in some cases more than one HLA allele is involved in increasing risk for the development of myositis. In addition, a growing number of protective factors, which are alleles seen in higher frequency in controls compared to myositis subjects, have been identified in myositis patients as a whole as well as in the various phenotypes. Thus, it very well may be that a combination of multiple genetic risk factors, along with the absence of protective factors, is important to allow for the expression of disease *(51)*.

Polymorphic determinants of genes encoding constant regions of immunoglobulin gamma heavy and kappa light chains (GM and KM loci on human chromosomes 14q32.33 and 2p12, respectively) have been associated with different immune responses in a variety of infectious and autoimmune diseases in various ethno-geographic populations *(52)*. GM and KM associations have been described in both Mesoamerican and Korean IIM populations *(37,38)*. Recently, additional associations have been seen in Caucasian and African American myositis populations and have been found to differ in some of the clinical and serologic subgroups (Table 2.4) *(50)*. While the physiologic mechanisms underlying these associations remain uncertain, several studies have identified higher serum titers of specific subclasses of IgG antibodies (i.e., IgG1, IgG2, IgG3) directed against antigenic epitopes of infectious disease agents or self-proteins in persons with specific GM and KM markers.

These candidate gene approaches have identified a number of alleles that increase or decrease risk for development of myositis and the associated subgroups. Due to the polygenic and complex nature of these risk factors and the additional roles of environmental and other factors, none of the current genetic risk factors can be used as a tool for accurately predicting development of disease. Yet, these factors are currently being studied in an attempt to decipher pathogenetic mechanisms. International collaborations are already under way utilizing genomewide association studies in large populations of well-defined patients to expand understanding of the genes linked to myositis and possibly develop novel diagnostic, pathogenic, and therapeutic approaches to the IIMs in the future.

**Table 2.4** A genetic classification of the idiopathic inflammatory myopathies[a]

| | All IIMs | PM | DM | IBM | JDM | Anti-Jo-1 | Anti-PL7 | Anti-Mi-2 | Anti-p155 | Anti-SRP |
|---|---|---|---|---|---|---|---|---|---|---|
| **HLA loci** | | | | | | | | | | |
| Ancestral haplotype | 8.1 | 8.1 | 8.1 | 8.1 | 8.1 | 8.1 | NA | NA | NA | NA |
| Other class I | B*0702 | B*44 C*0701 | A*68 B*15 | B*35 C*14 | NA | *C*04* | C*0304 | NA | NA | B*5001 |
| Other class II | DQA1*0301 | *DQA1*0201 DRB1*0401* | DQA1*0301 DQA1*01 | DRB1*0701 DQA1*03 DQA1*0201 | DQA1*0301 DQA1*0201 *DQA1*0201* | *DRB1*0701 DQA1*0201* | DRB1*1501 *DQA1*0501* | DRB1*0701 | DQA1*0301 | DQA1*0104 |
| **Immunoglobulin genes** | | | | | | | | | | |
| GM/KM markers | 3 23 5,13/1 | 3 23 5,13/1 | 3 23 5,13 | NA | 3 23 5,13/1,1 | 3 23 5,13 | 3 | NA | NA | NA |

[a]Information derived from (**39–41,43,45,46,50,58**); only data for Caucasians and the primary significant associations based on corrections for multiple comparisons or random forest evaluations are shown; alleles in italics are protective for the development of the phenotype. *PM* polymyositis; *DM* dermatomyositis; *IBM* inclusion body myositis; *JDM* juvenile DM; *anti-Jo-1* autoantibodies to histidyl-tRNA synthetase; *anti-PL7* autoantibodies to threonyl-tRNA synthetase; *anti-Mi-2* autoantibodies directed against chromodomain helicase DNA binding protein 4; *anti-p155* autoantibodies directed against transcriptional intermediary factor 1gamma; *anti-SRP* autoantibodies to the signal recognition particle; the 8.1 ancestral haplotype consists of HLA A*0101-B*0801-Cw*0701-DRB1*0301-DQA1*0501; *NA* not applicable (no significant associations seen)

**Acknowledgments** I am indebted to Paul Plotz, MD, Lisa Rider, MD, and Lori A. Love, MD, PhD, for many useful discussions in these areas. This work was supported by the intramural research program of the National Institute of Environmental Health Sciences, National Institutes of Health.

# References

1. Baer AN. Differential diagnosis of idiopathic inflammatory myopathies. Curr Rheumatol Rep 2006;8:178–87.
2. Bohan A, Peter JB, Bowman RL, Pearson CM. Computer-assisted analysis of 153 patients with polymyositis and dermatomyositis. Medicine (Baltimore) 1977;56:255–86.
3. Oddis CV, Rider LG, Reed AM, et al. International consensus guidelines for trials of therapies in the idiopathic inflammatory myopathies. Arthritis Rheum 2005;52:2607–15.
4. Griggs RC, Askanas V, DiMauro S, et al. Inclusion body myositis and myopathies. Ann Neurol 1995;38:705–13.
5. van der Meulen MF, Bronner IM, Hoogendijk JE, Burger H, van Venrooij WJ, Voskuyl AE, Dinant HJ, Linssen WH, Wokke JH, de Visser M. Polymyositis: an overdiagnosed entity. Neurology. 2003 Aug 12;61(3):316–21.
6. Miller FW, Rider LG, Plotz PH, et al. Polymyositis: an overdiagnosed entity. Neurology 2004;63:402.
7. Miller FW. Inflammatory myopathies: polymyositis, dermatomyositis, and related conditions. In: Koopman W, Moreland L, eds. *Arthritis and allied conditions: a textbook of rheumatology*. 15th ed. Philadelphia: Lippincott, Williams and Wilkins, 2004:1593–620.
8. Gerami P, Schope JM, McDonald L, Walling HW, Sontheimer RD. A systematic review of adult-onset clinically amyopathic dermatomyositis (dermatomyositis sine myositis): a missing link within the spectrum of the idiopathic inflammatory myopathies. J Am Acad Dermatol 2006;54:597–613.
9. Love LA, Leff RL, Fraser DD, et al. A new approach to the classification of idiopathic inflammatory myopathy: myositis-specific autoantibodies define useful homogeneous patient groups. Medicine (Baltimore) 1991;70:360–74.
10. Troyanov Y, Targoff IN, Tremblay JL, Goulet JR, Raymond Y, Senecal JL. Novel classification of idiopathic inflammatory myopathies based on overlap syndrome features and autoantibodies: analysis of 100 French Canadian patients. Medicine (Baltimore) 2005;84:231–49.
11. Rider LG, Miller FW. New perspectives on the idiopathic inflammatory myopathies of childhood. Curr Opin Rheumatol 1994;6:575–82.
12. Reed AM, Mason T. Recent advances in juvenile dermatomyositis. Curr Rheumatol Rep 2005; 7:94–8.
13. Pachman LM. Juvenile dermatomyositis: immunogenetics, pathophysiology, and disease expression. Rheum Dis Clin North Am 2002;28:579–602, vii.
14. Sigurgeirsson B, Lindelöf B, Edhag O, Allander E. Risk of cancer in patients with dermatomyositis or polymyositis. A population-based study. N Engl J Med 1992;326:363–7.
15. Hill CL, Zhang Y, Sigurgeirsson B, et al. Frequency of specific cancer types in dermatomyositis and polymyositis: a population-based study. Lancet 2001;357:96–100.
16. Chinoy H, Fertig N, Oddis CV, Ollier WE, Cooper RG. The diagnostic utility of myositis autoantibody testing for predicting the risk of cancer-associated myositis. Ann Rheum Dis 2007;66:1345–9.
17. Chahin N, Engel AG. Correlation of muscle biopsy, clinical course, and outcome in PM and sporadic IBM. Neurology 2008;70:418–24.
18. Engel AG, Franzini-Armstrong C. *Myology*. 3rd ed. New York: McGraw-Hill, 2004.
19. Yanmaz Alnigenis MN, Kolasinski SL, Kalovidouris AE. Focal myositis: a review of 100 previously published cases and a report of 2 new cases [letter]. Clin Exp Rheumatol 1999;17:631.

20. Noel E, Tebib J, Walch G, Vauzelle JL, Bouvier M. Focal myositis: a pseudotumoral form of polymyositis. Clin Rheumatol 1991;10:333–8.
21. Nuovo MA, Norman A, Chumas J, Ackerman LV. Myositis ossificans with atypical clinical, radiographic, or pathologic findings: a review of 23 cases. Skeletal Radiol 1992;21:87–101.
22. Gherardi RK, Coquet M, Cherin P, et al. Macrophagic myofasciitis: an emerging entity. Groupe d'Etudes et Recherche sur les Maladies Musculaires Acquises et Dysimmunitaires (GERMMAD) de l'Association Francaise contre les Myopathies (AFM). Lancet 1998;352:347–52.
23. Gunawardena H, Wedderburn LR, North J, et al. Clinical associations of autoantibodies to a p155/140 kDa doublet protein in juvenile dermatomyositis. Rheumatology (Oxford) 2008; 47:324–8.
24. Gunawardena H, Betteridge ZE, McHugh NJ. Newly identified autoantibodies: relationship to idiopathic inflammatory myopathy subsets and pathogenesis. Curr Opin Rheumatol 2008;20:675–80.
25. Fritzler MJ, Wiik A, Tan EM, et al. A critical evaluation of enzyme immunoassay kits for detection of antinuclear autoantibodies of defined specificities. III. Comparative performance characteristics of academic and manufacturers' laboratories. J Rheumatol 2003;30:2374–81.
26. Miller FW, Hess EV, Clauw DJ, et al. Approaches for identifying and defining environmentally associated rheumatic disorders. Arthritis Rheum 2000;43:243–9.
27. Gourley M, Miller FW. Mechanisms of disease: environmental factors in the pathogenesis of rheumatic disease. Nat Clin Pract Rheumatol 2007;3:172–80.
28. Takahashi K, Ogita T, Okudaira H, Yoshinoya S, Yoshizawa H, Miyamoto T. D-Penicillamine-induced polymyositis in patients with rheumatoid arthritis. Arthritis Rheum 1986;29:560–4.
29. Miller FW. Genetics of environmentally-associated rheumatic disease. In: Kaufman LD, Varga J, eds. *Rheumatic diseases and the environment*. London: Arnold, 1999:33–45.
30. Baer AN, Wortmann RL. Myotoxicity associated with lipid-lowering drugs. Curr Opin Rheumatol 2007;19:67–73.
31. Dourmishev AL, Dourmishev LA. Dermatomyositis and drugs. Adv Exp Med Biol 1999; 455:187–91.
32. Clark DW, Strandell J. Myopathy including polymyositis: a likely class adverse effect of proton pump inhibitors? Eur J Clin Pharmacol 2006;62:473–9.
33. Bannwarth B. Drug-induced myopathies. Expert Opin Drug Saf 2002;1:65–70.
34. O'Hanlon T, Koneru B, Bayat E, et al. Immunogenetic differences between Caucasian women with and those without silicone implants in whom myositis develops. Arthritis Rheum 2004;50:3646–50.
35. Shamim EA, Rider LG, Miller FW. Update on the genetics of the idiopathic inflammatory myopathies. Curr Opin Rheumatol 2000;12:482–91.
36. Rider LG, Gurley RC, Pandey JP, et al. Clinical, serologic, and immunogenetic features of familial idiopathic inflammatory myopathy. Arthritis Rheum 1998;41:710–9.
37. Rider LG, Shamim E, Okada S, et al. Genetic risk and protective factors for idiopathic inflammatory myopathy in Koreans and American whites: a tale of two loci. Arthritis Rheum 1999; 42:1285–90.
38. Shamim EA, Rider LG, Pandey JP, et al. Differences in idiopathic inflammatory myopathy phenotypes and genotypes between Mesoamerican Mestizos and North American Caucasians: ethnogeographic influences in the genetics and clinical expression of myositis. Arthritis Rheum 2002;46:1885–93.
39. Arnett FC, Reveille JD, O'Hanlon T. HLA-DRB1 alleles in a Caucasian population from Houston, TX USA. Hum Immunol 2004;1238–41.
40. O'Hanlon TP, Carrick DM, Arnett FC, et al. Immunogenetic risk and protective factors for the idiopathic inflammatory myopathies: distinct HLA-A, -B, -Cw, -DRB1 and -DQA1 allelic profiles and motifs define clinicopathologic groups in Caucasians. Medicine (Baltimore) 2005;84:338–49.
41. O'Hanlon TP, Carrick DM, Targoff IN, et al. Immunogenetic risk and protective factors for the idiopathic inflammatory myopathies: distinct HLA-A, -B, -Cw, -DRB1, and -DQA1 allelic profiles distinguish European American patients with different myositis autoantibodies. Medicine (Baltimore) 2006;85:111–27.

42. O'Hanlon TP, Rider LG, Mamyrova G, et al. HLA polymorphisms in African Americans with idiopathic inflammatory myopathy: allelic profiles distinguish patients with different clinical phenotypes and myositis autoantibodies. Arthritis Rheum 2006;54:3670–81.
43. Chinoy H, Salway F, Fertig N, et al. In adult onset myositis, the presence of interstitial lung disease and myositis specific/associated antibodies are governed by HLA class II haplotype, rather than by myositis subtype. Arthritis Res Ther 2005;8:R13.
44. Needham M, Mastaglia FL, Garlepp MJ. Genetics of inclusion-body myositis. Muscle Nerve 2007;35:549–61.
45. Wedderburn LR, McHugh NJ, Chinoy H, et al. HLA class II haplotype and autoantibody associations in children with juvenile dermatomyositis and juvenile dermatomyositis-scleroderma overlap. Rheumatology (Oxford) 2007;46:1786–91.
46. Mamyrova G, O'Hanlon TP, Monroe JB, et al. Immunogenetic risk and protective factors for juvenile dermatomyositis in Caucasians. Arthritis Rheum 2006;54:3979–87.
47. Chinoy H, Ollier WE, Cooper RG. Have recent immunogenetic investigations increased our understanding of disease mechanisms in the idiopathic inflammatory myopathies? Curr Opin Rheumatol 2004;16:707–13.
48. Chinoy H, Salway F, John S, et al. Interferon-gamma and interleukin-4 gene polymorphisms in Caucasian idiopathic inflammatory myopathy patients in UK. Ann Rheum Dis 2007;66:970–3.
49. Chinoy H, Platt H, Lamb JA, et al. The protein tyrosine phosphatase N22 gene is associated with juvenile and adult idiopathic inflammatory myopathy independent of the HLA 8.1 haplotype in British Caucasian patients 1. Arthritis Rheum 2008;58:3247–54.
50. O'Hanlon TP, Rider LG, Schiffenbauer A, et al. Immunoglobulin gene polymorphisms are susceptibility factors in clinical and autoantibody subgroups of the idiopathic inflammatory myopathies. Arthritis Rheum 2008;58:3239–46.
51. Gregersen PK. Modern genetics, ancient defenses, and potential therapies. N Engl J Med 2007;356:1263–6.
52. Dugoujon JM, Guitard E, Senegas MT. Gm and Km allotypes in autoimmune diseases. G Ital Cardiol 1992;22:85–95.
53. Miller FW. Classification and prognosis of inflammatory muscle disease. Rheum Dis Clin North Am 1994;20:811–26.
54. Bohan A, Peter JB, Bowman RL, Pearson CM. A computer-assisted analysis of 153 patients with polymyositis and dermatomyositis. Medicine 1977;56:255–86.
55. Dalakas MC, Hohlfeld R. Polymyositis and dermatomyositis. Lancet 2003;362:971–82.
56. Miller FW. Myositis-specific autoantibodies. Touchstones for understanding the inflammatory myopathies. JAMA 1993;270:1846–9.
57. Targoff IN. Myositis specific autoantibodies. Curr Rheumatol Rep 2006;8:196–203.
58. Targoff IN, Mamyrova G, Trieu EP, et al. A novel autoantibody to a 155-kd protein is associated with dermatomyositis. Arthritis Rheum 2006;54:3682–9.
59. Love LA, Miller FW. Noninfectious environmental agents associated with myopathies. Curr Opin Rheumatol 1993;5:712–8.
60. Okada S, Weatherhead E, Targoff IN, Wesley R, Miller FW. Global surface ultraviolet radiation intensity may modulate the clinical and immunologic expression of autoimmune muscle disease. Arthritis Rheum 2003;48:2285–93.
61. Seidler AM, Gottlieb AB. Dermatomyositis induced by drug therapy: a review of case reports. J Am Acad Dermatol 2008;59:872–80.
62. Gherardi RK, Authier FJ. Aluminum inclusion macrophagic myofasciitis: a recently identified condition. Immunol Allergy Clin North Am 2003;23:699–712.
63. Bassez G, Authier FJ, Lechapt-Zalcman E, et al. Inflammatory myopathy with abundant macrophages (IMAM): a condition sharing similarities with cytophagic histiocytic panniculitis and distinct from macrophagic myofasciitis. J Neuropathol Exp Neurol 2003;62:464–74.

# Chapter 3
# The Inflammatory Milieu: Cells and Cytokines

**Ann M. Reed and Thomas A. Griffin**

**Abstract** Idiopathic inflammatory myopathies (IIMs) are characterized by mononuclear inflammatory cell infiltrates in skeletal muscle with associated weakness and fatigue, although often the severity of inflammation does not correlate with clinical severity. Inflammation of other organs such as skin, lung, and gastrointestinal tract may also occur. IIMs are classified based on clinical, immunologic, and histopathologic features and include, but are not limited to, adult and juvenile dermatomyositis (DM and JDM, respectively), polymyositis (PM), and sporadic inclusion body myositis (IBM). Mononuclear cells are typically the major component of muscle inflammatory infiltrates in IIMs and include T lymphocytes (T cells), macrophages, dendritic cells (DCs), and B lymphocytes (B cells). Patterns of IIM inflammatory infiltrates include diffuse, endomysial, and perivascular. Endomysial infiltrates are composed primarily of T cells, with a high prevalence of CD8$^+$ T cells, and to a lesser extent CD4$^+$ T cells, DCs, and macrophages. These infiltrates typically surround muscle fibers that lack features of degeneration or necrosis. Perivascular infiltrates are composed mainly of CD4$^+$ T cells and include macrophages, DCs, and B cells. The importance of B cells is increasingly becoming appreciated, and their involvement is likely to be critical in pathologic processes, especially related to autoantibody production and formation of ectopic lymphoid aggregates. Histopathologic features and phenotypic variability of inflammatory infiltrates, localization of infiltrates, presence of rimmed vacuoles, and involvement of microvasculature all contribute to defining IIM subsets. While we do not yet fully understand the pathological processes involved in IIMs, we are gaining information and clarity at a rapid pace. With advances in immunological detection, gene expression, protein biomarkers, and imaging of immune responses, our understanding of the molecules, pathways, and cells involved in pathogenesis

A.M. Reed (✉)
Departments of Pediatrics and Medicine, Division of Rheumatology, Mayo Clinic College of Medicine, Rochester, MN, USA

T.A. Griffin
Department of Pediatrics, Division of Rheumatology, Cincinnati Children's Hospital Medical Center, Cincinnati, OH, USA

L.J. Kagen (ed.), *The Inflammatory Myopathies*,
DOI 10.1007/978-1-60327-827-0_3,
© Humana Press. a part of Springer Science+Business Media, LLC 2009

continues to improve. We have only just started to understand the orchestrated life of T cells, B cells, macrophages, and DCs in myositis; many questions remain unanswered on how a system that is perturbed on a daily basis involves a large-scale but localized abnormal immune reaction.

**Keywords** T lymphocytes • B lymphocytes • Dendritic cells • Macrophages • MHC • Cytokines • Chemokines • Type I interferons

# Introduction

Idiopathic inflammatory myopathies (IIMs) are characterized by mononuclear inflammatory cell infiltrates in skeletal muscle with associated weakness and fatigue, although often the severity of inflammation does not correlate with clinical severity. Inflammation of other organs, such as skin, lung, and gastrointestinal tract, may also occur. IIMs are classified based on clinical, immunologic, and histopathologic features and include, but are not limited to, adult and juvenile dermatomyositis (DM and JDM, respectively), polymyositis (PM), and sporadic inclusion body myositis (IBM).

Mononuclear cells are typically the major component of muscle inflammatory infiltrates in IIMs and include T lymphocytes (T cells), macrophages, dendritic cells (DCs), and B lymphocytes (B cells). Patterns of IIM inflammatory infiltrates include diffuse, endomysial, and perivascular *(1, 2)*. Endomysial infiltrates are composed primarily of T cells, with a high prevalence of CD8+ T cells, and to a lesser extent CD4+ T cells, DCs, and macrophages. These infiltrates typically surround muscle fibers that lack features of degeneration or necrosis. Perivascular infiltrates are composed mainly of CD4+ T cells and include macrophages, DCs, and B cells. The importance of B cells is increasingly becoming appreciated, and their involvement is likely to be critical in pathologic processes, especially related to autoantibody production and formation of ectopic lymphoid aggregates *(3, 4)*.

Histopathologic features and phenotypic variability of inflammatory infiltrates, localization of infiltrates, presence of rimmed vacuoles, and involvement of microvasculature all contribute to defining IIM subsets. Inflammatory infiltrates and muscle fiber involvement are typically spotty even when severe clinical disease is present. Thus, muscle inflammation may not be reliably detected on biopsy. In fact, there is only a weak correlation between inflammatory infiltrates on muscle biopsy and clinical weakness and fatigue. For these reasons, alternative concepts regarding muscle weakness and fatigue have evolved, including novel pathways of myofiber stress and involvement of extracellular matrix. For example, intrinsic myofiber processes independent of inflammation, such as endoplasmic reticulum (ER) stress and upregulation of major histocompatability complex (MHC) molecules, may play important pathogenic roles *(5, 6)*. Other stress responses may also be important and include changes in the extracellular matrix that involve matrix metalloproteinase alterations *(7–10)*.

While we do not yet fully understand the pathological processes involved in IIMs, we are gaining information and clarity at a rapid pace. With advances in immunological detection, gene expression, protein biomarkers, and imaging of immune responses, our understanding of the molecules, pathways, and cells involved in pathogenesis continues to improve. We have only just started to understand the orchestrated life of T cells, B cells, macrophages, and DCs in myositis. Many questions remain unanswered on how a system that is perturbed on a daily basis involves a large-scale, but localized, abnormal immune reaction.

## T Cells

The T cells primarily function in the recognition of antigens (typically peptides) presented by antigen-presenting cells (APC), particularly B cells, macrophages, and DCs. T cells are activated when antigen is presented by MHC molecules, which in humans are called human leukocyte antigens (HLAs) *(11)*. Subtypes of MHC proteins, specifically MHC classes I and II, differentiate the type of antigen that is presented and which T-cell subset responds. MHC class I peptide antigens are usually eight to ten amino acids long and derived from intracellular proteins, including those of intracellular pathogens, and when presented by MHC class I molecules they are primarily detected by $CD8^+$ (cytotoxic) T cells. In contrast, MHC class II molecules generally bind larger peptides that are derived from ingested extracellular proteins or intracellular proteins that are targeted to and degraded in endosomes. MHC class II peptide antigens are detected by $CD4^+$ (helper) T cells that can be subdivided into at least four subsets: $T_H1$, $T_H2$, $T_H17$, and T suppressor cells *(12)*. Pathogen-derived antigens, specifically those presented by macrophages and DCs in the presence of interleukin 2 (IL-2), interferon gamma (IFN-γ), and APC-derived IL-12 and cofactor IL-18, are thought to promote differentiation into $T_H1$ cells. Conversely, allergens and extracellular protein antigens tend to promote $T_H2$ cell differentiation in the presence of IL-4. The importance of $T_H17$ cells in inflammatory conditions has been uncovered. $T_H17$ cell differentiation occurs in the presence of IL-6 and transforming growth factor beta (TGF-β) *(13, 14)*. $T_H17$ cells are a major source of IL-17, which in vitro can act in concert with IL-1 to induce IL-6. IL-17 can also induce MHC class I expression in myocytes. $T_H17$ cells have been found with neutrophils in acute inflammatory infiltrates in a number of infections and autoimmune diseases. Last, TGF-β in the absence of IL-6 can direct the formation of T regulatory cells.

## T Cells in Myositis

T cells are typically the predominant cells in IIM inflammatory infiltrates. Endomysial infiltrates seen in PM and IBM consist primarily of cytotoxic $CD8^+$ T cells *(2, 15–21)* that surround nonnecrotic muscle fibers expressing MHC class I molecules *(1)*. These CD8⁺ T cells express perforin, which is hypothesized to cause myofiber injury and possibly necrosis *(22, 23)*. Granulysin is also expressed in both PM and IBM, and clinical steroid resistance is associated with the presence of CD8⁺ granulysin-expressing T cells in PM *(24)*.

The CD4⁺ T cells are the primary component of perivascular and perimysial infiltrates in DM and JDM. These CD4⁺ T cell infiltrates are associated with B cells, DCs, and macrophages *(4, 17, 18)*. Data suggest formation of neolymphoid structures in JDM muscle tissue where CD4⁺ mature and immature T cells are associated with B cells, including those in an activated state and with plasmacytoid dendritic cells (pDCs) (Fig. 3.1) *(3, 4)*. Interestingly, what had been thought to be CD4⁺ T$_H$1 cells have been identified, at least in part, as pDCs that express CD4, as well as other pDC markers CD123 and CD83, and they are CD11c– *(25, 26)*.

Further delineation of both T$_H$1 and T$_H$2 cells has involved characterization of CD28low or CD28null senescent T cells *(27)*. The loss of CD28 expression on T cells is the most consistent biological indicator of aging, and the frequency of CD28null T cells is a key indicator of immune incompetence with age. Human CD28null T cells are functionally active, long-lived lymphocytes that lack or have limited proliferative capacity. CD28null T cells are derived from CD28⁺ precursors that have undergone repeated stimulation, indicating that decreased expression of CD28 relates to T cell aging. In IIMs, a high frequency of CD4⁺ and CD8⁺ CD28null T cells are present in the circulation and in muscle tissue *(28–31)*.

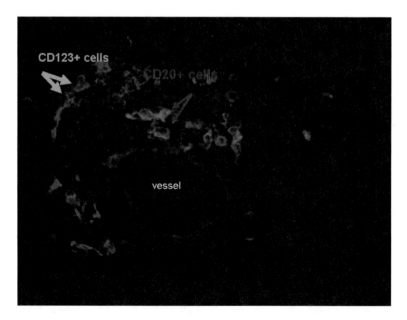

**Fig. 3.1** Plasmacytoid *DCs* (*green*) with B cells (*red*) in the perivascular region of a muscle biopsy from a patient with new-onset *JDM*

Immunohistochemical staining of muscle tissue from DM, PM, and IBM biopsies showed the presence of CTLA4, CD28, CD86, and CD40 on inflammatory cells. Low levels of CTLA4 and CD28 were observed on muscle cells; however, expression of CD28 and CTLA4 was upregulated in CD8$^+$ cells in PM and IBM *(30)*. In PM, the absolute number of circulating cytotoxic (CD8$^+$ CD28$^+$) T cells was selectively reduced *(15)*.

The CD4$^+$ T cell subtype $T_H17$, a producer of IL-17, has been demonstrated in muscle tissue of PM, JDM, and DM *(32–34)*. IL-17 can induce MHC class I expression in cultured myoblasts as well as IL-6 and cell signaling factors such as nuclear factor kappa B (NF-κB), c-fos, and c-jun *(32)*. Immunohistochemical staining shows an increase in IL-17 in CD4$^+$ T cells in the muscle tissue of JDM patients in both the perimysium and perivascular regions (Fig. 3.2).

The T cell markers CD45RO and CD45RA subdivide CD8$^+$ and CD4$^+$ T cells into primed memory and naïve T cells, respectively (Fig. 3.3) *(3, 35)*. In DM, PM, and IBM, at all sites of accumulation, the CD45RO$^+$ memory T cells were predominant, and the CD45RO/CD45RA ratio exceeded that in normal blood. In PM and IBM, the marked enrichment of endomysial memory T cells implicates these cells in pathogenesis. The enrichment of perivascular memory T cells in DM, JDM, and PM may be a result of enhanced transendothelial migration *(26)*. However, data support local maturation of T cells in neolymphoid structures where a large number of CD45RO$^+$ T cells are seen with a dense rim of CD45RA$^+$ T cells *(3, 16)*.

The T-cell receptor (TCR) restriction or expansion, or what has also been termed overusage, is seen in IIM muscle and lung tissue. This restriction is also seen in peripheral blood with expression of Vβ genes most commonly evaluated with individual differing patterns of restriction *(36–45)*. In one patient, a large fraction of microdissected T cells carried a common TCR-BV amino acid CDR3 complementary determining region 3 motif and conservative nucleotide exchanges in the CDR3 region, suggesting an antigen-driven response. In several cases, T-cell clones

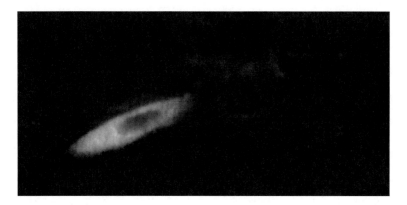

**Fig. 3.2**  IL-17 stained cells (*red*) in the perivascular inflammation in the muscle tissue with an associated blood vessel from a patient newly diagnosed with *JDM*

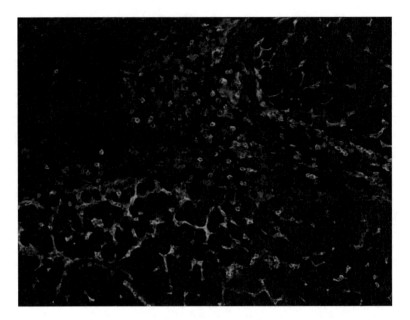

**Fig. 3.3** Ectopic lymphoid formation with CD45 RA⁺ (*red*), and CD4⁺ (*green*) cells. Non-*red* and -*green* cells are primarily CD20⁺ cells with blue-stained nuclei from a muscle biopsy of an individual with newly diagnosed JDM

were seen over time (several years) in CD8⁺ (but not CD4⁺) blood lymphocytes and in two patients' consecutive muscle biopsy specimens. During immunosuppressive therapy, oligoclonal CDR3-spectratype patterns tended to revert to polyclonal Gaussian distribution-like patterns, suggesting that CDR3 spectratyping may reflect ongoing T-cell clones in blood and target tissue that are disease related, the balance of which changes with disease improvement *(46)*.

## Dendritic Cells

Recent evidence has shown that DCs, the most potent APC, are present and exhibit increased activation in the inflamed muscle tissue of patients affected with IIMs, and these cells are likely of great importance in pathogenesis *(33, 47)*. The primary function of DCs is to capture and present protein antigens to naïve T cells. Because DCs are able to express both MHC class I and class II molecules, they are able to present antigens to both CD8⁺ and CD4⁺ T cells. Because of their central role in initiating immune responses while maintaining tolerance, impaired function of DCs might lead to breaking peripheral tolerance and initiation of immune responses to self-antigens.

Two phenotypically and functionally different DC subsets have been recognized in humans and mice on the basis of differential expression of myeloid (myeloid DC, mDC) and lymphoid lineage-associated markers (pDCs), as well as their differential responsiveness to maturation or differentiation stimuli *(48, 49)*. The mDCs are considered the most potent APCs. They are highly specialized in capturing antigens and triggering adaptive immune responses *(50, 51)*, whereas pDCs are involved in innate immune responses and are potent type I interferon-producing cells *(52)*.

## Dendritic Cells in Myositis

With recent advances in technology, specifically gene expression arrays and multiplex protein assays, it has been observed that a large number of differentially expressed genes in IIM tissues are induced by type I interferons *(53)*. This was initially observed in muscle tissue of JDM and DM subjects *(54–57)*. Upregulation of type I interferon-inducible genes has also been observed in peripheral blood of JDM and DM patients *(53, 58, 59)*. The source of type I interferon in muscle tissue may be the muscle itself; however, the identification of pDCs in IIM tissues makes pDCs the likely source of type I interferons in muscle, peripheral blood, and skin, where pDC-derived interferons may directly affect T-cell maturation and B-cell development into plasma cells. Several groups have reported distinct DC subsets in muscle biopsy specimens from IIM patients, and their role has begun to be elucidated. Immunohistochemical studies revealed that immature and mature DCs are present in PM, JDM, and DM muscle infiltrates, although the location differed between them, with a predominance of immature and mature DCs in lymphocytic aggregates and mature DCs in perivascular and endomysial areas *(33, 47)*.

Further delineation of DCs demonstrated the presence of increased numbers of mDCs in PM and IBM *(25, 60)*. Conversely, muscle biopsy specimens from children with newly diagnosed JDM contained mature CD123$^+$ pDCs, defined by expression of CD83 *(26)*. DCs in muscles from patients with DM and JDM are mainly located in perivascular regions, and they are mostly mature DCs, whereas in PM, DCs penetrate deeper into the muscle, surrounding or invading muscle fibers *(26, 47, 56)*. Mature DCs in IIM muscle appear to be associated with clusters of T and B cells adjacent to blood vessels, suggesting that transmigration of DCs through endothelium may provide access to lymph nodes to generate an autoimmune response *(26)*. Conversely, local expression of chemokines and their receptors is suggestive of lymphocyte maturation and ectopic lymphoid aggregation in IIM muscle tissue *(26)*. Nongranulomatous nodular accumulations of inflammatory cells were initially reported by De Bleecker et al. *(4)*, and they involved B-cell-rich centers surrounded by a T-cell-rich peripheral zone, resembling lymph nodes. The T-cell-rich zones have been shown to contain pDCs and follicular DCs with high endothelial venules (HEVs), suggestive of ectopic lymphoid formation *(3, 26)*. The ectopic lymphoid structures contained endothelium that frequently expressed intercellular adhesion molecule (ICAM-1), vascular cell adhesion molecule (VCAM-1), and to a lesser extent E-selectin, and there were immature T cells (CD45RA$^+$) close to the B cells and pDCs. This suggests that these structures may be involved in maturation of T cells and recruitment of additional inflammatory cells.

The mechanisms underlying sustained recruitment of inflammatory cells into muscle tissue are unknown. Chemokine receptor (CCl7) CCR7 and its ligands chenokine ligand (CCL19 and CCL21) are regarded as an essential chemokine system for DC migration into regional lymph nodes *(61, 62)*. Immunohistochemical analysis has demonstrated that CCR7 expression on mature DCs in PM *(47)*. By using the anatomic specificity of laser capture microdissection and reverse transcriptase polymerase chain reaction (RT-PCR) analysis, transcripts of CCL19 and CCL21 were also shown to be upregulated in mononuclear cells in JDM tissue *(16)*, mainly in JDM patients with inflammatory infiltrates organized as extranodal tissue *(26)*. This suggests that the expression of CCR7 and its ligands CCL19 and CCL21 might contribute to formation of lymphocytic aggregates where DCs mature and naïve T cells are primed. On the other hand, CCR7 messenger RNA (mRNA) was absent in immature DCs and is thought to be induced on maturation, probably reflecting a direct effect of DC activation through CD40 or TNFR. CD40 and its ligand CD40L have been shown to be essential for humoral immune responses in muscles of PM and DM *(62)*.

A key role for chenokine (C-X-C) receptor 4 (CXCR4) and its ligand CXCL12 in DC migration has been suggested *(63)*. In JDM, strong CXCR4 mRNA expression and protein expression of CXCR4 has been demonstrated on mature pDCs that were preferentially localized in perivascular aggregates of perimysium and endomysium *(26)*. pDCs are also located in the epidermis in DM patients' skin biopsies, whereas in systemic lupus erythematosus they are present in the dermis, suggesting a role in cutaneous pathogenesis in both of these disorders *(64)*.

The pDCs represent key effectors in innate immunity because of their unique capacity to secrete large amounts of type I interferons in response to viruses *(51)*, providing a unique link between innate and adaptive antiviral immunity. Increasing evidence suggests a pathogenic role for type I interferon-producing cells in myositis, whether from DCs or from myocytes themselves. The pathogenic role of type I interferons is most likely related to their many immunomodulatory effects. For example, IFN-α is known to stimulate differentiation of functionally efficient monocyte-derived DCs *(65, 66)* and to promote survival and differentiation of activated T cells *(67)* and B cells *(68)*. Type I interferons can upregulate MHC class I molecules, costimulatory molecules, and cytokine production *(66, 68, 69)* and through these might trigger an immune response.

Type I interferons may also induce differentiation of monocytes into DCs and induce transition of immature, tolerogenic mDCs to mature and potent APCs. Concomitantly, type I interferons can induce differentiation of B cells into plasma cells and lead to B-cell activity factor of the TNF family (BAFF) secretion by mDCs, a pivotal cytokine for autoreactive B-cell survival and antibody secretion, and lead to granulocyte-macrophage colony-stimulating factor (GM-CSF) secretion, a key cytokine for differentiation of neutrophils *(70, 71)*. Patients with IIMs have increased levels of BAFF associated with disease activity, anti-Jo-1 positivity, and interstitial lung disease (ILD), suggesting that BAFF is involved in at least some disease subsets of myositis *(71, 72)*. This raises the possibility that one mechanism by which type I interferons are involved in pathogenesis is through induction of BAFF in DCs and neutrophils.

# B Cells

During T-cell-dependent immune responses, antigen-activated B cells migrate into the primary follicles of peripheral lymph nodes and lymphoid tissues. These cells are induced to clonally expand, leading to formation of germinal centers. Germinal centerlike formations in tissues have been reported in autoimmune conditions, including thyroid tissue in autoimmune thyroid disease, salivary gland biopsies in Sjogren's syndrome, and rheumatoid arthritis synovium. B cells within germinal centers diversify their repertoire. Investigation of the VH regions of B cell receptors (BCRs) allows identification of the germline and indication of maturation. B-cell activation requires both binding of an antigen by BCRs and an interaction with antigen-specific T cells (CD4[+] T cells). CD4[+] T cells induce B-cell proliferation and direct the differentiation of clonally expanded progeny of naïve B cells into either plasma cells (antibody-producing cells) or memory B cells. Both cytokines from CD4[+] T cells and somatic hypermutation of V-region genes can influence antibody isotype switching and antibody-binding properties.

# B Cells in Myositis

Involvement of B cells in IIMs was once thought to be limited but is now believed to be influential and potentially involved in key immune responses. B cells are particularly present in perivascular infiltrates in JDM and DM *(17, 18)*. B-cell importance is suggested by up to 80% of patients with PM or DM, and a smaller proportion of patients with IBM, expressing myositis-specific autoantibodies.

CD138[+] plasma cells were observed in the endomysium of muscle tissue in PM and IBM. A substantial number of IIM subjects have autoantibody positivity, and gene expression assays showed immunoglobulin transcript prominence especially in PM and IBM *(73)*. Immunohistochemistry studies on muscle tissue showed the presence of B cells specifically in DM and JDM. B cells, including activated B cells, have been demonstrated in the lymphoid aggregates of JDM. These CD19[+] or CD20[+] cells are shown to be localized in tissue with surrounding T-cell and DC organization in a subset of subjects *(3)*. The presence of CD19[+] or CD20[+] cells in the tissue of IBM or PM is sparse; however, reports have shown a large number of CD138[+] plasma cells *(73)*. Clonal expansion of B cells that is seen in biopsies from DM, PM, and IBM suggests an antigen-driven process. The infiltrating B cells and plasma cells are clonally expanded, class switched, and have undergone somatic mutation *(73)*. Oligoclonal expansion of B cells using CDR3 variability has been observed in DM and IBM and appears to differ based on tissue location, suggesting local variability in B-cell expansion and antigen presentation.

# Macrophages

Macrophages are involved at all stages of immune responses. They provide innate immunity through early action prior to the development of T-cell responses. Thus, activated macrophages not only play a key role in host defense against infections and tumors but also can contribute to autoimmune diseases. Macrophages are important killer cells. For example, macrophages are able to kill or damage extracellular targets via antibody-dependent cell-mediated cytotoxicity. They also take part in the initiation of T-cell activation by processing and presenting antigen and are commonly seen in muscle tissue in IIMs. Macrophages in their activated state are able to produce more than 100 different chemokines and cytokines *(74)*.

# Macrophages in Myositis

Macrophages appear to play an important role in the pathogenesis of IIMs, yet they are the least-studied cell type in IIMs. Macrophages undergo functional and morphological changes during the inflammatory process, including sequential expression of cell surface markers *(75–77)*, production of cytokines and chemokines, and presentation of antigens to lymphocytes *(2, 58, 78, 79)*. For example, macrophages contribute to IL-18 expression in muscle tissue *(80)*. In PM and IBM, macrophages and cytotoxic T cells actively invading nonnecrotic muscle fibers expressed high levels of CXCL10 and CCL2 *(81)*. Certain $\beta$-chemokines, such as monocyte chemoattractant protein 1 (MCP-1), are upregulated in IIMs. Immunostaining was observed in endothelial cells in IBM with anti-CCR1 and anti-CD68, suggesting macrophage involvement *(82)*. The expression of 25F9 (an antibody that recognizes membrane-bound antigen on mature macrophages and thought to indicate maturation of monocytes to tissue macrophages) is found in the perimysium of DM and JDM patients. Muscle biopsies from PM subjects showed early activation markers 27E10 and MRP14 present on endomysial macrophages, both early and late in the disease process, and unaffected by treatment. These findings suggest that the role of macrophages may be different among disease subtypes and allows for their differentiation *(77)*.

# Natural Killer T Cells

Natural killer T (NKT) cells have been identified as subpopulations of CD4$^-$CD8$^-$ or CD4$^+$ T cells. NKT cells express both specific $\alpha\beta$ TCRs and NK markers in humans and mice *(83, 84)*. The majority of human NKT cells express TCR V24J18Vß11 and CD161 (NKR-P1A) on their surface *(85)*. Human NKT cells are believed to have regulatory effects on immune tolerance and autoimmunity, and the number of both CD4$^-$CD8$^-$ and CD4$^+$ NKT cells is selectively decreased in peripheral blood of patients with systemic lupus erythematosus, systemic sclerosis, rheumatoid arthritis, and Sjögren's syndrome *(85)*.

## NK Cells in Myositis

Little is known about the role of NK cells in IIMs; however, scattered NK cells are found in inflammatory infiltrates. Most of the autoaggressive cells are T cells and macrophages, but some are NK cells with an unclear contribution to disease *(19, 86)*. However, in peripheral blood a role is proposed even if it is not direct. The percentage of CD54$^+$ non-B cells (T cells and NK cells expressing CD54) is significantly lower in JDM patients *(87)*. Expression of CD161, an NKT cell marker, on peripheral blood CD8$^+$ T cells from patients with various rheumatic diseases (including DM and PM) is also decreased *(28)*. Other suggestions that NK cells play a role in IIMs involve killer cell immunoglobulin-like receptors (KIRs), a group of polymorphic receptors expressed on NK cells and subsets of T cells *(88)*. Polymorphisms of KIRs (like MHC molecules) are associated with protection and susceptibility in infection, pregnancy, autoimmunity, and transplantation. A decrease in the 2DL1 inhibitory KIR, with a corresponding lack of the associated ligand HLA-C, is seen in JDM.

## Muscle and Endothelial Cell Involvement

Traditional APC exist in the muscle infiltrates in IIMs; however, evidence suggests that muscle fibers themselves may serve an immune function, and promote an autoimmune response, via antigen presentation. Upregulation of MHC class I molecules is known to occur early in the disease process and may be seen prior to presence of any inflammatory infiltrates *(89–91)*. Specifically, HLA-G is expressed in inflamed muscle and is proposed to provide a protective effect from autoreactive lysis directed by inhibition of NK cells on healthy muscle tissue *(92)*. The subtypes HLA-G1 and HLA-G5 inhibit the priming of antigen-specific and memory T-cell immune responses. HLA-G is not the only inhibitory protein expressed by muscle tissue. The B7-costimulatory molecule, B7-H1, is an inducible protein in muscle that can directly inhibit CD4$^+$ and CD8$^+$ T-cell activation in interactions of muscle and T cells *(93)*. Muscle cells themselves are thought to be actively involved in the recruitment of inflammatory cells. Cultured myoblasts express IL-1 and IL-6 constitutively, while IL-1 and TNF-$\alpha$ are detected after treatment with proinflammatory cytokines, and IL-8 and RANTES are expressed when MCP-1 is used for induction. This suggests that muscle cells are immunologically active during times of inflammation and may themselves be stimuli for immune responses, possibly secondary to stress responses.

Upregulation of MHC class I molecules in skeletal muscle of IIMs and in a mouse model of myositis that is driven by skeletal muscle MHC class I upregulation appears to induce an ER stress response that involves the unfolded protein response and the ER overload response (5, 6). MHC class I folding and assembly in the ER involve a number of chaperones, including calnexin, calreticulin, ERp57, tapasin, and GRP78. In the mouse model of myositis, misfolding of MHC class I heavy chains triggers the ER stress response since myofibers are ill equipped to handle excessive production of proteins that must be processed in the ER.

There is evidence that muscle fibers in inflammatory myopathies undergo apoptosis and display upregulation of inducible and neuronal nitric oxide synthase (NOS). While inducible NOS is upregulated on the sarcolemma of all kinds of muscle fibers, neuronal NOS is increased in the sarcoplasm of damaged as well as atrophic muscle fibers; however, no myositis disease-specific patterns have been identified. Enhanced expression of NOS with production of nitric oxide may contribute to oxidative stress mediating muscle fiber damage and muscle fiber necrosis, representing the predominant cell death mechanism in myositis. Also, inflammatory cells show numerous DNA-fragmentation-positive nuclei and expression of apoptosis-related proteins, including the Fas "death receptor," Fas (CD95/APO-1), and Bcl-2, indicating that apoptosis plays a role in the regulation of the inflammatory cellular response (94, 95).

Another novel nonimmune mechanism in muscle fiber damage in myositis is the DNA-binding protein high-mobility group box 1 (HMGB1) chromosomal protein, which is ubiquitously expressed and actively released from macrophages/monocytes. When released, HMGB1 has potent proinflammatory effects and induces TNF$\alpha$ and IL-1. HMGB1 is expressed in muscle tissue in PM and DM and is decreased after 3-6 months of treatment (96). The role of HMGB1 in the disease mechanisms of myositis still needs to be determined.

A morphological structural change in the microcirculation of DM and JDM muscle tissue is the loss of capillaries, even in early cases without detectable inflammatory infiltrates (97, 98). The disturbed microcirculation in muscle tissue includes changes in endothelial cells, specifically activated high endothelium venules, which may be present even prior to onset of inflammatory infiltrates (3, 20). High endothelium venules are present in neolymphoid structures (3, 99) and are proposed to be present in secondary lymphoid tissues. Disturbances in microcirculation are hypothesized to contribute to tissue hypoxia, metabolic alterations, and subsequent increased expression of endothelial adhesion molecules (100, 101). Notably, neovascularization was greater in JDM than other IIMs (102).

Changes in the muscle expression of key adhesion molecules show a consistent (but not complete) concordance with changes in and status of muscle function in IIM patients (100). ICAM-1 expression in vessels is seen more often in JDM; however, ICAM-1 expression in myofibers is present in PM and DM. VCAM-1 expression in vessels is significantly greater in PM and DM, while VCAM-1 expression in muscle fibers is almost absent. These findings emphasize the importance of adhesion molecules in the pathophysiology of IIMs, corroborating microvascular involvement in these diseases (103). Other factors that may affect muscle fibers include inducible costimulator ligand (ICOSL), a member of the B7 family of costimulatory molecules related to B7.1/2, which regulates CD4[+] as well as CD8[+]

T-cell responses via interaction with its receptor, ICOS, on activated T cells. ICOSL expression is markedly increased in muscle fibers in IIM, showing that muscle fibers themselves may be an active contributor or initiator of the inflammatory process *(104)*.

Not only is muscle tissue thought to possess immune regulation capabilities, but also skin shows signs of immunoreactivity. Increased expression of ICAM-1 is seen in IIMs on endothelial cells, inflammatory cells, and focally grouped keratinocytes in contact with subepidermal inflammatory infiltrates. Expression of VCAM-1 was predominant on endothelial cells of the upper reticular dermis and dermal stellate-shaped cells. E-selectin (endothelial leukocyte adhesion molecule 1) was mainly detected in blood vessels of the papillary dermis and upper reticular dermis, sometimes independent of inflammation *(105)*. This pattern of adhesion molecule expression is not unique to IIMs but is similar to that described in other immune-mediated skin disorders.

Further evidence that suggests myositis autoantigens contribute to muscle fibers being an active participant in the immune response and involves high levels of autoantigens expressed in myositis muscle. Specifically, increased autoantigen expression correlates with a differentiation state, such that myositis autoantigen expression is increased in cells that have features of regenerating muscle cells and in cultured myoblasts *(106)*. These data implicate regenerating muscle cells rather than mature myofibers as the source of ongoing antigen supply in autoimmune myositis.

## Cytokines and Chemokines

The IIMs involve complex inflammatory milieus in affected skeletal muscle and skin. The immune effector cells that participate in this inflammation are likely to be influenced and regulated by cytokines and chemokines. While many cytokines and chemokines have been detected in affected tissues, evidence for a direct role in disease pathogenesis is lacking for most. This review focuses on several key cytokines that may play central roles in IIM pathogenesis and for which therapeutic inhibition has either been applied or contemplated, thereby actually testing their role in disease.

## Type I Interferons

Type I interferons comprise members of the IFN-α family, with at least 13 different functional IFN-α proteins and a single IFN-β protein *(107)*. Type I interferons are particularly important in coordinating innate and adaptive immune responses to viruses and other intracellular infections. Notable actions of type I interferons include upregulation of MHC class I expression, activation of NK cell cytotoxicity, promotion of activated T-cell survival, induction of many proinflammatory cytokines and chemokines, and support of DC maturation. There has been mounting evidence in support of an important pathogenic role for type I interferons in each form of IIM, especially DM and JDM *(108)*.

Type I interferons are notoriously difficult to detect due to their strong potency, which requires only small amounts of cytokine for large downstream effects, and their ability to produce long-term consequences after only brief exposures. For example, type I interferons are required to initiate an animal model of psoriasis via transient strong expression early in disease, whereas upregulated expression of genes induced by type I interferons, such as IRF-7, persists long after expression of type I interferons has subsided *(109)*. In fact, most evidence for type I interferon action in IIMs comes not from their detection but rather from demonstration of their actions. This lack of detection leads to uncertainty regarding the cellular origins of type I interferons, although observation of pDCs in inflammatory infiltrates in both affected muscle and skin *(26, 33, 56, 64, 102, 110)* makes these cells leading candidates for type I interferon production as they are known to be capable of producing large amounts of these cytokines *(111)*.

The first clear evidence for type I interferon action in JDM was provided by Tezak et al. *(57)*, who noted induction of many type I interferon-responsive genes by global gene expression profiling of affected skeletal muscle tissue from four untreated JDM patients. These findings were confirmed when this cohort was extended to 21 JDM patients *(112)*. Similarly, a number of other investigators have demonstrated upregulation of type I interferon-responsive genes in muscle tissue of adults with DM *(55, 56, 113–115)*. The most extensive of these studies *(25)* investigated muscle tissue gene expression profiling in 53 patients with various forms of IIMs. They found a strong type I interferon signature in DM, with 12 of the 14 most upregulated genes being type I interferon inducible. They also found much weaker, but still present, type I interferon signatures in PM and IBM. This study not only detected type I interferon action via gene expression but also demonstrated expression of MxA, a type I interferon-inducible antiviral protein, in DM myofibers and vessel endothelium *(56)*. Expression of MxA protein in muscle vasculature in DM was also demonstrated by Eloranta et al. *(110)*. MxA has also been detected in affected skin in DM, suggesting a similar role for type I interferons in both skin and muscle inflammation *(116)*.

The possibility that type I interferons play an important role in IIM pathogenesis has led to several studies that examined type I interferon action in circulating white blood cells. Assessment of type I interferon signatures in peripheral blood may not only provide insight into disease pathogenesis but also provide readily accessible biomarkers for monitoring disease activity. For example, O'Connor et al. *(54)* demonstrated increased mRNA expression of MxA in peripheral blood mononuclear cells in JDM and found that MxA expression appeared to correlate with muscle disease activity. Likewise, Baechler et al. *(53, 58)* found upregulation of type I interferon-inducible genes in peripheral blood cells of 10 of 12 patients with either DM or JDM, and the magnitude of the type I interferon signature appeared to correlate with disease activity. These authors also detected elevated levels of several type I interferon-inducible chemokines (IP-10, MCP-1, and MCP-2) in the blood of patients with the greatest degree of disease activity. Walsh et al. *(59)* demonstrated type I interferon signatures in peripheral blood mononuclear cells in both DM and PM (but not IBM), which correlated with disease activity and response to treatment. Bilgic et al. *(34)* further expanded the association of disease activity with type I interferon gene and protein expression (I-TAC, IP-10, MCP-1, MCP-2), as well as with the IL-17 pathway components (IL-17 and IL-6), and suggested these markers of disease are sensitive to monitor disease activity in DM and JDM). These several studies demonstrate that type I interferon action is evident in blood cells in many IIM patients, which may be a useful means of assessing disease activity.

The mechanism by which type I interferons contribute to disease pathogenesis remains uncertain, although several possibilities exist. Type I interferons may exert pathogenic influence via induction of other proinflammatory cytokines and chemokines. For example, expression of IL-15 (which is type I interferon inducible and T-cell activating) has been found to be increased in affected myofibers *(62, 117)*. Likewise, Fall et al. *(118)* have demonstrated increased expression of type I interferon-inducible α-type CXC chemokines (IP-10, MIG, and I-TAC), which may play a role in angiostasis in affected tissues. Upregulation of these chemokines may also be involved in recruiting CXCR3$^+$ lymphocytes to sites of inflammation in affected muscle and skin *(116, 119–121)*. In addition, several type I interferon-inducible β-type CC chemokines have been detected in IIM tissues, including MCP-1, MCP-2, MIP-1, and MIP-1 *(58, 78, 82, 119, 122)*.

Other than induction of proinflammatory cytokines and chemokines, type I interferons may contribute to disease pathogenesis by inducing excessive expression of MHC class I molecules in affected myofibers. Normal myofibers typically express little MHC class I, whereas upregulation of MHC class I has been widely demonstrated in IIM myofibers *(89–91, 123–125)*. Direct involvement of excessive MHC class I expression in mediating disease was supported by a mouse model of self-sustaining myositis that is induced by overexpression of an MHC class I molecule (H-2K$^b$) exclusively in myofibers *(5)*. Nagaraju et al. *(6)* demonstrated that excessive MHC class I expression both in this model and in PM and DM tissues is associated with activation of an ER stress response, which appears to be due to overloading of the ER with proteins that myofibers are not normally prepared to handle. It is suggested that a chronic ER stress response in affected myofibers may perpetuate disease by causing myofiber injury and apoptosis, which in turn provoke further type I interferon production, MHC class I overexpression, and ER stress.

In summary, there is evidence for type I interferon action in each of the IIMs, especially DM and JDM. The pathogenic effects of type I interferons are potentially numerous and include induction of other proinflammatory cytokines and chemokines and induction of excessive MHC class I expression. The evidence for a pathogenic role of type I interferons is currently indirect and correlative, with direct evidence awaiting future therapeutic trials of type I interferon inhibition in IIM patients.

# Tumor Necrosis Factor-α

Tumor necrosis factor alpha is an important immunoregulatory cytokine that has the potential to mediate many of the pathological processes observed in IIMs, including facilitation of inflammatory cell migration and infiltration, local activation of lymphocytes and macrophages, induction of MHC class I molecules in muscle fibers, promotion of muscle fiber atrophy, and upregulation of adhesion molecule expression (particularly ICAM-1) *(126)*. A possible role for TNFα in the pathogenesis of IIMs was first suggested by demonstration of TNF production in affected tissues. Tews and Goebel *(127)* detected variable TNFα production in both inflammatory cells in affected muscle and in muscle fibers themselves in IIMs, while Lepidi et al. *(128)* detected increased TNFα mRNA expression in most IIM tissues. Tateyama et al. *(129)* demonstrated the presence of TNFα[+] macrophages and lymphocytes in some but not all PM muscle tissue, and they also found that the presence of TNFα[+] cells appeared to correlate with a greater abundance of atrophic muscle fibers. Caproni et al. *(121)* detected TNFα in DM skin tissue. A genetic susceptibility involving TNFα was suggested by Fedcyna et al. *(130)*, who detected greater amounts of muscle fiber TNFα in JDM patients with a TNF promoter polymorphism, which Pachman et al. *(131)* found to be associated with prolonged disease. Indirect evidence of TNFα action was provided by De Bleeker et al. *(78)*, who detected expression of TNF receptors in affected tissues, including endothelium in DM. Interestingly, TNFα and its p55 receptor were prominently expressed in regenerating muscle fibers, raising the possibility that TNFα plays a role in mediating regeneration rather than having a direct pathological role. TNFα and its soluble receptors have also been detected in the blood of patients with IIMs and correlated with disease activity *(132, 133)*. In summary, many investigators have detected TNFα expression in IIMs, but its pathogenic role is difficult to ascertain from these observational studies.

The role of TNFα in IIMs has been more directly assessed by observing responses to therapeutic agents that inhibit TNFα action, including etanercept, infliximab, and adalimumab. Dastmalchi et al. *(134)* treated 13 refractory IIM patients with infliximab in an open trial and observed few responders compared to a number with flares. In addition, they typically observed no improvement in inflammatory infiltrates on repeat muscle biopsies and found evidence for increased type I interferon activity in most patients. Iannone et al. *(135)* treated five active DM patients with etanercept in an open trial, and all worsened. Conversely, Riley et al. *(136)* treated five refractory JDM patients with infliximab in an open trial, and all improved, including some with improvement in calcinosis. Likewise, several single case reports have been made of favorable responses to either infliximab or etanercept in PM *(137–139)*. Barohn et al. *(140)* found little if any improvement in patients with IBM treated with etanercept, and Hengstman et al. *(141)* found inconsistent responses to infliximab in DM and PM. In fact, there are reports of myositis developing in patients treated with anti-TNFα agents for other autoimmune diseases *(142, 143)*. Thus, while there are a few anecdotal reports of favorable responses to TNFα blockade, most investigators have observed inconsistent results that suggest TNFα does not play a critical role in the pathogenesis of IIMs. It may even have a counterregulatory role considering the many patients that flared with anti-TNFα treatment.

## Interleukin 1

There are three genes in the IL-1 family: IL-1α, IL-1β, and IL-Ra (receptor antagonist). IL-1α and IL-1β are potent proinflammatory cytokines that have been consistently detected in myositis tissue. These IL-1s may play an important role in IIM pathogenesis, not only by driving the action of inflammatory cells but also by producing negative effects on muscle function.

A number of investigators have detected prominent expression of IL-1α and IL-1β in IIM tissues *(125, 127, 128, 144)*. Schmidt et al. *(145)* demonstrated particularly high levels of a number of proinflammatory chemokines and cytokines, including IL-1β, in IBM tissue. They also demonstrated the ability of IL-1β to upregulate amyloid precursor protein in cultured myotubes and showed colocalization of amyloid deposits with Il-1β expression in IBM tissue, suggesting a direct link between IL-1β action and pathogenic amyloid deposition.

The potential of IL-1 to act in concert with other cytokines to amplify inflammation in IIM tissues is exemplified by the work of Chevrel et al. *(32)*, who demonstrated expression of both IL-1β and IL-17 in PM and DM muscle tissues. They further demonstrated that these two cytokines had additive effects on muscle cells and tissue with regard to induction of downstream chemokines and cytokines, such as IL-6, upregulation of MHC class I expression, and upregulation of a number of "inflammatory" cell surface markers, including several adhesion molecules. Chevrel et al. *(146)* also demonstrated a similar additive action of IL-1β and TNFα in muscle tissues and cells with regard to several processes that are observed in myositis muscle: IL-6 production, NF-κB nuclear translocation, and MHC class I induction. In addition, they noted that these actions were inhibited by their respective soluble receptors, lending support to the use of such inhibitors in the treatment of myositis. Additional correlative evidence for a role in disease pathogenesis was the observation by Lundberg et al. *(100)* of decreased IL-1 expression in DM and PM tissue after corticosteroid treatment. Grundtman et al. *(147)* demonstrated expression of IL-1 receptors in PM and DM muscle, including expression on inflammatory cells, endothelial cells, and myofibers. Notably, they also detected colocalized expression of IL-1α with IL-1 receptors in endothelial cells and all three IL-1s with IL-1 receptors in inflammatory cells. Son et al. *(148)* detected elevated serum protein and PBMC mRNA for IL-1Ra in patients with PM and DM that correlated with disease activity. Likewise, significantly elevated levels of IL-1Ra were detected in all three types of IIM tissue by Baird and Montine *(149)*.

Therapeutic experience with IL-1 inhibition is currently minimal, although there is an anecdotal report of a patient with refractory PM/antisynthetase syndrome who had a dramatic and sustained response to treatment with the IL-1 inhibitor anakinra *(150)*.

Further trials with IL-1 inhibitors will be important in directly assessing the role of IL-1 in IIM.

# Conclusion

Many cytokines and chemokines have been detected in IIM tissues, but their roles in disease pathogenesis remain largely hypothetical. Biologic medications that inhibit the action of specific cytokines have been and will be important for directly assessing the roles of targeted molecules in IIM patients. Animal models of myositis offer valuable approaches for assessing the role of key cytokines and chemokines in disease processes. Undoubtedly, knowledge regarding the role of cytokines and chemokines in IIMs will continue to expand rapidly and ultimately serve the goal of improving the outcomes of patients with IIMs.

# References

1. Dalakas MC, Hohlfeld R. Polymyositis and dermatomyositis. Lancet 2003;362(9388):971–82.
2. Dalakas MC, Sivakumar K. The immunopathologic and inflammatory differences between dermatomyositis, polymyositis and sporadic inclusion body myositis. Curr Opin Neurol 1996;9(3):235–9.
3. López de Padilla CM, Vallejo AN, Lacomis D, McNallan KT, Reed AM. Extra-nodal lymphoid microstructures in inflamed muscle and disease severity of new-onset juvenile dermatomyositis. Arthritis Rheum 2009; 60(4):1160–72.
4. De Bleecker JL, Engel AG, Butcher EC. Peripheral lymphoid tissue-like adhesion molecule expression in nodular infiltrates in inflammatory myopathies. Neuromuscul Disord 1996;6(4):255–60.
5. Nagaraju K, Raben N, Loeffler L, et al. Conditional up-regulation of MHC class I in skeletal muscle leads to self-sustaining autoimmune myositis and myositis-specific autoantibodies. Proc Natl Acad Sci U S A 2000;97(16):9209–14.
6. Nagaraju K, Casciola-Rosen L, Lundberg I, et al. Activation of the endoplasmic reticulum stress response in autoimmune myositis: potential role in muscle fiber damage and dysfunction. Arthritis Rheum 2005;52(6):1824–35.
7. Choi YC, Dalakas MC. Expression of matrix metalloproteinases in the muscle of patients with inflammatory myopathies. Neurology 2000;54(1):65–71.
8. Schoser BG, Blottner D, Stuerenburg HJ. Matrix metalloproteinases in inflammatory myopathies: enhanced immunoreactivity near atrophic myofibers. Acta Neurol Scand 2002;105(4):309–13.
9. Kieseier BC, Schneider C, Clements JM, et al. Expression of specific matrix metalloproteinases in inflammatory myopathies. Brain 2001;124(Pt 2):341–51.
10. Hurnaus S, Mueller-Felber W, Pongratz D, Schoser BG. Serum levels of matrix metalloproteinases-2 and -9 and their tissue inhibitors in inflammatory neuromuscular disorders. Eur Neurol 2006;55(4):204–8.
11. Thorsby E. Invited anniversary review: HLA associated diseases. Hum Immunol 1997; 53(1):1–11.
12. Tesmer LA, Lundy SK, Sarkar S, Fox DA. Th17 cells in human disease. Immunol Rev 2008;223:87–113.

13. Bettelli E, Korn T, Oukka M, Kuchroo VK. Induction and effector functions of T(H)17 cells. Nature 2008;453(7198):1051–7.
14. Dong C. TH17 cells in development: an updated view of their molecular identity and genetic programming. Nat Rev Immunol 2008;8(5):337–48.
15. Iannone F, Cauli A, Yanni G, et al. T-lymphocyte immunophenotyping in polymyositis and dermatomyositis. Br J Rheumatol 1996;35(9):839–45.
16. Engel AG, Arahata K. Mononuclear cells in myopathies: quantitation of functionally distinct subsets, recognition of antigen-specific cell-mediated cytotoxicity in some diseases, and implications for the pathogenesis of the different inflammatory myopathies. Hum Pathol 1986;17(7):704–21.
17. Arahata K, Engel AG. Monoclonal antibody analysis of mononuclear cells in myopathies. I: quantitation of subsets according to diagnosis and sites of accumulation and demonstration and counts of muscle fibers invaded by T cells. Ann Neurol 1984;16(2):193–208.
18. Arahata K, Engel AG. Monoclonal antibody analysis of mononuclear cells in myopathies. V: identification and quantitation of T8+ cytotoxic and T8+ suppressor cells. Ann Neurol 1988;23(5):493–9.
19. Arahata K, Engel AG. Monoclonal antibody analysis of mononuclear cells in myopathies. IV: cell-mediated cytotoxicity and muscle fiber necrosis. Ann Neurol 1988;23(2):168–73.
20. Emslie-Smith AM, Arahata K, Engel AG. Major histocompatibility complex class I antigen expression, immunolocalization of interferon subtypes, and T cell-mediated cytotoxicity in myopathies. Hum Pathol 1989;20(3):224–31.
21. Hohlfeld R, Goebels N, Engel AG. Cellular mechanisms in inflammatory myopathies. Baillieres Clin Neurol 1993;2(3):617–35.
22. Orimo S, Koga R, Goto K, et al. Immunohistochemical analysis of perforin and granzyme A in inflammatory myopathies. Neuromuscul Disord 1994;4(3):219–26.
23. Goebels N, Michaelis D, Engelhardt M, et al. Differential expression of perforin in muscle-infiltrating T cells in polymyositis and dermatomyositis. J Clin Invest 1996;97(12):2905–10.
24. Ikezoe K, Ohshima S, Osoegawa M, et al. Expression of granulysin in polymyositis and inclusion-body myositis. J Neurol Neurosurg Psychiatry 2006;77(10):1187–90.
25. Greenberg SA, Pinkus JL, Pinkus GS, et al. Interferon-alpha/beta-mediated innate immune mechanisms in dermatomyositis. Ann Neurol 2005;57(5):664–78.
26. Lopez de Padilla CM, Vallejo AN, McNallan KT, et al. Plasmacytoid dendritic cells in inflamed muscle of patients with juvenile dermatomyositis. Arthritis Rheum 2007;56(5):1658–68.
27. Vallejo AN. CD28 extinction in human T cells: altered functions and the program of T-cell senescence. Immunol Rev 2005;205:158–69.
28. Mitsuo A, Morimoto S, Nakiri Y, et al. Decreased CD161+ CD8+ T cells in the peripheral blood of patients suffering from rheumatic diseases. Rheumatology (Oxford) 2006;45(12):1477–84.
29. Nagaraju K, Raben N, Villalba ML, et al. Costimulatory markers in muscle of patients with idiopathic inflammatory myopathies and in cultured muscle cells. Clin Immunol 1999;92(2):161–9.
30. Murata M, Dalakas MC. Expression of the costimulatory molecule BB-1, the ligands CTLA-4 and CD28, and their mRNA in inflammatory myopathies. Am J Pathol 1999;155(2):453–60.
31. Grundtman C, Malmstrom V, Lundberg IE. Immune mechanisms in the pathogenesis of idiopathic inflammatory myopathies. Arthritis Res Ther 2007;9(2):208.
32. Chevrel G, Page G, Granet C, Streichenberger N, Varennes A, Miossec P. Interleukin-17 increases the effects of IL-1 beta on muscle cells: arguments for the role of T cells in the pathogenesis of myositis. J Neuroimmunol 2003;137(1-2):125–33.
33. Page G, Sattler A, Kersten S, Thiel A, Radbruch A, Miossec P. Plasma cell-like morphology of Th1-cytokine-producing cells associated with the loss of CD3 expression. Am J Pathol 2004;164(2):409–17.
34. Bilgic HYS, McNallan KT, Wilson JC, et al. IL-6 and IFN-regulated genes and chemokines as biomarkers of disease activity in dermatomyositis. Arthritis Rheum 2008;(accepted for publication).
35. de Bleecker JL, Engel AG. Immunocytochemical study of CD45 T cell isoforms in inflammatory myopathies. Am J Pathol 1995;146(5):1178–87.

36. O'Hanlon TP, Dalakas MC, Plotz PH, Miller FW. The alpha beta T-cell receptor repertoire in inclusion body myositis: diverse patterns of gene expression by muscle-infiltrating lymphocytes. J Autoimmun 1994;7(3):321–33.

37. O'Hanlon TP, Dalakas MC, Plotz PH, Miller FW. Predominant TCR-alpha beta variable and joining gene expression by muscle-infiltrating lymphocytes in the idiopathic inflammatory myopathies. J Immunol 1994;152(5):2569–76.

38. O'Hanlon TP, Dalakas MC, Plotz PH, Miller FW. The alpha beta T-cell receptor repertoire in idiopathic inflammatory myopathies: distinct patterns of gene expression by muscle-infiltrating lymphocytes in different clinical and serologic groups. Ann N Y Acad Sci 1995;756:410–3.

39. O'Hanlon TP, Messersmith WA, Dalakas MC, Plotz PH, Miller FW. Gamma delta T cell receptor gene expression by muscle-infiltrating lymphocytes in the idiopathic inflammatory myopathies. Clin Exp Immunol 1995;100(3):519–28.

40. Mizuno K, Yachie A, Nagaoki S, et al. Oligoclonal expansion of circulating and tissue-infiltrating $CD8^+$ T cells with killer/effector phenotypes in juvenile dermatomyositis syndrome. Clin Exp Immunol 2004;137(1):187–94.

41. Bradshaw EM, Orihuela A, McArdel SL, et al. A local antigen-driven humoral response is present in the inflammatory myopathies. J Immunol 2007;178(1):547–56.

42. Englund P, Wahlstrom J, Fathi M, et al. Restricted T cell receptor BV gene usage in the lungs and muscles of patients with idiopathic inflammatory myopathies. Arthritis Rheum 2007;56(1):372–83.

43. Reed AM, Geyer SM, Maurer M, McNallan K, Pachman L, Wettstein P. T cell receptor repertoire restriction in active juvenile dermatomyositis. Ann Rheumatol 2008.

44. Benveniste O, Cherin P, Maisonobe T, et al. Severe perturbations of the blood T cell repertoire in polymyositis, but not dermatomyositis patients. J Immunol 2001;167(6):3521–9.

45. Benveniste O, Herson S, Salomon B, et al. Long-term persistence of clonally expanded T cells in patients with polymyositis. Ann Neurol 2004;56(6):867–72.

46. Hofbauer M, Wiesener S, Babbe H, et al. Clonal tracking of autoaggressive T cells in polymyositis by combining laser microdissection, single-cell PCR, and CDR3-spectratype analysis. Proc Natl Acad Sci U S A 2003;100(7):4090–5.

47. Page G, Chevrel G, Miossec P. Anatomic localization of immature and mature dendritic cell subsets in dermatomyositis and polymyositis: interaction with chemokines and Th1 cytokine-producing cells. Arthritis Rheum 2004;50(1):199–208.

48. Thomas R, Lipsky PE. Dendritic cells: origin and differentiation. Stem Cells 1996; 14(2):196–206.

49. Ardavin C. Origin, precursors and differentiation of mouse dendritic cells. Nat Rev Immunol 2003;3(7):582–90.

50. Reid SD, Penna G, Adorini L. The control of T cell responses by dendritic cell subsets. Curr Opin Immunol 2000;12(1):114–21.

51. Colonna M, Trinchieri G, Liu YJ. Plasmacytoid dendritic cells in immunity. Nat Immunol 2004;5(12):1219–26.

52. Jego G, Palucka AK, Blanck JP, Chalouni C, Pascual V, Banchereau J. Plasmacytoid dendritic cells induce plasma cell differentiation through type I interferon and interleukin 6. Immunity 2003;19(2):225–34.

53. Baechler EC, Batliwalla FM, Reed AM, et al. Gene expression profiling in human autoimmunity. Immunol Rev 2006;210:120–37.

54. O'Connor KA, Abbott KA, Sabin B, Kuroda M, Pachman LM. MxA gene expression in juvenile dermatomyositis peripheral blood mononuclear cells: association with muscle involvement. Clin Immunol 2006;120(3):319–25.

55. Raju R, Dalakas MC. Gene expression profile in the muscles of patients with inflammatory myopathies: effect of therapy with IVIg and biological validation of clinically relevant genes. Brain 2005;128(Pt 8):1887–96.

56. Greenberg SA, Bradshaw EM, Pinkus JL, et al. Plasma cells in muscle in inclusion body myositis and polymyositis. Neurology 2005;65(11):1782–7.

57. Tezak Z, Hoffman EP, Lutz JL, et al. Gene expression profiling in DQA1*0501+ children with untreated dermatomyositis: a novel model of pathogenesis. J Immunol 2002;168(8):4154–63.
58. Baechler EC, Bauer JW, Slattery CA, et al. An interferon signature in the peripheral blood of dermatomyositis patients is associated with disease activity. Mol Med 2007;13(1-2):59–68.
59. Walsh RJ, Kong SW, Yao Y, et al. Type I interferon-inducible gene expression in blood is present and reflects disease activity in dermatomyositis and polymyositis. Arthritis Rheum 2007;56(11):3784–92.
60. Greenberg SA, Pinkus GS, Amato AA, Pinkus JL. Myeloid dendritic cells in inclusion-body myositis and polymyositis. Muscle Nerve 2007;35(1):17–23.
61. Marsland BJ, Battig P, Bauer M, et al. CCL19 and CCL21 induce a potent proinflammatory differentiation program in licensed dendritic cells. Immunity 2005;22(4):493–505.
62. Sugiura T, Kawaguchi Y, Harigai M, et al. Increased CD40 expression on muscle cells of polymyositis and dermatomyositis: role of CD40-CD40 ligand interaction in IL-6, IL-8, IL-15, and monocyte chemoattractant protein-1 production. J Immunol 2000;164(12):6593–600.
63. Kabashima K, Sugita K, Shiraishi N, Tamamura H, Fujii N, Tokura Y. CXCR4 engagement promotes dendritic cell survival and maturation. Biochem Biophys Res Commun 2007;361(4):1012–6.
64. McNiff JM, Kaplan DH. Plasmacytoid dendritic cells are present in cutaneous dermatomyositis lesions in a pattern distinct from lupus erythematosus. J Cutan Pathol 2008;35(5):452–6.
65. Paquette RL, Hsu NC, Kiertscher SM, et al. Interferon-alpha and granulocyte-macrophage colony-stimulating factor differentiate peripheral blood monocytes into potent antigen-presenting cells. J Leukoc Biol 1998;64(3):358–67.
66. Marrack P, Kappler J, Mitchell T. Type I interferons keep activated T cells alive. J Exp Med 1999;189(3):521–30.
67. Marrack P, Kappler J. The T cell and its receptor. Sci Am 1986;254(2):36–45.
68. Ruuth K, Carlsson L, Hallberg B, Lundgren E. Interferon-alpha promotes survival of human primary B-lymphocytes via phosphatidylinositol 3-kinase. Biochem Biophys Res Commun 2001;284(3):583–6.
69. Kadowaki N, Ho S, Antonenko S, et al. Subsets of human dendritic cell precursors express different toll-like receptors and respond to different microbial antigens. J Exp Med 2001; 194(6):863–69.
70. Zhang X, Park CS, Yoon SO, et al. BAFF supports human B cell differentiation in the lymphoid follicles through distinct receptors. Int Immunol 2005;17(6):779–88.
71. Krystufkova O, Vallerskog T, Barbasso Helmers S, et al. Increased serum levels of B-cell activating factor (BAFF) in subsets of patients with idiopathic inflammatory myopathies. Ann Rheum Dis 2008;epub ahead of print.
72. McNallan K GE, Baechler EC, Peterson EJ, Osborn T, Crowson CS, Reed AM. ∆BAFF, a diagnostic tool in the early events of autoimmunity. Arthritis Rheum 2008;58:S442.
73. Greenberg SA, Bradshaw EM, Pinkus JL, Pinkus GS, Burlesm T, Dse B, Breyoli LS, O'Conner KC, Amato AA. Plasma cells in muscle in inclusion body myositis and polymyositis. Neurology 2005; 65:1782–1787
74. Mantovani A, Sica A, Sozzani S, Allavena P, Vecchi A, Locati M. The chemokine system in diverse forms of macrophage activation and polarization. Trends Immunol 2004;25(12):677–86.
75. Schulz-Schaeffer WJ, Bruck W, Puschel K. Macrophage subtyping in the determination of age of injection sites. Int J Legal Med 1996;109(1):29–33.
76. O'Laughlin S, Braverman M, Smith-Jefferies M, Buckley P. Macrophages (histiocytes) in various reactive and inflammatory conditions express different antigenic phenotypes. Hum Pathol 1992;23(12):1410–8.
77. Rostasy KM, Piepkorn M, Goebel HH, Menck S, Hanefeld F, Schulz-Schaeffer WJ. Monocyte/macrophage differentiation in dermatomyositis and polymyositis. Muscle Nerve 2004;30(2):225–30.
78. Confalonieri P, Bernasconi P, Megna P, Galbiati S, Cornelio F, Mantegazza R. Increased expression of beta-chemokines in muscle of patients with inflammatory myopathies. J Neuropathol Exp Neurol 2000;59(2):164–9.

79. De Bleecker JL, Meire VI, Declercq W, Van Aken EH. Immunolocalization of tumor necrosis factor-alpha and its receptors in inflammatory myopathies. Neuromuscul Disord 1999;9(4): 239–46.

80. Tucci M, Quatraro C, Dammacco F, Silvestris F. Increased IL-18 production by dendritic cells in active inflammatory myopathies. Ann NY Acad Sci 2007;1107:184–92.

81. De Paepe B, Creus KK, De Bleecker JL. Chemokine profile of different inflammatory myopathies reflects humoral versus cytotoxic immune responses. Ann N Y Acad Sci 2007;1109:441–53.

82. Civatte M, Bartoli C, Schleinitz N, Chetaille B, Pellissier JF, Figarella-Branger D. Expression of the beta chemokines CCL3, CCL4, CCL5 and their receptors in idiopathic inflammatory myopathies. Neuropathol Appl Neurobiol 2005;31(1):70–9.

83. Sandberg JK, Fast NM, Palacios EH, et al. Selective loss of innate CD4(+) V alpha 24 natural killer T cells in human immunodeficiency virus infection. J Virol 2002;76(15):7528–34.

84. Nakamura T, Takahashi K, Fukazawa T, et al. Relative contribution of CD2 and LFA-1 to murine T and natural killer cell functions. J Immunol 1990;145(11):3628–34.

85. Kojo S, Adachi Y, Keino H, Taniguchi M, Sumida T. Dysfunction of T cell receptor AV24AJ18+, BV11+ double-negative regulatory natural killer T cells in autoimmune diseases. Arthritis Rheum 2001;44(5):1127–38.

86. Figarella-Branger D, Pellissier JF, Bianco N, Devictor B, Toga M. Inflammatory and non-inflammatory inclusion body myositis. Characterization of the mononuclear cells and expression of the immunoreactive class I major histocompatibility complex product. Acta Neuropathol 1990;79(5):528–36.

87. O'Gorman MR, Bianchi L, Zaas D, Corrochano V, Pachman LM. Decreased levels of CD54 (ICAM-1)-positive lymphocytes in the peripheral blood in untreated patients with active juvenile dermatomyositis. Clin Diagn Lab Immunol 2000;7(4):693–7.

88. McNallan K, Crowson C, Reed AM. Absence of killer Ig-like inhibitory receptor with the associated HLA ligand in juvenile dermatomyositis. Hum Immunol 2008;submitted.

89. Li CK, Varsani H, Holton JL, Gao B, Woo P, Wedderburn LR. MHC class I overexpression on muscles in early juvenile dermatomyositis. J Rheumatol 2004;31(3):605–9.

90. van der Pas J, Hengstman GJ, ter Laak HJ, Borm GF, van Engelen BG. Diagnostic value of MHC class I staining in idiopathic inflammatory myopathies. J Neurol Neurosurg Ps 2004;75(1):136–9.

91. Nagaraju K. Role of major histocompatibility complex class I molecules in autoimmune myositis. Curr Opin Rheumatol 2005;17(6):725–30.

92. Wiendl H, Mitsdoerffer M, Hofmeister V, et al. The non-classical MHC molecule HLA-G protects human muscle cells from immune-mediated lysis: implications for myoblast transplantation and gene therapy. Brain 2003;126(Pt 1):176–85.

93. Wiendl H, Mitsdoerffer M, Schneider D, et al. Human muscle cells express a B7-related molecule, B7-H1, with strong negative immune regulatory potential: a novel mechanism of counterbalancing the immune attack in idiopathic inflammatory myopathies. FASEB J 2003;17(13):1892–4.

94. Behrens L, Bender A, Johnson MA, Hohlfeld R. Cytotoxic mechanisms in inflammatory myopathies. Co-expression of Fas and protective Bcl-2 in muscle fibres and inflammatory cells. Brain 1997;120(Pt 6):929–38.

95. Tews DS, Goebel HH. Cell death and oxidative damage in inflammatory myopathies. Clin Immunol Immunopathol 1998;87(3):240–7.

96. Ulfgren AK, Grundtman C, Borg K, et al. Down-regulation of the aberrant expression of the inflammation mediator high mobility group box chromosomal protein 1 in muscle tissue of patients with polymyositis and dermatomyositis treated with corticosteroids. Arthritis Rheum 2004;50(5):1586–94.

97. Emslie-Smith AM, Engel AG. Microvascular changes in early and advanced dermatomyositis: a quantitative study. Ann Neurol 1990;27(4):343–56.

98. Kissel JT, Mendell JR, Rammohan KW. Microvascular deposition of complement membrane attack complex in dermatomyositis. N Engl J Med 1986;314(6):329–34.

99. Girard JP, Springer TA. High endothelial venules (HEVs): specialized endothelium for lymphocyte migration. Immunol Today 1995;16(9):449–57.

100. Lundberg I, Kratz AK, Alexanderson H, Patarroyo M. Decreased expression of interleukin-1alpha, interleukin-1beta, and cell adhesion molecules in muscle tissue following corticosteroid treatment in patients with polymyositis and dermatomyositis. Arthritis Rheum 2000;43(2):336–48.
101. Park JH, Vansant JP, Kumar NG, et al. Dermatomyositis: correlative MR imaging and P-31 MR spectroscopy for quantitative characterization of inflammatory disease. Radiology 1990;177(2):473–9.
102. Nagaraju K, Rider LG, Fan C, et al. Endothelial cell activation and neovascularization are prominent in dermatomyositis. J Autoimmune Dis 2006;3:2.
103. Sallum AM, Kiss MH, Silva CA, et al. Difference in adhesion molecule expression (ICAM-1 and VCAM-1) in juvenile and adult dermatomyositis, polymyositis and inclusion body myositis. Autoimmun Rev 2006;5(2):93–100.
104. Wiendl H, Mitsdoerffer M, Schneider D, et al. Muscle fibres and cultured muscle cells express the B7.1/2-related inducible co-stimulatory molecule, ICOSL: implications for the pathogenesis of inflammatory myopathies. Brain 2003;126(Pt 5):1026–35.
105. Hausmann G, Mascaro JM, Jr., Herrero C, Cid MC, Palou J, Mascaro JM. Cell adhesion molecule expression in cutaneous lesions of dermatomyositis. Acta Derm Venereol 1996;76(3):222–5.
106. Casciola-Rosen L, Nagaraju K, Plotz P, et al. Enhanced autoantigen expression in regenerating muscle cells in idiopathic inflammatory myopathy. J Exp Med 2005;201(4):591–601.
107. Theofilopoulos AN, Baccala R, Beutler B, Kono DH. Type I interferons (alpha/beta) in immunity and autoimmunity. Annu Rev Immunol 2005;23:307–36.
108. Griffin TA, Reed AM. Pathogenesis of myositis in children. Curr Opin Rheumatol 2007; 19(5):487–91.
109. Nestle FO, Conrad C, Tun-Kyi A, et al. Plasmacytoid predendritic cells initiate psoriasis through interferon-alpha production. J Exp Med 2005;202(1):135–43.
110. Eloranta ML, Barbasso Helmers S, Ulfgren AK, Ronnblom L, Alm GV, Lundberg IE. A possible mechanism for endogenous activation of the type I interferon system in myositis patients with anti-Jo-1 or anti-Ro 52/anti-Ro 60 autoantibodies. Arthritis Rheum 2007;56(9):3112–24.
111. Siegal FP, Kadowaki N, Shodell M, et al. The nature of the principal type 1 interferon-producing cells in human blood. Science 1999;284(5421):1835–7.
112. Bakay M, Wang Z, Melcon G, et al. Nuclear envelope dystrophies show a transcriptional fingerprint suggesting disruption of Rb-MyoD pathways in muscle regeneration. Brain 2006; 129(Pt 4):996–1013.
113. Greenberg SA, Sanoudou D, Haslett JN, et al. Molecular profiles of inflammatory myopathies. Neurology 2002;59(8):1170–82.
114. Zhou X, Dimachkie MM, Xiong M, Tan FK, Arnett FC. cDNA microarrays reveal distinct gene expression clusters in idiopathic inflammatory myopathies. Med Sci Monit 2004; 10(7):BR191–7.
115. Tian L, Greenberg SA, Kong SW, Altschuler J, Kohane IS, Park PJ. Discovering statistically significant pathways in expression profiling studies. Proc Natl Acad Sci U S A 2005;102(38):13544–9.
116. Wenzel J, Schmidt R, Proelss J, Zahn S, Bieber T, Tuting T. Type I interferon-associated skin recruitment of CXCR3+ lymphocytes in dermatomyositis. Clin Exp Dermatol 2006;31(4):576–82.
117. Sugiura T, Harigai M, Kawaguchi Y, et al. Increased IL-15 production of muscle cells in polymyositis and dermatomyositis. Int Immunol 2002;14(8):917–24.
118. Fall N, Bove KE, Stringer K, et al. Association between lack of angiogenic response in muscle tissue and high expression of angiostatic ELR-negative CXC chemokines in patients with juvenile dermatomyositis: possible link to vasculopathy. Arthritis Rheum 2005;52(10):3175–80.
119. Liprandi A, Figarella-Branger D, Daniel L, Lepidi H, Bartoli C, Pellissier JF. Expression of adhesion molecules in idiopathic inflammatory myopathies. Immunohistochemical study of 17 cases. Ann Pathol 1999;19(1):12–18.
120. De Paepe B, De Keyzer K, Martin JJ, De Bleecker JL. Alpha-chemokine receptors CXCR1–3 and their ligands in idiopathic inflammatory myopathies. Acta Neuropathol 2005;109(6):576–82.

121. Caproni M, Torchia D, Cardinali C, et al. Infiltrating cells, related cytokines and chemokine receptors in lesional skin of patients with dermatomyositis. Br J Dermatol 2004;151(4):784–91.

122. De Bleecker JL, De Paepe B, Vanwalleghem IE, Schroder JM. Differential expression of chemokines in inflammatory myopathies. Neurology 2002;58(12):1779–85.

123. Bartoccioni E, Gallucci S, Scuderi F, et al. MHC class I, MHC class II and intercellular adhesion molecule-1 (ICAM-1) expression in inflammatory myopathies. Clin Exp Immunol 1994;95(1):166–72.

124. Englund P, Nennesmo I, Klareskog L, Lundberg IE. Interleukin-1alpha expression in capillaries and major histocompatibility complex class I expression in type II muscle fibers from polymyositis and dermatomyositis patients: important pathogenic features independent of inflammatory cell clusters in muscle tissue. Arthritis Rheum 2002;46(4):1044–55.

125. Dorph C, Englund P, Nennesmo I, Lundberg IE. Signs of inflammation in both symptomatic and asymptomatic muscles from patients with polymyositis and dermatomyositis. Ann Rheum Dis 2006;65(12):1565–71.

126. Michaelis D, Goebels N, Hohlfeld R. Constitutive and cytokine-induced expression of human leukocyte antigens and cell adhesion molecules by human myotubes. Am J Pathol 1993;143(4):1142–9.

127. Tews DS, Goebel HH. Cytokine expression profile in idiopathic inflammatory myopathies. J Neuropathol Exp Neurol 1996;55(3):342–7.

128. Lepidi H, Frances V, Figarella-Branger D, Bartoli C, Machado-Baeta A, Pellissier JF. Local expression of cytokines in idiopathic inflammatory myopathies. Neuropathol Appl Neurobiol 1998;24(1):73–9.

129. Tateyama M, Nagano I, Yoshioka M, Chida K, Nakamura S, Itoyama Y. Expression of tumor necrosis factor-alpha in muscles of polymyositis. J Neurol Sci 1997;146(1):45–51.

130. Fedczyna TO, Lutz J, Pachman LM. Expression of TNFalpha by muscle fibers in biopsies from children with untreated juvenile dermatomyositis: association with the TNFalpha-308A allele. Clin Immunol 2001;100(2):236–9.

131. Pachman LM, Liotta-Davis MR, Hong DK, et al. TNFalpha-308A allele in juvenile dermatomyositis: association with increased production of tumor necrosis factor alpha, disease duration, and pathologic calcifications. Arthritis Rheum 2000;43(10):2368–77.

132. Hassan AB, Fathi M, Dastmalchi M, Lundberg IE, Padyukov L. Genetically determined imbalance between serum levels of tumour necrosis factor (TNF) and interleukin (IL)-10 is associated with anti-Jo-1 and anti-Ro52 autoantibodies in patients with poly- and dermatomyositis. J Autoimmun 2006;27(1):62–8.

133. Shimizu T, Tomita Y, Son K, Nishinarita S, Sawada S, Horie T. Elevation of serum soluble tumour necrosis factor receptors in patients with polymyositis and dermatomyositis. Clin Rheumatol 2000;19(5):352–9.

134. Dastmalchi M, Grundtman C, Alexanderson H, et al. A high incidence of disease flares in an open pilot study of infliximab in patients with refractory inflammatory myopathies. Ann Rheum Dis 2008; 67(12):1670–7.

135. Iannone F, Scioscia C, Falappone PC, Covelli M, Lapadula G. Use of etanercept in the treatment of dermatomyositis: a case series. J Rheumatol 2006;33(9):1802–4.

136. Riley P, McCann LJ, Maillard SM, Woo P, Murray KJ, Pilkington CA. Effectiveness of infliximab in the treatment of refractory juvenile dermatomyositis with calcinosis. Rheumatology (Oxford) 2008;47(6):877–80.

137. Labioche I, Liozon E, Weschler B, Loustaud-Ratti V, Soria P, Vidal E. Refractory polymyositis responding to infliximab: extended follow-up. Rheumatology (Oxford) 2004;43(4):531–2.

138. Uthman I, El-Sayad J. Refractory polymyositis responding to infliximab. Rheumatology (Oxford) 2004;43(9):1198–9.

139. Sprott H, Glatzel M, Michel BA. Treatment of myositis with etanercept (Enbrel), a recombinant human soluble fusion protein of TNF-alpha type II receptor and IgG1. Rheumatology (Oxford) 2004;43(4):524–6.

140. Barohn RJ, Herbelin L, Kissel JT, et al. Pilot trial of etanercept in the treatment of inclusion-body myositis. Neurology 2006;66(2 Suppl 1):S123–4.

141. Hengstman GJ, De Bleecker JL, Feist E, et al. Open-label trial of anti-TNF-alpha in dermato- and polymyositis treated concomitantly with methotrexate. Eur Neurol 2008; 59(3-4):159–63.
142. Liozon E, Ouattara B, Loustaud-Ratti V, Vidal E. Severe polymyositis and flare in autoimmunity following treatment with adalimumab in a patient with overlapping features of polyarthritis and scleroderma. Scand J Rheumatol 2007;36(6):484–6.
143. Ramos-Casals M, Brito-Zeron P, Munoz S, et al. Autoimmune diseases induced by TNF-targeted therapies: analysis of 233 cases. Medicine (Baltimore) 2007;86(4):242–51.
144. Lundberg I, Ulfgren AK, Nyberg P, Andersson U, Klareskog L. Cytokine production in muscle tissue of patients with idiopathic inflammatory myopathies. Arthritis Rheum 1997;40(5):865–74.
145. Schmidt J, Barthel K, Wrede A, Salajegheh M, Bahr M, Dalakas MC. Interrelation of inflammation and APP in sIBM: IL-1 beta induces accumulation of beta-amyloid in skeletal muscle. Brain 2008;131(Pt 5):1228–40.
146. Chevrel G, Granet C, Miossec P. Contribution of tumour necrosis factor alpha and interleukin (IL) 1beta to IL6 production, NF-kappaB nuclear translocation, and class I MHC expression in muscle cells: in vitro regulation with specific cytokine inhibitors. Ann Rheum Dis 2005;64(9):1257–62.
147. Grundtman C, Salomonsson S, Dorph C, Bruton J, Andersson U, Lundberg IE. Immunolocalization of interleukin-1 receptors in the sarcolemma and nuclei of skeletal muscle in patients with idiopathic inflammatory myopathies. Arthritis Rheum 2007; 56(2):674–87.
148. Son K, Tomita Y, Shimizu T, Nishinarita S, Sawada S, Horie T. Abnormal IL-1 receptor antagonist production in patients with polymyositis and dermatomyositis. Intern Med 2000;39(2):128–35.
149. Baird GS, Montine TJ. Multiplex immunoassay analysis of cytokines in idiopathic inflammatory myopathy. Arch Pathol Lab Med 2008;132(2):232–8.
150. Furlan A, Botsios C, Ruffatti A, Todesco S, Punzi L. Antisynthetase syndrome with refractory polyarthritis and fever successfully treated with the IL-1 receptor antagonist, anakinra: a case report. Joint Bone Spine 2008;75(3):366–7.

# Chapter 4
# Juvenile Dermatomyositis: An Update on Clinical and Laboratory Findings

Lauren M. Pachman

**Abstract** The clinical and laboratory findings in juvenile dermatomyositis (JDM) are impacted by the duration of the chronic inflammation, which may not be reversible, making prompt diagnosis and institution of effective therapy imperative. With symptoms greater than 4 months, the child is more likely to have muscle enzymes within the normal range, chronic skin changes, decreased nailfold capillary end-row loops, with associated impaired bioavailability of orally administered prednisone (and perhaps other substances), thus providing the rationale for the intravenous route of administration of methylprednisolone. Diagnostic testing of resistant cases includes myositis-specific antibodies, which may identify children at risk for persistent disease, as well as interstitial pulmonary fibrosis. Chronic inflammation is often cutaneous and is accompanied by the development of dystrophic calcification, decreased bone density, and partial lipodystrophy with the potential of the metabolic syndrome. Great strides have been made in the characterization of the inflammation induced by type 1 interferon (IFN-$\alpha$/$\beta$), which shares features of the systemic lupus erythematosus (SLE)-like signature on gene expression profiling. Environmental influences, such as season of birth, ultraviolet exposure, as well as human leukocyte antigen (HLA)-related genetic factors DR3*0301, DQA*0501, and DAQ*0301, appear to contribute to disease susceptibility. Although the TNF-$\alpha$ A polymorphism at the $-308$ promoter region is associated with increased TNF-$\alpha$ production, augmenting the severity of the inflammatory process, sporadic reports of use of inhibitors of TNF-$\alpha$ have not been encouraging. Several biomarkers, such as the absolute number of circulating CD3-negative natural killer cells and serum levels of interferon alpha (IFN-$\alpha$) or interleukin 17 (IL-17) are under consideration as indicators of immune reactivity. Inasmuch as it appears that 40% of the children may heal vascular damage, the disease course could be considered as either unicyclic or nonunicyclic. The

L.M. Pachman
Division of Rheumatology, Children's Memorial Hospital, Northwestern University's Feinberg School of Medicine, FOCIS/CMRC Center of Excellence in Clinical Immunology, Cure JM Program of Excellence in Juvenile Myositis, Chicago, IL, USA

L.J. Kagen (ed.), *The Inflammatory Myopathies*,
DOI 10.1007/978-1-60327-827-0_4,
© Humana Press, a part of Springer Science + Business Media, LLC 2009

mainstay of therapy remains the corticosteroids with the use of methotrexate at diagnosis; hydroxychloroquine, mycophenolate mofetil (MMF), and intravenous immunoglobulin each appear to help diminish cutaneous symptoms, and the use of adequate doses of cyclosporine early in the development of calcifications may help their resolution. Other biologic interventions are currently under investigation. Overall, the outlook for children with JDM has markedly improved since the 1990's, but much more information is needed about disease etiology and pathogenesis to be able to intercept the inflammatory process more effectively.

**Keywords** Juvenile dermatomyositis • Interferon-alpha • TNF-alpha • Disease duration

## Historical Background and Overview

Although we now recognize juvenile dermatomyositis as the most common of the pediatric inflammatory myopathies, the major symptoms of characteristic rash and symmetrical proximal weakness were united into the diagnosis of a specific clinical entity only relatively recently. They were independently described by Wagner *(1)* and Hepp *(2)*, but Unverricht *(3)* stressed that these two defining clinical components were essential to the diagnosis. All three physicians' names were combined as late as 1967 in published case reports of children with these symptoms *(4)*. Because the term *JDM* was in use as an abbreviation for juvenile diabetes mellitus, *JDMS* was selected to indicate children with juvenile dermatomyositis (approximately 1979–1997). When the designations of type 1 and type 2 diabetes, which were based on new knowledge of disease pathophysiology, gained acceptance *(5)*, the term *JDM* could then be employed to identify children with juvenile dermatomyositis, in parallel with the term used for adults with dermatomyositis (DM).

This review focuses on evidence concerning clinical and laboratory features of children reported to have both the characteristic rash of JDM and symmetrical proximal muscle weakness. We now recognize that these criteria still define a very heterogeneous population although the pediatric patients fulfill the classical criteria of Bohan and Peter *(6)* for definite/probable JDM. For a more comprehensive discussion of disease classification, serologic findings, the inflammatory milieu, and muscle biopsy data, as well as modes of assessment, please refer to the specific chapters related to these subjects presented in this text.

## Demographic Data

Classified as a rare disease, a National New-Onset JDM Registry sponsored by the National Institutes of Health established the yearly incidence of JDM as 3.2 cases per million children under the age of 18 *(7)*, compared with a yearly incidence of

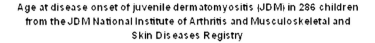

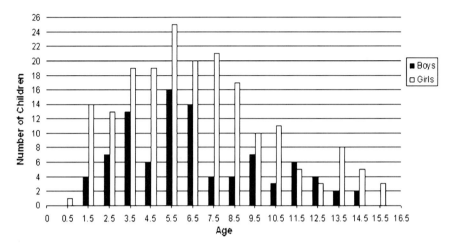

Fig. 4.1 Bar graph representing the age at the time of the first symptom, either rash or weakness, in children diagnosed with juvenile dermatomyositis *(12)*. The open bars represent girls; the solid bars depict boys

1.9 per million children under the age of 16 reported for the United Kingdom *(8,9)*. Unlike systemic lupus erythematosus (SLE) or the overlap syndromes, there does not appear to be an increased incidence of specifically defined JDM in the black population in either geographic region. For the New Onset JDM Research Registry, the ethnicity distribution of 395 newly diagnosed children with rash and weakness was white (75%), Hispanic (11%), black (10%), and Asian (2%) *(8,9,10)*, which is similar to Great Britain *(8)*, but differs in other parts of the world *(11–14)*. There is a female predominance: 2.3:1 in the United States *(7)* compared with a 2.2:1 ratio in the United Kingdom *(9)* and a 4.5:1 ratio in Taiwan *(13)*, in contrast to Japan *(12)*, as well as Saudi Arabia, where more boys than girls with JDM were reported (1:1.3) *(14)*. With respect to age at the time of the first definitive JDM symptom, rash, or weakness, more than 25% of the patients in the U.S. registry were age 4 or younger *(13)*, similar to data from Great Britain (Fig. 4.1) *(8)*.

## Risk Factors for JDM: Overview

Ancestral gene associations with autoimmune disease in general, and the inflammatory myopathies in particular, are discussed in Chap. 2. Studies of monozygotic twins indicated that the concordance rates for most autoimmune diseases are low in general *(15)*, despite sporadic reports of monozygotic twins with JDM *(16)*, suggesting significant participation of epigenetic factors rather than straightforward patterns of genetic inheritance related to human leukocyte antigen (HLA) *(17)*. Although familial DM is rare *(18)*, it has been recognized for over a decade that the children with inflammatory myopathies have strong family pedigrees documenting multigenerational autoimmunity *(19)*.

More recently, attention has turned to environmental risk factors and their interaction with specific genetic markers. These environmental risk factors include occupational exposure, previous drug exposure, vaccines, infectious agents, and ultraviolet (UV) light. Although administration of vaccines (most notably hepatitis B) has been reported before the onset of a modified case of JDM *(20)*, it is difficult to prove causality. Macrophage myositis has been implicated after administration of vaccines when aluminum hydroxide was identified in electron micrographs of muscle from the affected patient *(21)*. Finally, there is a brief report of the clinical features of patients given vaccines before developing an inflammatory myopathy *(22)*.

## Ultraviolet Light as an Environmental Risk Factor

It is well known that sun exposure can precipitate or reactivate both the cutaneous and muscle symptoms of JDM *(23)*. Increased sun exposure (as determined by latitude of residence) is associated with an increased incidence of Mi-2, an antihelicase antibody, in sera from children with JDM *(24)*. The antigen Mi-2 is a component of the multisubunit protein complex, which substantially contributes to nucleosome remodeling *(25)* and appears to increase with increasing UV intensity *(26)*. In fact, the overall relative incidence of adults with DM increases with decreasing latitude and increasing intensity of UV light *(27)*, which suggests that there may be a continuum between juvenile polymyositis (JPM) and JDM in children as well. Children with polymyositis, when exposed to excessive UVB may develop characteristics of DM *(28)*. Patients with DM and photosensitivity (similar to those with SLE) may have a lower threshold of sensitivity to develop erythema when exposed to UVB, which is known to elicit interferon alpha (IFN-$\alpha$) *(29)*. This sensitivity may be augmented by the tumor necrosis factor alpha (TNF-$\alpha$) 308A allele that appears to enable keratinocytes to produce more TNF-$\alpha$ on exposure to UVB *(30)*.

## Infection as an Environmental Risk Factor

Investigation of patterns of infection in association with the first detection of the symptoms, as in other autoimmune diseases *(31)*, has been fruitful in JDM. A U.S. national study of 286 children with new onset of the symptoms of JDM documented that, in the 3 months before the first symptom of JDM, 57% of the patients had upper respiratory complaints, 30% gastrointestinal complaints, and of these, 63% were given antibiotics *(10)*, and 19% had contact with a sick animal, suggesting a possible vector *(10)*. In a Canadian study, preceding upper respiratory complaints were identified in 24 of 30 children with JDM *(32)*. Monozygotic twins were reported to have severe upper respiratory infections 1 week before they both displayed symptoms of JDM *(16)*.

In an early case-control study (1967–1972) of 48 children with myositis, an antecedent group A beta hemolytic streptococcal infection was reported for 20 cases of myositis, compared with 13 children in the control group *(33)*. Furthermore, a documented streptococcal infection elicited recurrence of JDM symptoms and necrotizing vasculitis *(34)*, suggesting that this microbe played a role in disease pathogenesis. This line of investigation was pursued by Massa et al. *(35)* in an investigation of HLA-binding peptide motifs, which identified two overlapping epitopes of the streptococcal M5 type protein and their counterparts, derived from homologous regions of human skeletal heavy chain myosin. JDM disease activity was highly associated with T-cell reactivity to the myositis-specific peptides as determined by lymphocyte proliferation, cytotoxicity, and cytokine release. Oligoclonality and largely overlapping T-cell receptor (TCR) Vβ gene usage in the responding cell population were documented as well *(35)*. These studies identifying a potential self-antigen in some, but not all, patients with active JDM suggested that it might be a target for specific immunotherapy *(35)*. Studies of T-cell expansion confirmed CD8[+] T-cell oligoclonality in JDM muscle inflammatory infiltrates *(36)*, as well as increased levels of somatic mutant frequencies to an unidentified antigen in peripheral blood from children with JDM compared with age-matched controls *(37)*. Peripheral blood studies documented a selective depletion of CD3-negative CD56[+]/CD16[+] natural killer cells that was highly associated with inflammatory muscle disease at diagnosis and with cutaneous disease activity over 36 months, suggesting that this assay might be a potential biomarker for disease activity *(38)*.

Another group of potential infectious antigens are the Coxsackie virus B members of the enterovirus group. A case-control antibody study tested sera obtained within 4 months of the first definite symptom in 12 new onset children with JDM who lived in the northern Midwest. These sera were compared with 24 regional, age-matched controls with juvenile idiopathic arthritis and 2,192 children hospitalized with viral syndromes. This study documented an increase in complement-fixing antibodies to Coxsackie Virus B (CVB) B1, B2, and B4 and an increase in type-specific neutralizing antibody to CV B2, B4, and B5, thus providing evidence of specific serologic response to B2 and B4 antigenic stimulation using both methods *(39)*. There were no other significant differences between test and controls to 13 other CV viral antigens, hepatitis B surface antigen, or *Mycoplasma pneumoniae* *(39)*. Testing for specific neutralizing antibody in adults with DM showed elevated titers to CV B antigens *(40)*. In a subsequent U.S. national case-control study (1989–1992), an increase in antibody titers to enterovirus, but not to specific Coxsackie virus B antigens, was measured in 80 children with JDM and their playmates but not in children from the same region who had juvenile arthritis *(41)*. These data provide evidence to suggest an antigenic response to CVB antigens, which may fluctuate over the years, may be influenced by the length of time from the onset of the first symptom of JDM to the time of testing and may vary with the geographic region of the country.

There are conflicting reports of detection of enteroviral/CV B antigens for the examination of skeletal muscle from patients with inflammatory myopathy (seven JDM) showed that five were positive for CV B RNA by reverse transcriptase polymerase chain reaction (RT-PCR) and slot-blot hybridization *(42)*. This finding is in contrast to work by a different team, who tested adult diagnostic biopsies (ten polymyositis, five DM) using PCR and Southern blot analysis without identi-fication of enterovirus or encephalomyocarditis antigen *(43)*. Their experimental design included a murine model positive control by which exposure to enteroviral antigen produced clinical myositis *(44)*. When muscle biopsies from 20 untreated children with JDM were tested, a search for viral-related RNA or bacterial DNA was not successful *(45)*. At the moment, despite active and continued speculation about the role of environmental agents that might serve to start the inflammatory cascade found in JDM, no specific agents (or shared antigens) have been consistently identified as causative agents in the etiology of JDM *(46)*.

## Seasonality: Associations with Disease Onset and Birth of Children with JDM

The onset of symptoms of 11 of 12 children with JDM who lived in the central Midwestern states was reported to occur between June and January. These children also had elevated complement-fixing titers to CV B as noted in the preceding section *(39)*. This apparent seasonality was confirmed in a national study of 79 children (1989–1992) who had a peak of disease onset peak symptoms in the months from June to September *(47)*. In a subsequent study, seasonality was not verified in a larger nationwide study of 323 children diagnosed with JDM, but without serological subcharacterization regarding myositis-associated or -specific antibodies (MAAs or MSAs, respectively) *(10)*. A Toronto study also identified spring as the time of peak onset of symptoms since 1991 in 120 children with inflammatory myopathies, including those who were classified as having amyopathic JDM *(48)*. Thus, although there appears to be a trend toward increased onset of JDM symptoms in the spring or summer in the northern part of the continent of North America, this observation is still under active investigation and may vary not only by latitude and extent of exposure to UVB but also by year.

In contrast, the season of birth appears to be a contribution factor to JDM disease susceptibility. A large, well-controlled study of the season of birth of 307 children with JDM showed that birth dates of Hispanic children with JDM peaked in mid-October, compared with the uniform distribution birthdays of Hispanic children without JDM ($p=0.002$). Children negative for the p155 antibody (discussed in Chap. 10) had a mean birth date of July 5, while those positive for this antibody did not have a significant localization in the calendar year *(49)*. HLA antigens were also grouped by time of year of birth. An HLA antigen on chromosome 6, DQA1*0501, was linked to births centering about August 7, while those negative for this antigen were grouped about April 14 ($p = 0.039$) *(49)*.

It was conjectured that a specific season of birth of infants who went on to develop JDM might be associated with increased exposure to a particular antigen that was prevalent at that time of year *(49)*.

## Diagnostic Criteria for Juvenile Dermatomyositis

The diagnosis of JDM should be considered when the child develops an unexplained, persistent rash on the face or over the joints, complains of muscle weakness or pain, or has increasing trouble with the activities of daily living that require functional proximal musculature. The criteria that are still the most utilized are those of Bohan and Peter *(6)*, in which category IV contains children with either myositis alone or myositis with the characteristic rash. Children with JDM are clearly differentiated from patients with these symptoms who also have other connective tissue diseases, in which the "natural history of such heterogeneous myopathic syndromes is surely influenced by the underlying concomitant disorder" *(6)*. Table 4.1 presents the criteria currently required for the definitive diagnosis of JDM and presents some of the advantages and problems that accompany each of these criteria. Despite their imperfections, the classification criteria originally proposed by Bohan and Peter are still widely used in the diagnosis of children with inflammatory myopathy: symmetrical proximal muscle weakness, characteristic rash, elevated serum levels of muscle-derived enzymes, a muscle biopsy that is characteristic of an inflammatory myopathy, and an electromyograph (EMG) that is characteristic of an inflammatory myopathy not a neuropathy (discussed in Chap. 2). Some examples of the characteristic rash include a malar rash that crosses the bridge of the nose as well as telangiectasia of capillaries on the eyelids (Fig. 4.2a). The vasculitis may be associated with ulceration, often in the area of the medial as well as the lateral canthus of the eye (shown in Fig. 4.2b), and dilated capillaries at the edge of the nailfold, with progressive dropout of the end-row capillary loops (Fig. 4.2c). Another common cutaneous feature is thickened papules (alligator skin) on the dorsum of the hand over the MCP (metacarpal phalyngeal) and PIP (proximal interphalyngeal) joints (Fig. 4.2d). The T2-weighted image with fat suppression will often identify symmetrical change and thickened fascia around inflamed muscle groups (see Chap. 8) and provides a guide for the diagnostic muscle biopsy. The muscle biopsy provides critical documentation of the extent of tissue damage and gives an indication of the chronicity of the process, with increased fibrosis and capillary occlusion in addition to the classical perifascicular atrophy and inflammatory infiltrate (see Chap. 6).

Other diagnostic modalities were proposed by an international consensus conference to evaluate children with inflammatory myopathy, including serologic testing for MSAs and MAAs as well as nailfold capillary microscopy (Table 4.2) *(50)*. MSAs were not identified until 1991, when Love et al. *(51)* proposed that they classified subgroups of idiopathic inflammatory myopathies (IIMs) (also see Chaps 2 and 10). In U.S. children with IIMs, the frequency of these MSAs is on the order of 10–30%. The recently described anti-p-155 autoantibody was documented in about 30% of children and adults with JDM and DM, respectively. In adults, DM

**Table 4.1** Bohan and Peter Criteria *(6)*

| | | Advantages (+) and problems (−) |
|---|---|---|
| 1. Characteristic rashes | | |
| Scaly erythematous eruptions over the metacarpal-phalangeal or interphalangeal joints (Grotton's papules) | − | May be subtle and initially intermittent, related to sun exposure |
| Periorbital purplish discoloration (heliotrope rash) | − | Gottron's papules seen in overlap syndromes |
| Erythematous scaly rashes over the face, neck (V sign), upper back, and arms (shawl sign) and extensor tendons (linear extensor erythema) and other extensor surfaces | + | In full-blown state, rash is diagnostic |
| 2. Symmetric, often progressive, proximal muscle weakness | | |
| | − | Difficult to test reliably in children under the age of 4 |
| | + | Childhood Myositis Assessment Scale (CMAS) reliably measures both strength and endurance |
| 3. Elevations of serum levels of muscle-associated enzymes | | |
| Creatine kinase (CK) | − | Often normalize within 4.5 months; selected elevation of one-fourth of enzymes |
| Aldolase | − | Lack of method standardization |
| Lactate dehydrogenase (LDH) | − | Aldolase often not performed |
| Transaminases (ALT/SGPT and AST/SGOT) | + | If positive, helps to establish diagnosis |
| | + | Used to follow patient's response to therapy early in disease course |
| 4. Characteristic, electromyographic (EMG) triad seen in myositis | | |
| Short-duration, small, low-amplitude polyphasic potentials | | May be normal if unaffected muscle is tested |
| Fibrillation potentials, seen even at rest | | Invasive and painful |
| Bizarre, high-frequency repetitive discharges | | Differentiates neuropathy from myopathy |
| 5. Evidence of chronic inflammation in muscle biopsy | | |
| Necrosis of type I and type II muscle fibers | − | May not reflect degree of inflammation if not magnetic resonance imaging (MRI) directed |
| Degeneration and regeneration of myofibers with variation in myofiber size | − | Invasive and expensive |
| Interstitial of perivascular mononuclear cells | + | Provides clear evidence of type of inflammation, early vascular changes, tissue damage, disease pathophysiology |

*AST* Aspartate aminotransferase; *ALT* alanine aminotransferase

was highly linked to a concurrent malignancy *(52)*. In Great Britain, 23% of children with JDM were positive for this antibody, which was associated with specific clinical characteristics: more cutaneous involvement, Gottron's papules, ulcerations, and edema, with periorbital swelling and rash over the small and large joints *(53)*. The next most

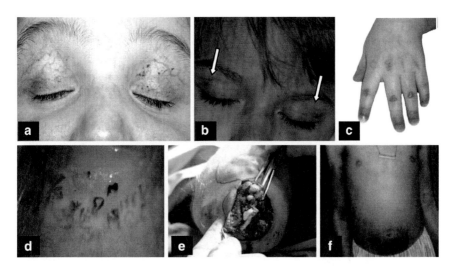

**Fig. 4.2** (**a**) The rash of JDM crosses the bridge of the nose, and in active vasculitis, the capillaries on the eyelids may develop telangiectasia as illustrated here. (**b**) Infarcts of the lateral aspect of both eyelids in a child with vasculitic JDM (*arrow*). (**c**) Gottron's papules over the PIPs and MCPs as well as erythema of the nailfold margin in a child with newly diagnosed JDM. (**d**) Nailfold capillary dropout with residual dilated and tortuous microvasculature and increased cuticle associated with decreased vascularity. (**e**) Interoperative photograph of the removal of calcifications from subcutaneous fat. (**f**) Evidence of acanthosis nigricans in a boy with long-standing symptoms of JDM

**Table 4.2**   Additional parameters for diagnosis *(50)*

| | Advantages (+) and problems (−) | |
|---|---|---|
| 1. Nailfold capillaroscopy | − | Methods of data collection, interpretation not yet standardized |
| | + | Provides a sequential record for examination |
| 2. Magnetic resonance imaging | − | Requires sedation for younger child; may not identify early, primarily vascular changes; edema not specific for JDM |
| | + | When pattern is symmetrical and typical, identifies affected tissue |
| 3. Myositis-specific antibodies | − | Expensive; not easily available; long turnaround time |
| | + | Identifies subgroups of children with specific clinical course |
| 4. Indicators of immune activation | − | Not widely available; may not be disease specific |
| | + | More sensitive indicators of disease flare before clinical symptoms |

common MSA in childhood is anti-Mi-2, an antihelicase antibody, found in about 10% of children *(24)*. Children with this MSA may have an initially mild disease course, which may be followed by interstitial pulmonary involvement in later years.

In children with polymyositis, other antibodies are more common: JO-1 antigen *(54)* and anti-SRP *(55)*. Each defines a subgroup of children who may have symptoms of myositis and pulmonary interstitial fibrosis that may be resistant to therapy.

## Physical Signs of Children with JDM at Diagnosis

At diagnosis, children with JDM are more likely to be below their age-related percentiles for height and weight, which is directly related to the chronicity of the inflammatory process prior to diagnosis *(56)*. The NIAMS New Onset Registry study of 162 untreated children with definite or probable JDM showed that older children were more likely to present with dysphagia ($p = 0.017$), fever ($p = 0.022$), and arthritis ($p < 0.001$) at diagnosis, while the longer the period of untreated inflammation was, the more likely that dystrophic calcifications would develop ($p = 0.006$). Several reviews compiled information concerning the diagnosis of children with myositis *(57, 58)* as well as our current concepts of the immunologic mechanisms involved in disease pathophysiology *(59)*. Table 4.3 presents the dominant clinical features of children with JDM *(59)*. Some of the clinical challenges are briefly reviewed here.

**Table 4.3** Clinical features of patients with juvenile dermatomyositis

Constitutional
  Fever: 16–65%
  Adenopathy: 20%
  Lethargy: 10%
Pulmonary
  Dyspnea: 7–43%
Gastrointestinal
  Dysphonia or dysphagia: 18–44%
  Gastrointestinal symptoms: 22–37%
Musculoskeletal
  Weakness: 95%
  Myalgia or arthralgia: 25–73%
  Arthritis: 23–58%
  Contractures: 26–27%
  Raynaud's disease: 9–14%
Cutaneous
  Gottron's papules: 57–100%
  Heliotrope rash: 66–100%
  Nailfold capillary changes: 91%
  Malar or facial rash: 42–73%
  Mouth ulcers: 35%
  Skin ulcers: 23–30%
  Limb edema: 11–32%
  Calcinosis: 6–30%
  Lipodystrophy: 10–14%

*Source:* From **Ref. 59**. Reprinted from *The Lancet*. Used with permission from Elsevier

## Gastrointestinal

A life-threatening symptom of JDM is difficulty swallowing for fluid may come out the nose, or produce choking, as a result of loss of smooth muscle peristaltic waves in the lower two-thirds of the esophagus. In its most severe form, there is penetration of the airway, with entry into the larynx, often associated with subsequent pneumonia. Penetration of the airway can be documented by a very thin preparation of barium given as a rehabilitation cookie swallow. Children with milder esophageal impairment may demonstrate pooling of the barium in the valeculae. Often, the child will complain of heartburn, even prior to the administration of corticosteroids, and testing for esophageal reflux may be positive, particularly when core strength is diminished. Palatal weakness may be assessed by asking the child to say the letter "E" to ascertain change in voice quality because acquisition of a more nasal tone is often an associated finding. Penetration of the airway is cause for admission to the hospital to control the symptoms of inflammation effectively and to forestall aspiration pneumonia.

A common gastrointestinal complaint is constipation, often early in the disease course, which is also a reflection of decreased smooth muscle tone. It is not unusual for the child to complain of early satiety, claiming to be full after a few bites of food only to be hungry a few hours later. This may occur in either the untreated child or one with active symptoms not yet responsive to therapy. Another increasingly recognized complaint is that of abdominal cramping, which may be associated with concomitant celiac disease *(60)*.

## Unusual Cutaneous Components of JDM

In addition to the classical findings detailed in Chap. 13, children may present with massive anasarca *(61)* and panniculitis *(62, 63)*, which like SLE, may occur on the scalp, arms, thighs, and buttocks *(64)*. The clinical and therapeutic aspects of cutaneous involvement in JDM are reviewed elsewhere *(65)*.

## Cardiac and Pulmonary Complications

Cardiac involvement in untreated children with JDM may be indicated early in the disease course by tachycardia or a right bundle branch block pattern on electrocardiogram *(66)* and occasionally later in the disease course by dilated myocardiopathy *(67)*. Severe muscle weakness in children with myositis may mask respiratory compromise for they may not be able to move about and they also have limited lung funtion. Pulmonary complaints may become apparent as the child regains muscle strength and endurance, only to be limited by shortness of breath. Children who are weak and who test positive for antibody against the Jo-1 antigen may or may not have inflammatory skin manifestations. They may also have evidence of interstitial fibrosis, or honeycombing, on high-resolution computed tomography (CT) of the chest accompanied by decreased diffusion studies of the lung *(68)*. On the other hand, children who are positive for SRP often have muscle disease that is refractory to medical therapy and frequently develop severe progressive interstitial fibrosis of the lung early in their disease course *(55)*.

## *Decreased Peripheral Vascular Perfusion*

It is not uncommon for children with JDM to have loss of end-row capillary loops on nailfold capillaroscopy (Fig. 4.2d) *(69)*. They may complain that their hands and feet are so cold that they must wear socks and gloves to bed at night. Other vulnerable areas are the tip of the nose and the pinnae of the ears. The decreased perfusion of the digits is often associated with minor cutaneous infections, such as paronyechae, which often respond to topical antibiotics, such as mupirocin, but may require intravenous administration of antibiotics to eliminate the infection. Because these local cutaneous infections are usually positive for staphylococcal or streptococcal organisms, they may precipitate the flare of systemic disease if they are not promptly treated.

## Muscle Histopathology in the Pediatric Inflammatory Myopathies

Induction of major histocompatibility complex (MHC) class I antigen on the muscle fibers has long been recognized as one of the early signs of inflammatory response in affected muscle *(70, 71)* and is considered as a possible diagnostic test to differentiate inflammatory myopathy from the dystrophies of childhood *(72)*. It is only recently that the range of inflammatory changes in morphologically normal pediatric muscle have been quantified *(73)*, thus permitting comparisons with muscle biopsy data from children with definite or probable JDM. An international consensus conference scored muscle biopsies from 33 children with untreated JDM for capillary loss, inflammatory cells, and the muscle domain (including muscle fiber damage, perifascicular atrophy, expression of neonatal myosin degeneration or regeneration), and increase in connective tissue, with the goal of uncovering predictors of disease course *(74)*. Biopsies of affected muscle in children with untreated JDM contained increased mononuclear cells positive for CD3 (pan T cell), $p < 0.002$; CD68 (monocytes/macrophages, some dendritic cells $p < 0.002$); CD20 (B cells, $p < 0.004$), and neonatal myosin ($p < 0.002$) *(74)*, which is present in regenerating muscle *(75)*.

Another group proposed, after a study of 72 biopsies, that the child's subsequent clinical course could be predicted by the muscle biopsy findings, but they did not factor into the analysis the duration of untreated disease prior to the muscle biopsy *(76)* or define the immune composition of the muscle biopsy components that appear to be associated with cytotoxicity and tissue damage. There is histological evidence that polymyositis and JDM may be part of a disease continuum. Only one in five children diagnosed with JPM had muscle pathology consistent with JPM, the rest had characteristic features of JDM, vascular involvement, and perifasicular atrophy *(48)*, and the clinical course of JPM may evolve into that of JDM (see the next section).

## Type 1 Interferon-Induced Genetic Response in Muscle and Blood from Children with JDM

The tantalizing data from the studies of the symptoms of infection preceding the first definite symptom of JDM suggest that either an elusive agent or a shared epitope (perhaps following the molecular mimicry pathway) in a supportive genetic setting may stimulate the immune response cascade leading to symptoms of JDM. Substantiating support for this premise is derived from evidence, first reported in 2002, concerning the florid type 1 interferon (IFN-$\alpha/\beta$) response identified in gene expression profile studies of diagnostic muscle biopsy samples from untreated children with active JDM symptoms *(77)*. Peripheral blood mononuclear cells were used to identify upregulation of type 1 IFN-induced genes, which appeared to correlate with muscle inflammation but not the continued skin involvement over time *(78)*. Increased selective expression of IFN-$\alpha$-induced genes peripheral blood mononuclear cells from patients with DM (both adult and pediatric) was confirmed *(79)*. This observation was extended to document that the peripheral blood mononuclear cells from 30 to 50% of children with active symptoms of classical JDM had an SLE-like type 1 IFN gene expression profile signature *(80)*. Further supporting data came from examination of the sera of 84% of untreated patients with JDM, which detected levels of IFN-$\alpha$, significantly associated with the TNF-$\alpha$-308 A allele and which declined to control levels with the institution of effective therapy *(81)*.

Children presenting with polymyositis had undetectable levels of IFN-$\alpha$, but one child (MSA negative) with biopsy-confirmed polymyositis and disease resolution, off all medication for 2 years, had intense sun exposure and developed a limited rash of JDM and recurrence of profound weakness with elevation of muscle-derived enzymes 3 months later. Sequential serological studies documented the development of elevated circulating levels of IFN-$\alpha$, comparable to that measured in JDM, in contrast to very low levels measured in matched children with JPM. The serum level of IFN-$\alpha$ gradually declined as the child's symptoms responded to therapy *(28)*.

## Commonalities and Differences Between Children with JDM and SLE

Further studies of gene expression profile data from peripheral blood showed that children with JDM who had both a JDM signature as well as an SLE-like signature also had very low levels of antibody to three SLE-like antigens: Ro 56, Ro 60, and SSA *(82)*.

Previous studies had firmly documented that, in contrast to children with SLE, children with JDM did not have evidence of polyclonal B cell activation. Of a panel of 14 tissue and cellular antigens, the only antibody identified in 80% of children with JDM was a speckled antinuclear antibody with an average titer of 1:320 *(83)*. Furthermore, symptoms of inflammatory myopathy, including skin manifestations, develop in children who have a congenital immunodeficiency in immunoglobulin production *(84, 85)*, suggesting that B cells may not necessarily be a critical factor in JDM disease pathophysiology even though they are clearly part of the activated immune response in the inflammatory myopathy *(86)*. This evidence propelled an ongoing clinical trial of antibody to CD20, a B-cell antigen, in patients with IIMs.

## Impact of Duration of Untreated Disease at Diagnosis on Physical and Laboratory Findings as Well as Gene Expression Profile Data

We are just beginning to identify some of the long-term effects of chronic, unsuppressed inflammation in children with JDM and the impact of inflammation on the evolution of the disease pathophysiology.

### *Physical Findings*

The length of the interval of time between the first definite symptom of JDM, rash or weakness, and diagnostic testing plays a critical role in disease pathophysiology. As noted, children with JDM are frequently shorter and lighter in weight than their age-related healthy counterparts *(56)*. Children who have a sudden onset of weakness often come to diagnosis within several weeks of trouble, but children with a persistent rash often wait for a much longer time to obtain medical care. The rash of JDM, not the muscle weakness, is accompanied by loss of end-row capillary loops on nailfold capillaroscopy, suggesting that there are significant differences in the pathophysiology of the inflammatory process in muscle compared with the pathophysiology in inflamed skin *(87)*.

### *Diagnostic Laboratory Testing*

Muscle enzyme elevation is one of the criteria for diagnosis of an inflammatory myopathy, including JDM, but children who have a moderately prolonged interval of time, 4.5 months or more, between their first symptom and diagnostic testing may have muscle enzymes that are well within the normal range (Table 4.4) *(56)*.

**Table 4.4**   Cut points of untreated JDM that optimally differentiate the children with normal and nonnormal muscle enzymes ($n = 126$)

| Enzyme | Children with normal values | Children with nonnormal values | Cut point of untreated JDM, in months[a] | $P$ value |
|---|---|---|---|---|
| CK | 33 (26%) | 93 | 4.65 | <0.01 |
| LDH | 16 (13%) | 110 | 2.53 | <0.01 |
| Aldolase | 22 (17%) | 104 | 4.65 | <0.01 |
| SGOT/AST | 21 (17%) | 105 | 3.68 | <0.01 |

*Source:* From **Ref. 56**. Reprinted from *The Journal of Pediatrics*. Used with permission from Elsevier

[a]Children with duration of untreated JDM (in months) greater than these cut points are classified as having normal enzyme values. Those with duration of untreated disease less than or equal to these cut points are classified as having a nonnormal (high) enzyme value

## Bone Density

At diagnosis (for those over the age of 4), the age-adjusted Z score is often much lower than expected (*88*) and is associated with an elevated RANKL (Receptor activator of nuclear factor kappa B ligand)- OPG (Osteoprotegerin) ratio, indicating osteoclastic activation (*89*). Furthermore, it is not uncommon to have low levels of osteocalcin, indicating decreased bone turnover, despite normal serum concentrations of ionized calcium and parathyroid hormone (*90*). In addition, in JDM absorption of calcium is decreased, which is exacerbated by administration of corticosteroids, thus making administration of vitamin D and calcium (see the section on supplemental therapies) imperative in children with growing bones.

## Microvascular Changes

The capillary loop structures in the nailfolds are easily accessible for examination in children, including those with JDM (*91, 92*). Prolonged cutaneous inflammation of JDM is associated with progressive loss of end-row capillary loops as quantitated by capillary microscopy (Fig. 4.2d) (*69*). Children seen early in their disease course but who meet the criteria of probable or definite JDM may have normal numbers of end-row capillary loops at diagnosis, but capillary loss is documented on sequential examination (*93*). This capillary loss persists as long as 36 months after start of therapy in approximately 60% of children, but the remaining 40% show clear evidence of revascularization so that the microvasculature recovers to approach the normal range. At 36 months after diagnosis, children who had a unicyclic course had documentation of increased regeneration of end-row capillary loops ($p$-0.007) and improvement of the disease activity score (DAS) for skin (DAS skin, $p <$ 0.001). These data suggest that classification of the disease course of JDM might be reduced to two variables—unicyclic or nonunicyclic (*87*)—rather than the three options of unicyclic, intermittent, or continuous disease course (*94*).

## *Pattern of Cell Death*

Chronic inflammation appears to alter the mechanism and distribution of muscle and endothelial cell death. In diagnostic muscle biopsies from 14 untreated children with JDM, symptoms longer than 2 months were associated with a greater number of FAS (Apoptosis Stimulating Fragment)-positive cells in the perivascular region, indicating endothelial cell death. In the muscle, there was increased caspase 3 and nuclei positive for TUNEL (terminal deoxynucleotidyl transferase biotin-dUTP nick end labeling) within the laminin layer of the muscle cell, indicating apoptosis, compared with biopsies from children with short disease duration of less than 2 months. Children who were weaker came to diagnosis more rapidly and had overall more TUNEL-positive cells, indicating muscle death, and lack of caspase 3 staining, suggesting a necrotic rather than an apoptotic process *(95)*.

## *Dystrophic Calcifications*

The young age of the child, persistent chronic inflammation, and local injury all contribute to the development of dystrophic calcifications. The deposits may develop over the elbows, buttocks, and thighs, at sites of pressure, as well as over the patella and behind knees (Fig. 4.2e). In older children with active inflammation, calcifications increase in fat, often at the tail of the breast or in the abdomen at the belt line. In some children who test negative for Pm (polymyositis)/Scl (scleroderma), small calcifications occur on the palmar surface of the digits, similar to those seen in defined scleroderma.

Clearly, these deposits are a consequence of the chronicity and local intensity of the inflammatory response, often fueled by the proinflammatory cytokine TNF-$\alpha$. Both muscle fibers *(96)* and peripheral blood mononuclear cells from children with JDM positive for the TNF-$\alpha$-308 A polymorphism are more likely to produce more TNF-$\alpha$ than tissues that are negative for this allele. In addition, children positive for the TNF-$\alpha$-308 A polymorphism are more likely to have a chronic disease course as well as dystrophic calcifications *(97)*. These calcifications contain an uneven distribution of the mineral hydroxyapatite, as identified by X-ray diffraction and micro-CT. Areas of the body subjected to external pressure contain more densely packed calcifications *(98)*.

A contributing factor to the development of dystrophic calcifications is chronic cutaneous inflammation in the very young child *(99)*, who may also have less fetuin-A *(100)* to retard his or her development *(101)*. One of the components of dystrophic calcifications, matrix gammacarboxyglutamate (GLA) protein (MGP), is excreted in the urine of children with JDM at twice the rate of healthy children. Those who had JDM with calcifications excreted MGP at three times the normal values *(102)*. Immunohistochemical studies of muscle stained for various forms of MGP (unphosphorylated, phosphorylated, carboxylated, and noncarboxylated) showed a higher display of phosphorylated MGP in the muscle of JDM patients who had dystrophic calcification than children with JDM without calcific deposits or children with muscular dystrophy *(103)*.

Immunohistochemical studies of the calcifications themselves have documented the presence of members of the SIBLING (small integrin-binding ligand N-linked glycoprotein) family in different regions of the deposits *(104)*. As the calcifications are mobilized, they may drain, either as extrusions of ricelike grains or more liquid, seeping out as "milk of calcium." It is not uncommon for areas of chronic inflammation and necrosis to develop a calcified rim that surrounds fluid containing high levels of hydroxyapatite and that may attract infection with atypical mycobacterium, requiring additional specific therapy.

## *Partial Lipodystrophy*

Children who have prolonged active symptoms of JDM are at risk for developing partial lipodystrophy (PLD), which is characterized by loss of subcutaneous fat (particularly over the proximal muscles and buccal area), resulting in a hypermuscular appearance, menstrual irregularities in girls, and elevated triglycerides, leading to an incipient metabolic syndrome, associated with acanthosis nigricans (Fig. 4.2e). Assessment of abnormalities in fat distribution in children has been performed by measuring skinfold thickness with calipers *(105)* or by determining the trunk-to-limb ratio of fat distribution using DXA (Dual X-ray absorptiometry)-derived values *(106)*. Unlike adults, in which the DXA was able to detect differences in localized or generalized loss of fat *(107)*, use of this modality in children with PLD was not sensitive enough to confirm the clinical impressions *(106)*. Of note, in these children (all under 18), PLD was associated with duration of untreated disease and loss of nailfold capillary end-row loops *(106)*.

## Chronic Inflammation and Gene Expression Profile Data

Chronic inflammation alters the genes that are upregulated in muscle biopsies from untreated children with JDM. Muscle biopsies from untreated children with active symptoms of either long or short duration display a marked upregulation of genes induced by type 1 IFN-$\alpha$. For example, a gene that helps resists viral invasion, myxovirus A (MXA), was upregulated 96-fold (Fig. 4.3) *(77)*. When biopsies were tested for gene expression profiles using the variable of long duration compared with short duration of symptoms, disease lasting 2 months or more was associated with a significant increase in genes associated with vascular remodeling *(108)*, noted previously *(109)*, as well as a marked increase in mature plasmacytoid dendritic cells as defined by the immunohistochemical markers, DC (Dendritic Cell) Lamp and BDCA2 (C-type lectin uniquely expressed by human plasmacytoid dendritic cells (pDCs)) *(108)*. Examination of sequential samples of peripheral blood mononuclear cells from children with untreated JDM by quantitative RT-PCR showed marked

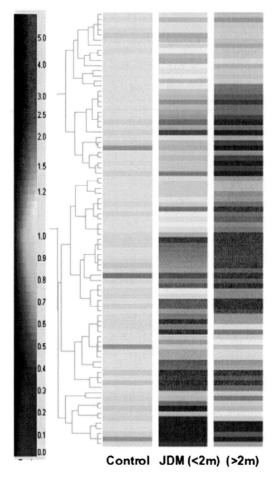

**Fig. 4.3** Comparison of gene expression profiles from diagnostic muscle biopsies from 19 girls with JDM with disease duration longer than 2 months with 3 girls who had symptoms for 2 months or less, showing differences in levels of expression. Vascular remodeling genes were upregulated biopsies from children with longer disease duration (From **Ref. *108***. Reprinted from BMC Immunology. Used with permission from Biomed Central, see Creative Commons at http:// creativecommons.org/licenses/by/3.0)

upregulation of the IFN-α-induced gene MXA, which was highly associated with muscle rather than skin inflammation, again suggesting that there were two separate potential pathways for disease pathogenesis in muscle and in skin. By 10 years after diagnosis, the level of MXA gene expression returned to that of age-matched control *(78)*. Further examination of the immune response has documented a central role of CD 17⁺ Tregs in directing the immune response pathway in patients with DM, suggesting that IL-17 might serve as a biomarker for disease activity (see Chap. 3) *(110)*.

# Diagnostic Evaluation

Several specific evaluation tools to standardize the examiner's observations have been carefully studied, both in Europe by the Pediatric Rheumatology International Trials Organization (PRINTO) *(111, 112)* and by the International Myositis Assessment and Clinical Studies Group (IMACS) in North America *(113)*. These tools include a validated overall DAS with subscores for skin and muscle *(114)*, evaluation of both strength and endurance on muscle testing *(115)*, measures of cutaneous involvement in JDM *(116, 117)*, and validation of a health assessment questionnaire *(118)*. These and other measures of disease activity and damage are discussed more fully in Chap. 15.

# Differential Diagnosis of JDM

It was not unusual for the child to be seen by three to five physicians before referral to a pediatric rheumatologist; the median time interval between first symptom and diagnosis was 3.0 months (range 0.5–20 months) *(119)*. Although the general differential diagnosis for all IIMs is considered in Chap. 14, other types of inflammatory myopathies in children must be considered to differentiate them from JDM (Table 4.5). In addition, children with other conditions can present with symptoms of rash, weakness, or both (Table 4.6).

**Table 4.5**  Clinical classification of juvenile idiopathic inflammatory myopathies

|  | Important features |
|---|---|
| Dermatomyositis | Characteristic skin rashes of Gottron's papules on extensor surfaces and heliotrope discoloration over eyelids; it may have many systemic manifestations in addition to proximal weakness and accounts for 85% of juvenile IIMs |
| Myositis associated with another autoimmune disease (overlap myositis) | Overlap with scleroderma most common in children, but any autoimmune disease may be associated with myositis; seen in 3–10% of juvenile IIMs |
| Polymyositis | Characteristic skin rashes are absent and might have severe weakness; seen in 2–8% of juvenile IIMs |
| Amyopathic dermatomyositis | Typical juvenile dermamyositis skin rashes without muscle involvement for at least 2 years; rare in children; rather mild muscle inflammation is often present but missed; calcinosis or arthritis might be seen |
| Focal myositis | Most often presents as an enlarging mass within the affected muscle, which is usually painful or tender to palpation; most common sites of involvement are the thighs and calves, followed by the neck; few case reports in children |

(continued)

**Table 4.5** (continued)

| | Important features |
|---|---|
| Orbital myositis | A form of focal myositis involving the extraocular muscles; presents with orbital pain worsened by eye movement; diplopia, proptosis, conjunctival injection, periorbital edema, and globe retraction with narrowing of the palpebral fissure are commonly associated symptoms; reported in more than 30 children |
| Inclusion body myositis | Characterized by slowly progressive proximal and distal weakness, low serum creatine kinase, and rimmed vacuoles on trichrome stain of muscle biopsy; few case reports in children |
| Cancer-associated myositis | Myositis develops within 2 years of a diagnosis of cancer; solid organ tumors, lymphoma, and leukemia reported; only a few case reports in children, mainly with atypical cases of juvenile dermatomyositis; routine screening for malignancy is neither needed nor cost-effective in the assessment of childhood myositis |
| Granulomatous myositis | Granulomas prominent in muscle biopsy, often with distal weakness; mainly idiopathic or related to sarcoidosis in pediatric cases; few cases reported in children |
| Macrophagic myofasciitis | Myositis of the deltoids or quadriceps, which is predominantly macrophagic; childhood cases might also present with hypotonia, developmental delay, and failure to thrive; intramuscular injection of aluminum-containing vaccines might be the cause; increasing number of childhood cases reported over the past decade since the 1990's |
| Eosinophilic myositis | Prominent eosinophilic infiltrates on muscle biopsy, associated with peripheral eosinophilia; eosinophilic polymyositis generally needs treatment with corticosteroids; some reports in children; however, some cases identified as muscular dystrophy, with calpain-3 mutations |

*Source:* Feldman, et al. *(59)*. Reprinted from The Lancet. Used with permission from Elsevier

**Table 4.6** Differential diagnosis of childhood idiopathic inflammatory myopathies

| | Condition |
|---|---|
| Weakness alone | |
| Muscular dystrophies | Limb-girdle dystrophies, dystrophinopathies, fascioscapulohumeral dystrophy, other dystrophies |
| Metabolic myopathies | Muscle glycogenoses (glycogen storage diseases), lipid storage disorders, mitochondrial myopathies |
| Endocrine myopathies | Hypothyroidism, hyperthyroidism, Cushing's syndrome or exogenous steroid myopathy, diabetes mellitus |
| Drug-induced myopathy | Consider in patients taking any of the following drugs or biologic therapies: statins, interferon $\alpha$, glucocorticoids, hydroxychloroquine, diuretics, amphotericin b, caine anesthetics, growth hormone, cimetidine, and vincristine |
| Neuromuscular transmission disorders | Myasthenia gravis |
| Motor neuron disorder | Spinal muscular atrophy |

(continued)

**Table 4.6**  (continued)

|  | Condition |
|---|---|
| Weakness with or without rash |  |
| Viral | Enterovirus, influenza, Coxsackie virus, echovirus, parvovirus, poliovirus, hepatitis B, human T-lymphotropic virus 1 |
| Bacterial and parasitic organisms | Staphylococcus, streptococcus, toxoplasmosis, trichinosis, *Lyme borreliosis* |
| Other rheumatic conditions | Systemic lupus erythematosus, scleroderma, juvenile idiopathic arthritis, mixed connective tissue disease, idiopathic vasculitis |
| Other inflammatory conditions | Inflammatory bowel disease, celiac disease |
| Rash without weakness | Psoriasis, eczema, allergy |

*Source:* From **Ref. 59**. Reprinted from *The Lancet*. Used with permission from Elsevier
In many of these conditions, diagnosis is facilitated by muscle biopsy; muscle biopsy should be strongly considered in the absence of rashes of typical juvenile dermatomyositis. For further information, see http://www.neuro.wustl.edu/neuromuscular/index.html

# Therapy of JDM

It was not until the 1950s that the fate of children who contracted this disease was characterized *(120)*: One-third died; one-third were designated as "crippled" (often by calcifications and secondary loss of range of motion), and one-third survived *(121)*. However, there are special considerations that apply to children with respect to both the indications for specific therapy and their consequences, which may modify recommendations for adults with IIMs reviewed in Chap. 18.

## *Corticosteroid Therapy*

It is well known that cortisone was administered to children with myopathies *(121)*, with improvement in their symptoms *(122)*. However, there is little objective evidence concerning the indications and efficacy of dose, route, and frequency of the administration of corticosteroids and their interactions in the context of newer immune-modifying agents. The early studies recommended giving oral prednisone at daily doses as high as 2 mg/kg, often with the consequences of growth retardation, gastric ulcers, spinal cord compression factures, posterior lens cataracts, and induction of diabetes-associated metabolic abnormalities *(123, 124)*. The addition of methotrexate to the child's steroid regimen at the diagnosis of JDM may allow more aggressive tapering of the corticosteroids *(125)*.

The route of administration of the corticosteroids is of importance for high doses (30 mg/kg) of intravenous methylprednisolone (IVMP) given early in the disease course was associated with a marked decrease in the development of dystrophic calcifications *(126, 127)*. The evidence for decreased bioavailability of steroids taken by mouth in children with active JDM was provided by a pharmacokinetic study comparing IVMP and orally administered prednisone at 1 mg/kg. This study documented the association of lack of absorption of oral prednisone in children with loss of nailfold capillary end-row loops. Children with fewer end-row capillary loops absorbed far less oral prednisone than children with a normal number of end-row loops *(128)*. Once absorbed, corticosteroids may induce a metallic taste, which can be ameliorated by sour hard candy, such as lemon drops.

## Methotrexate

As noted, methotrexate is often a steroid-sparing drug, but in children there are two other major considerations: (1) Their faster metabolic rate may necessitate higher doses per unit weight than conventionally given to adults *(129)*, and (2) decreased drug absorption by mouth often makes another route of administration (subcutaneous or intravenous) more effective. The minimum effective dose of methotrexate is 15 mg/m$^2$. Some children complain of nausea, which may be so debilitating that they cannot tolerate this drug despite antiemetics. The adverse consequences of this medication are similar to that found in adults and are reviewed in Chap. 18.

## Cyclosporine A

Again, bioavailability plays a critical role in effective therapy. Use of cyclosporine A (CSA), with starting doses at 3 mg/kg, divided every 12 h, may help mobilize dystrophic calcium deposits as well as suppress chronic cutaneous inflammation. The availability of CSA levels, which should be obtained 1 h before the next dose of the drug, is useful to monitor absorption, with the goal to attain blood levels between 80 and 110 μg/dl. The drug levels often fluctuate with capillary inflammation, drug absorption, and change in the child's weight as the child responds to therapy.

## Intravenous Gamma Globulin

Long suggested as a relatively nontoxic therapy for children with JDM *(130, 131)*, reports of steroid sparing in children *(132)* were followed by data suggesting that use of immunoglobulin preparations poor in immunoglobulin A (IgA) would result in fewer adverse reactions *(133)*. This observation is similar to that of children with primary B-cell immunodeficiency disease who require replacement IgG for lifesaving protection. It is of note that administration of intravenous IgG may also be required for replacement in children with JDM if their B-cell activity has been sufficiently suppressed to lower the IgG level so that it is no longer protective and the child has frequent infections. Another indication for intravenous IgG in JDM might be persistent skin involvement; the rash may clear for a few weeks after administration but may return once the exogenous immunoglobulin levels have waned.

## Mycophenolate Mofetil

Children with SLE and JDM may have elevated circulating levels of IFN-$\alpha$ and may share components of a florid type 1 IFN signature *(80)* as well as antibodies found in SLE *(82)*. This provided the rationale for the use of mycophenolate mofetil (MMF) in children with JDM for it had been found to be effective in some patients with SLE *(134, 135)* as well as in adults with DM *(136)*. The results of a 2-year study of more than 50 children with JDM, using an initial dose of 20 mg/kg divided twice daily, showed improvement in scores for skin involvement with relatively few adverse reactions *(137)*.

## Cyclophosphamide

Cyclophosphamide may be useful in intractable cases for which rapid control of the inflammatory response is needed and to mitigate the progression of interstitial fibrosis *(138)*. It may be administered intravenously in conjunction with corticosteroids, but for most of our patients with defined JDM without interstitial fibrosis, this therapy is not required (see Chap. 18).

## Hydroxychloroquine

As in adults, the steroid-sparing drug hydroxychloroquine appears to be effective in the treatment of cutaneous involvement in children with JDM *(139)*. As the relationship between JDM and cardiovascular disease is clarified, it may be found to be protective in this patient population as in adults with SLE *(140)*. A small percentage of children develop diarrhea or abdominal pain with this medication, which resolves with discontinuation of the drug. More commonly, the small child has trouble with swallowing the large pills, and this becomes an obstacle to therapy.

## Supplemental Therapies and Care

Avoidance of direct sun exposure and the heat of the day and frequent application of sunscreen (minimally at a sun protection factor [SPF] of 30) are basic directions for parents of children with JDM. All children with JDM should be given supplemental vitamin D and calcium; for the smaller child, 400 IU of vitamin D and 600 mg of calcium are given. For the child over 25 kg, at least 800 IU of vitamin D and 1,200 mg of calcium are given to counteract the effect of oral prednisone (which blocks absorption of calcium from the gastrointestinal tract). Another steroid consequence, especially in the adolescent, is acne, which may respond to topical preparations of clindamycin as well as other more routine measures. Omeprazole or lansoprazole in appropriate doses to prevent gastric irritation is also part of the regimen for each child given corticosteroids. In children given methotrexate, folic acid at 1 mg/day usually modifies the severity of oral ulcers, which if they do develop may respond to a higher dose of folic acid. The rash of JDM may be quite pruritic and associated with hives, which often are diminished by the use of H2 blockers such as cetirizine in age-appropriate dosage. Because of the possibility of spinal cord compression fractures, we suggest avoidance of trampoline use or jumping rope. The use of two sets of books, one for home and one for school, helps the child with proximal muscle weakness to cope with school; elevator passes are helpful until the child can climb stairs easily.

## Outcomes of JDM

There are few comprehensive studies of the long-term outcomes of children diagnosed with JDM *(141–143)*. Those that have been published reviewed the course of a diverse group of children who may not have been characterized with modern diagnostic testing tools. Mortality associated with JDM has markedly decreased since the 1960's, from 30% *(121)* to less than 2–3% *(141)* (or 1%, depending on the reporting site) and is primarily cardiopulmonary in nature *(144)*. In the past 10 years, morbidity associated with this illness, previously thought to be primarily disability secondary to joint contractures with or without calcinosis or cardiopulmonary disease in adults *(143, 145)*, is just beginning to be recognized in the pediatric population as age-specific data are acquired from studies of well-defined patient cohorts. Morbidity secondary to PLD *(107)*, associated with insulin resistance, is discussed in Chap. 15 and is clearly associated with persistent skin inflammation, which in turn is associated with nailfold capillary dropout, suggesting that tissue hypoxia and chronic inflammation are critical factors in promoting the adverse outcomes in JDM.

Physical findings in 197 children with JDM at 36 months after diagnosis included vasculitis (24%), persistent rash (46%), and weakness (23%), while fewer children had both rash and weakness (15%). In addition, 9% had arthritis, and 34% had calcifications *(146)*. Arthritis, a presenting complaint in over 60% of children, may also reappear as the immunosuppressive therapy is tapered and is nonerosive and responsive to medical intervention *(147)*. A follow-up study based in Taiwan indicated that 25% of patients were able to discontinue medical therapy successfully *(13)*. In a study of outcome in Hungary of 44 children with JDM, the disease course was monophasic in 59% of children, and 35% of the children developed calcification *(148)*.

In India, after delay in start of therapy (mean of 1.18 years), a monocyclic course was seen in 73% of the 33 cases, calcinosis developed in 27%, and there were two deaths (6%) suggesting that ethnicity and environment influenced disease outcome *(149)*. A brief report of adults who previously had symptoms of JDM two decades or more before an intensive cardiovascular study documented abnormal thickening of the carotid intima media complex ($p = 0.03$) and a trend toward decreased brachial artery change on relaxation ($p = 0.09$). These results documented that cardiovascular impairment was significantly more extensive in adults who had JDM in childhood, and who had not been as aggressively treated as we do now, than controls matched for age and body mass index *(145)*.

## Summary and Hopes for the Future

Since the 1990's, an increased collaborative research effort focused on the clinical and laboratory aspects of the pediatric inflammatory myopathies has yielded new insights into the pathophysiology of this group of diseases in children. The recognition of the impact of the disease evolution has strengthened the impetus for early diagnosis and aggressive intervention. The interplay of genetic and environmental factors is of importance at disease initiation, but we have yet to learn about factors that perpetuate the inflammation. Further definition of MAAs and MSAs may help to delineate separate but related clinical entities, which may have different organ involvement and distinct outcomes. Chronic skin involvement, once thought to be a relatively benign component of JDM, may be a harbinger of dystrophic calcifications and increased morbidity. In the near future, targeted investigations will more clearly define the immunological pathways of the inflammatory process, thus providing guidance to effective means of intervention.

**Acknowledgment**   This work was supported in part by NIH/NIAMS R01 AR48289, the Cure JM Foundation, and Macie's Miracle Foundation. I would like to acknowledge the expert collaboration and assistance of Kelli Day.

## References

1.  Wagner E. Em fall von acuter polymyositis. Dtsch Arch Klin Med 1886;40:241–7.
2.  Hepp P. Ueber Psendotrichiose, eine besondere Form von acuter parenchymatöser Polymyositis. Berliner Klinische Wochenschrift 1887;24:389–91.
3.  Unverricht H. Dermatomyositis acuta. Dtsch Med Wochenschr 1881;17:41.
4.  Spiessens H, Wellens W. [Wagner-Hepp-Unverricht disease (dermatomyositis). Analytical study of personal observations]. Ned Tijdschr Geneeskd 1967;111(11):485–90.
5.  American Diabetes Association. Report of the expert committee on the diagnosis and classification of diabetes mellitus. Diabetes Care 1987;20:1183–97.
6.  Bohan A, Peter J. Polymyositis and dermatomyositis (first of two parts). N Engl J Med 1975;292(7):344–7.
7.  Mendez E, Lipton R, Dyer A, et al. Incidence of juvenile dermatomyositis (JDM) 1995–98: results from the NIAMS Registry. Arthritis Care Res 2003;49:300–5.

8. Symmons D, Sills J, Davis S. The incidence of juvenile dermatomyositis: results from a nation-wide study. Br J Rheumatol 1995;34(8):732–6.

9. McCann L, Juggins A, Maillard S, et al. The Juvenile Dermatomyositis National Registry and Repository (UK and Ireland)—clinical characteristics of children recruited within the first 5 yr. Rheumatology (Oxford) 2006;45(8):1255–60.

10. Pachman L, Lipton R, Ramsey-Goldman R, et al. History of infection before the onset of juvenile dermatomyositis: results from the National Institute of Arthritis and Musculoskeletal and Skin Diseases Research Registry. Arthritis Rheum 2005;53(2):166–72.

11. Hiketa T, Matsumoto Y, Ohashi M, Sakaki R. Juvenile dermatomyositis: a statistical study of 114 patients with dermatomyositis. J Dermatol 1992;19:19:470–6.

12. Kobayashi S, Higuchi K, Tamaki H, et al. Characteristics of juvenile dermatomyositis in Japan. Acta Paediatr Jpn 1997;39(2):257–62.

13. Chiu S, Yang Y, Wang L, Chiang B. Ten-year experience of juvenile dermatomyositis: a retrospective study. J Microbiol Immunol Infect 2007;40(1):68–73.

14. Shehata R, Al-Mayouf S, al-Dalaan A, al-Mazaid A, al-Balaa S, Bahabri S. Juvenile dermatomyositis: clinical profile and disease course in 25 patients. Clin Exp Rheumatol 1999;17(1):115–8.

15. Salvetti M, Ristori G, Bomprezzi R, Pozzilli P, Leslie RD. Twins: mirrors of the immune system. Immunol Today 2000;21(7):342–7.

16. Harati Y, Niakan E, Bergman E. Childhood dermatomyositis in monozygotic twins. Neurology 1986;36(5):721–3.

17. Ballestar E, Esteller M, Richardson B. The epigenetic face of systemic lupus erythematosus. J Immunol 2006;176(12):7143–7.

18. Plamondon S, Dent P, Reed A. Familial dermatomyositis. J Rheumatol 1999;26 (12):2691–2.

19. Ginn L, Lin J, Plotz P, et al. Familial autoimmunity in pedigrees of idiopathic inflammatory myopathy patients suggests common genetic risk factors for many autoimmune diseases. Arthritis Rheum 1998;41(3):400–5.

20. Altman A, Szyper-Kravitz M, Shoenfeld Y. HBV vaccine and dermatomyositis: is there an association? Rheumatol Int 2008;28(6):609–12.

21. Gherardi R, Coquet M, Cherin P, et al. Macrophagic myofasciitis lesions assess long-term persistence of vaccine-derived aluminium hydroxide in muscle. Brain 2001;124(Pt 9):1821–31.

22. Shamim E, Rider L, Perez M, Cawkwell G, Wise R, Miller F. Demographic and clinical features of patients who develop myositis following immunization. Arthritis Rheum 1998;41:S204.

23. Dourmishev L, Meffert H, Piazena H. Dermatomyositis: comparative studies of cutaneous photosensitivity in lupus erythematosus and normal subjects. Photodermatol Photoimmunol Photomed 2004;20(5):230–4.

24. Rider L, Miller F, Targoff I, et al. A broadened spectrum of juvenile myositis: myositis-specific autoantibodies in children. Arthritis Rheum 1994;37:1534–8.

25. Wang H, Zhang Y. Mi2, an auto-antigen for dermatomyositis, is an ATP-dependent nucleosome remodeling factor. Nucleic Acids Res 2001;29(12):2517–21.

26. Okada S, Weatherhead E, Targoff I, Wesley R, Miller F. Global surface ultraviolet radiation intensity may modulate the clinical and immunologic expression of autoimmune muscle disease. Arthritis Rheum 2003;48(8):2285–93.

27. Hengstman G, van Venrooij W, Vencovsky J, Moutsopoulos H, van Engelen B. The relative prevalence of dermatomyositis and polymyositis in Europe exhibits a latitudinal gradient. Ann Rheum Dis 2000;59(2):141–2.

28. Pachman L, Niewold T, Kanucki S, Morgan G, Geraci N, Chen Y. Decreased type-1 interferon in sera of untreated children with juvenile polymyositis (JPM) compared with juvenile dermatomyositis (JDM) matched for short disease duration. Arthritis Rheum 2008;58(9):S225.

29. Reefman E, Kuiper H, Limburg P, Kallenberg C, Bijl M. Type I interferons are involved in the development of UVB-induced inflammatory skin lesions in systemic lupus erythematosus (SLE) patients. Ann Rheum Dis 2007;67:11–8.

30. Silverberg N, Paller A, Pachman L. THF-alpha-308 polymorphism (AA, AG) is associated with increased UVB induced keratinocyte TNF-alpha production in vitro. Arthritis Rheum 1999;42:137.

31. Rose NR. Mechanisms of autoimmunity. Semin Liver Dis 2002;22(4):387–94.
32. Manlhiot C, Liang L, Tran D, Bitnun A, Tyrrell P, Feldman B. Assessment of an infectious disease history preceding juvenile dermatomyositis symptom onset. Rheumatology (Oxford) 2008;47(4):526–9.
33. Koch M, Brody J, Gillespie M. Childhood polymyositis: a case-controlled study. Am J Epidemiol 1976;104:627–31.
34. Martini A, Ravelli A, Albani S, et al. Recurrent juvenile dermatomyositis and cutaneous necrotizing arteritis with molecular mimicry between streptococcal type 5 M protein and human skeletal myosin. J Pediatr 1992;121(5 Pt 1):739–42.
35. Massa M, Costouros N, Mazzoli F, et al. Self-epitopes shared between human skeletal myosin and *Streptococcus phylogenes* M5 protein are targets of immune responses in active juvenile dermatomyositis. Arthritis Rheum 2002;46:3015–25.
36. Mizuno K, Yachie A, Nagaoki S, et al. Oligoclonal expansion of circulating and tissue-infiltrating CD8 + T cells with killer/effector phenotypes in juvenile dermatomyositis syndrome. Clin Exp Immunol 2004;137(1):187–94.
37. Abramson L, Albertini R, Pachman L, Finette B. Association among somatic HPRT mutant frequency, peripheral blood T-lymphocyte clonality, and serologic parameters of disease activity in children with juvenile onset dermatomyositis. Clin Immunol 1999;91(1):61–7.
38. Pachman L, Geraci N, Morgan G, et al. Absolute number of circulating CD3-CD56 + /CD16+ natural killer (NK) cells, a potential biomarker of disease activity in juvenile dermatomyositis (JDM). Arthritis Rheum 2008;58(9):S225,#157.
39. Christensen M, Pachman L, Schneiderman R, Patel D, Friedman J. Prevalence of coxsackie B virus antibodies in patients with juvenile dermatomyositis. Arthritis Rheum 1986;29:1365–70.
40. Nishikai M. Coxsackievirus infection and the development of polymyositis/dermatomyositis. Rheumatol Int 1994;14(2):43–6.
41. Pachman L, Hayford J, Hochberg M, et al. New-onset juvenile dermatomyositis: comparisons with a healthy cohort and children with juvenile rheumatoid arthritis. Arthritis Rheum 1997;40(8):1526–33.
42. Bowles N, Dubowitz V, Sewry C, Archard L. Dermatomyositis, polymyositis, and Coxsackie-B-virus infection. Lancet 1987;1(8540):1004–7.
43. Jongen P, Zoll G, Beaumont M, Melchers W, van de Putte L, Galama J. Polymyositis and dermatomyositis: no persistence of enterovirus or encephalomyocarditis virus RNA in muscle. Ann Rheum Dis 1993;52(8):575–8.
44. Jongen P, Heessen F, ter Laak H, Galama J, Gabreels F. Coxsackie B1 virus-induced murine myositis: relationship of disease severity to virus dose and antiviral antibody response. Neuromuscul Disord 1994;4(1):17–23.
45. Pachman L, Litt D, Rowley A, et al. Lack of detection of enteroviral RNA or bacterial DNA in MRI directed muscle biopsies from 20 children with active untreated juvenile dermatomyositis. Arthritis Rheum 1995;38:1513–18.
46. Bradshaw E, Orihuela A, McArdel S, et al. A local antigen-driven humoral response is present in the inflammatory myopathies. J Immunol 2007;178(1):547–56.
47. Pachman L, Hayford J, Chung A, et al. Juvenile dermatomyositis at diagnosis: clinical characteristics of 79 children. J Rheumatol 1998;25(6):1198–204.
48. Ramanan A, Feldman B. Clinical features and outcomes of juvenile dermatomyositis and other childhood onset myositis syndromes. Rheum Dis Clin North Am 2002;28:833–57.
49. Vegosen L, Weinberg C, O'Hanlon T, Targoff I, Miller F, Rider L. Seasonal birth patterns of myositis subgroups suggest an etiologic role for early environmental exposures. Arthritis Rheum 2007;56(8):2719–28.
50. Brown V, Pilkington C, Feldman B, Davidson J. An international consensus survey of the diagnostic criteria for juvenile dermatomyositis (JDM). Rheumatology (Oxford) 2006;45(8):990–33.
51. Love L, Leff R, Fraser D, et al. A new approach to the classification of idiopathic inflammatory myopathy: myositis-specific autoantibodies define useful homogeneous patient groups. Medicine (Baltimore) 1991;70:360–74.

52. Targoff I, Mamyrova G, Trieu E, et al. A novel autoantibody to a 155-kd protein is associated with dermatomyositis. Arthritis Rheum 2006;54(11):3682–9.
53. Gunawardena H, Wedderburn L, North J, et al. Clinical associations of autoantibodies to a p155/140 kDa doublet protein in juvenile dermatomyositis. Rheumatology (Oxford) 2008;47(3):324–8.
54. Rider L, Targoff I, Taylor-Albert E, et al. Anti-Jo-1 autoantibodies define a clinically homogenous subset of childhood idiopathic inflammatory myopathy (IIM). Arthritis Rheum 1995;38:S362.
55. Rouster-Stevens K, Pachman L. Autoantibody to signal recognition particle in African American girls with juvenile polymyositis. J Rheumatol 2008;35(5):927–9.
56. Pachman L, Abbott K, Sinacore J, et al. Duration of illness is an important variable for untreated children with juvenile dermatomyositis. J Pediatr 2006;148(2):247–53.
57. Pilkington C, Wedderburn L. Paediatric idiopathic inflammatory muscle disease: recognition and management. Drugs 2005;65(10):1355–65.
58. Rider L, Pachman L, Miller F, Bollar H. Myositis and you, a guide to dermatomyositis for patients, families and healthcare providers. Washington, DC: Myositis Association, 2008.
59. Feldman B, Rider L, Reed A, Pachman L. Juvenile dermatomyositis and other idiopathic inflammatory myopathies of childhood. Lancet 2008;371(9631):2201–12.
60. Falcini F, Porfirio B, Lionetti P. Juvenile dermatomyositis and celiac disease. J Rheumatol 1999;26 (6):1419–20.
61. Mitchell J, Dennis G, Rider L. Juvenile dermatomyositis presenting with anasarca: a possible indicator of severe disease activity. J Pediatr 2001;138(6):942–5.
62. Chao Y, Yang L. Dermatomyositis presenting as panniculitis. Int J Dermatol 2000;39(2):141–4.
63. Lee M, Lim Y, Choi J, Sung K, Moon K, Koh J. Panniculitis showing membranocystic changes in the dermatomyositis. J Dermatol 1999;26(9):608–10.
64. Ghali F, Reed A, Groben P, McCauliffe D. Panniculitis in juvenile dermatomyositis. Pediatr Dermatol 1999;16(4):270–2.
65. Barrio V, Callen J, Paller A. Skin rashes and sun protection. In: Rider L, Pachman L, Miller F, Bollar H, eds. Myositis and you: a guide to juvenile dermatomyositis for patients, families and healthcare providers. Washington, DC: Myositis Association, 2008:217–25.
66. Pachman L, Cooke N. Juvenile dermatomyositis: a clinical and immunologic study. J Pediatr 1980;96(2):226–34.
67. Archard L, Richardson P, Olsen E, Dubowitz V, Sewry C, Bowles N. The role of Coxsackie B viruses in the pathogenesis of myocarditis, dilated cardiomyopathy and inflammatory muscle disease. Biochem Soc Symp 1987;53:51–62.
68. Chmiel J, Wessel H, Targoff I, Pachman L. Pulmonary fibrosis and myositis in a child with anti-Jo-1 antibody. J Rheumatol 1995;22(4):762–5.
69. Smith R, Sundberg J, Shamiyah E, Dyer A, Pachman L. Skin involvement in juvenile dermatomyositis is associated with loss of endrow nailfold capillary loops. J Rheumatol 2004;31(8):1644–49.
70. Topaloglu H, Muntoni F, Dubowitz V, Sewry C. Expression of HLA class I antigens in skeletal muscle is a diagnostic marker in juvenile dermatomyositis. J Child Neurol 1997;12(1):60–3.
71. Hohlfeld R, Goebels N, Engel AG. Cellular mechanisms in inflammatory myopathies. Baillieres Clin Neurol 1993;2(3):617–35.
72. Civatte M, Schleinitz N, Krammer P, et al. Class I MHC detection as a diagnostic tool in noninformative muscle biopsies of patients suffering from dermatomyositis (DM). Neuropathol Appl Neurobiol 2003;29(6):546–52.
73. Varsani H, Newton K, Li C, Harding B, Holton J, Wedderburn L. Quantification of normal range of inflammatory changes in morphologically normal pediatric muscle. Muscle Nerve 2008;37(2):259–61.
74. Wedderburn L, Varsani H, Li C, et al. International consensus on a proposed score system for muscle biopsy evaluation in patients with juvenile dermatomyositis: a tool for potential use in clinical trials. Arthritis Rheum 2007;57(7):1192–201.

75. Winter A, Borenmann A. NCAM, vimentin and neonatal myosin heavy chain expression in human muscle diseases. Neuropathol Appl Neurobiol 1999;25:417–24.
76. Miles L, Bove K, Lovell D, et al. Predictability of the clinical course of juvenile dermatomyositis based on initial muscle biopsy: a retrospective study of 72 patients. Arthritis Rheum 2007;57:1183–91.
77. Tezak Z, Hoffman E, Lutz J, et al. Expression profiling in DQA1*0501 children with juvenile dermatomyositis: a novel model of pathogenesis. J Immunol 2002;168:4154–63.
78. Connor K, Abbott K, Sabin B, Kuroda M, Pachman L. MxA gene expression in juvenile dermatomyositis peripheral blood mononuclear cells: association with muscle involvement. Clin Immunol 2006;120(3):319–25.
79. Baechler E, Bauer J, Slattery C, et al. An interferon signature in the peripheral blood of dermatomyositis patients is associated with disease activity. Mol Med 2007;13(1-2):59–68.
80. Pascual V, Patel P, McVicker V, Abbott K, Gurhsahaney A, Pachman L. Peripheral blood mononuclear cell gene expression profiles in children with juvenile dermatomyositis/polymyositis (JDM/JPM) share type-1 interferon (IFN) signatures with systemic lupus erythematosus (SLE) but are distinct. Arthritis Rheum 2006;54:S695.
81. Niewold T, Kariuki S, Morgan G, Geraci N, Shrestha S, Pachman L. Serum interferon alpha activity is associated with biological markers of disease activity and severity in juvenile dermatomyositis. Arthritis Rheum 2008;58(9):S501.
82. Balboni I, Patel P., Limb C, et al. Autoantigen microarray analysis of autoantibody profiling of juvenile dermatomyositis sera: reveals a SLE-like type I interferon signature reactivity to RNA-containing autoantigens in a subgroup of patients. Arthritis Rheum 2007;54:S787.
83. Pachman L, Friedman J, Maryjowski M, et al. Immunogenetic studies in juvenile dermatomyositis III: study of antibody to organ-specific and nuclear antigens. Arthritis Rheum 1985;28(2):151–7.
84. Thyss A, el Baze P, Lefebvre J, Schneider M, Ortonne J. Dermatomyositis-like syndrome in X-linked hypogammaglobulinemia. Case-report and review of the literature. Acta Derm Venereol 1990;70(4):309–13.
85. Webster A, Tripp J, Hayward A, et al. Echovirus encephalitis and myositis in primary immunoglobulin deficiency. Arch Dis Child 1973;53:33–7.
86. DeBleeker J, Engel A, Butcher E. Peripheral lymphoid tissue-like adhesion molecule expression in nodular infiltrates in inflammatory myopathies. Neuromuscul Disord 1996;6(4):255–60.
87. Christen-Zaechs S, Seshadri R, Sundberg J, Paller A, Pachman L. Juvenile dermatomyositis: persistent association of nailfold capillaroscopy changes and skin involvement over 36 months with duration of untreated disease. Arthritis Rheum 2008;58:571–6.
88. Perez M, Abrams S, Koenning G, Stuff J, O'Brien K, Ellis K. Mineral metabolism in children with dermatomyositis. J Rheumatol 1994;21(12):2364–9.
89. Rouster-Stevens K, Langman C, Price H, et al. RANKL:osteoprotegerin ratio and bone mineral density in children with untreated juvenile dermatomyositis. Arthritis Rheum 2007;56(3):977–83.
90. Reed A, Haugen M, Pachman L, Langman C. Abnormalities in serum osteocalcin values in children with chronic rheumatic diseases. J Pediatr 1990;116(4):574–80.
91. Silver R, Maricq H. Childhood dermatomyositis: serial microvascular studies. Pediatrics 1989;83:278–83.
92. Ingegnoli F, Zeni S, Gerloni V, Fantini F. Capillaroscopic observations in childhood rheumatic diseases and healthy controls. Clin Exp Rheumatol 2005;23(6):905–11.
93. Ostrowski R, Sullivan C, Morgan G, Seshadri R, Morgan G, Pachman L. Normal nailfold end row loops are associated with a shorter duration of untreated disease in children with juvenile dermatomyositis. Arthritis Rheum 2008;58(9):S255–6.
94. Spencer C, Hanson V, Singsen B, Bernstein B, Kornreich H, King K. Course of treated juvenile dermatomyositis. J Pediatr 1984;105:399–408.
95. Zhao Y, Fedczyna T, McVicker V, Caliendo J, Li H, Pachman L. Apoptosis in the skeletal muscle of untreated children with juvenile dermatomyositis: impact of duration of untreated disease. Clin Immunol 2007;125:165–72.

96. Fedczyna T, Lutz J, Pachman L. Expression of TNF-a by muscle fibers in biopsies from untreated children with juvenile dermatomyositis: association with the TNF-a-308A allele. Clin Immunol 2001;100:236–9.

97. Pachman L, Liotta-Davis M, Hong D, et al. TNF-alpha-308A allele in juvenile dermatomyositis: association with increased production of tumor necrosis factor alpha, disease duration, and pathologic calcifications. Arthritis Rheum 2000;43(10):2368–77.

98. Stock S, Ignatiev K, Lee P, Abbott K, Pachman L. Pathological calcification in juvenile dermatomyositis (JDM): microCT and synchrotron X-ray diffraction reveal hydroxyapatite with varied microstructures. Calcif Tissue Res 2004;45:248–56.

99. Pachman L, Veis A, Stock S, et al. Composition of calcifications in children with juvenile dermatomyositis: association with chronic cutaneous inflammation. Arthritis Rheum 2006;54(10):3345–50.

100. Marhaug G, Shah V, Shroff R, et al. Age-dependent inhibition of ectopic calcification: a possible role for fetuin-A and osteopontin in patients with juvenile dermatomyositis with calcinosis. Rheumatology (Oxford) 2008;47(7):1031–7.

101. Schafer C, Heiss A, Schwarz A, et al. The serum protein alpha 2-Heremans-Schmid glycoprotein/fetuin-A is a systemically acting inhibitor of ectopic calcification. J Clin Invest 2003;112(3):357–66.

102. Lian J, Pachman L, Gundberg C, Partridge REH, Maryjowski M. Gamma carboxyglutamate excretion and calcinosis in juvenile dermatomatomyositis. Arthritis Rheum 1982;22:1094.

103. van Summeren M, Spliet W, van Royen-Kerkhof A, et al. Calcinosis in juvenile dermatomyositis: a possible role for the vitamin K-dependent protein matrix Gla protein. Rheumatology (Oxford) 2008;47(3):267–71.

104. Urganus AL, Zhao YD, Pachman LM. Juvenile dermatomyositis calcifications selectively displayed markers of bone formation. Arthritis Rheum 2009;501–508.

105. Verma S, Singh S, Bhalla A, Khullar M. Study of subcutaneous fat in children with juvenile dermatomyositis. Arthritis Rheum 2006;55(4):564–8.

106. Scaleci J, Zhao Y-D, Morgan G, Sullivan C, Seshadri R, Pachman LM. Descriptive analysis of the clinical features of patients with juvenile dermatomyositis and partial lipodystrophy. Arthritis Rheum 2008;58(9):S231.

107. Bingham A, Mamyrova G, Rother K, et al. Predictors of acquired lipodystrophy in juvenile-onset dermatomyositis and a gradient of severity. Medicine (Baltimore) 2008;87(2):70–86.

108. Chen Y, Shi R, Geraci N, Shrestha S, Gordish-Dressman H, Pachman L. Duration of chronic inflammation alters gene expression in muscle from untreated girls with juvenile dermatomyositis. BMC Immunol 2008;9:43.

109. Nagaraju K, Rider L, Fan C, et al. Endothelial cell activation and neovascularization are prominent in dermatomyositis. J Autoimmune Dis 2006;3:2.

110. Bilgic H, Ytterberg S, McNallan K, et al. IL-17 and IFN-regulated genes and chemokines as biomarkers of disease activity in inflammatory myopathies. Arthritis Rheum 2008;58(9):S922.

111. Ruperto N, Ravelli A, Murray K, Lovell D, Andersson-Gare B, et al. Preliminary core sets of measures for disease activity and damage for juvenile systemic lupus erythematosus and juvenile dermatomyositis. Rheumatology (Oxford) 2003;42:1452–9.

112. Ruperto N, Ravelli A, Pistorio A, et al. The provisional Paediatric Rheumatology International Trials Organization/American College of Rheumatology/European League Against Rheumatism Disease activity core set for the evaluation of response to therapy in juvenile dermatomyositis: a prospective validation study. Arthritis Rheum 2008;58:4–13.

113. Rider L, Giannini E, Brunner H, et al. International consensus on preliminary definitions of improvement in adult and juvenile myositis. Arthritis Rheum 2004;50(7):2281–90.

114. Bode R, Klein-Gitelman M, Miller M, Lechman T, Pachman L. Disease activity score for children with juvenile dermatomyositis (JDM): reliability and validity evidence. Arthritis Care Res 2003;49:7–15.

115. Huber A, Feldman B, Rennebohm R, et al. Validation and clinical significance of the Childhood Myositis Assessment Scale for assessment of muscle function in the juvenile idiopathic inflammatory myopathies. Arthritis Rheum 2004;50(5):1595–603.

116. Jain M, Smith M, Cintas H, Koziol D, Wesley R, Harris-Love M, Lovell D, Rider LG, Hicks J. Intra-rater and inter-rater reliability of the 10-point Manual Muscle Test (MMT) of strength in children with juvenile idiopathic inflammatory myopathies (JIIM). Phys Occup Ther Pediatr 2006;26(3):5–17.

117. Huber A, Lachenbruch P, Dugan E, Miller F, Rider L. Alternative scoring of the Cutaneous Assessment Tool in juvenile dermatomyositis: results using abbreviated formats. Arthritis Rheum 2008;59(3):352–6.

118. Huber A, Hicks J, Lachenbruch P, et al. Validation of the Childhood Health Assessment Questionnaire in the juvenile idiopathic myopathies. Juvenile Dermatomyositis Disease Activity Collaborative Study Group. J Rheumatol 2001;28(5):1106–11.

119. Pachman L, Hayford J, Chung A, et al. Juvenile dermatomyositis at diagnosis: clinical characteristics of 79 children. J Rheumatol 1998;25:1198–204.

120. Wedgewood R, Cook C, Cohen J. Dermatomyositis; report of 26 cases in children with a discussion of endocrine therapy in 13. Pediatrics 1953;12(4):447–66.

121. Bitnum S, Daeschner C, Travis L, Dodge W, Hopps H. Dermatomyositis. J Pediatr 1964;64:101–31.

122. Sullivan D, Cassidy J, Petty R. Dermatomyositis in the pediatric patient. Arthritis Rheum 1977;20(2 Suppl):327–31.

123. Oddis C, Rider L, Reed A, et al. International consensus guidelines for trials of therapies in the idiopathic inflammatory myopathies. Arthritis Rheum 2005;52(9):2607–15.

124. Rider L, Pilkington C, Malleson P. Long term therapies of juvenile myositis. In: Rider L, Pachman L, Miller F, Bollar H, eds. Myositis and you: a guide to juvenile dermatomyositis for patients, families and healthcare providers. Washington, DC: Myositis Association, 2007:1595–1603.

125. Ramanan A, Campbell-Webster N, Ota S, et al. The effectiveness of treating juvenile dermatomyositis with methotrexate and aggressively tapered corticosteroids. Arthritis Rheum 2005;52(11):3570–8.

126. Fisler R, Liang M, Fuhlbrigge R, Yalcindag A, Sundel R. Aggressive management of juvenile dermatomyositis results in improved outcome and decreased incidence of calcinosis. J Am Acad Dermatol 2002;47:505–11.

127. Callen A, Pachman L, Hayford J, Chung A, Ramsey-Goldman R. Intermittent high-dose intravenous methylprednisolone (IV pulse) therapy prevents calcinosis and shortens disease course in juvenile dermatomyositis (JDMS). Arthritis Rheum 1994;37:R10.

128. Rouster-Stevens K, Gursahney A, Ngai K, Daru J, Pachman L. Pharmacokinetic study of oral prednisolone compared to intravenous methylprednisolone in patients with juvenile dermatomyositis. Arthritis Care Res 2008;59:222–6.

129. Wallace C, Sherry D. Preliminary report of higher dose methotrexate treatment in juvenile rheumatoid arthritis. J Rheumatol 1992;19:1604–7.

130. Lang B, Laxer R, Murphy G, Silverman E, Roifman C. Treatment of dermatomyositis with intravenous gammaglobulin. Am J Med 1991;91:169–72.

131. Tsai M, Lai C, Lin S, Chiang B, Chou C, Hsieh K. Intravenous immunoglobulin therapy in juvenile dermatomyositis. Chung-Hua Min Kuo Hsiao Erh Ko i Hsueh Hui Tsa Chih 1997;38(2):111–5.

132. Al-Mayouf S, Laxer R, Schneider R, Silverman E, Feldman B. Intravenous immunoglobulin therapy for juvenile dermatomyositis: efficacy and safety. J Rheumatol 2000;27(10):2498–503.

133. Manlhiot C, Tyrrell P, Liang L, Atkinson A, Lau W, Feldman B. Safety of intravenous immunoglobulin in the treatment of juvenile dermatomyositis: adverse reactions are associated with immunoglobulin A content. Pediatrics 2008;121(3):e626–30.

134. D'Cruz D, Khamashta M, Hughes G. Systemic lupus erythematosus. Lancet 2007;369(9561):587–96.

135. Mok C. Mycophenolate mofetil for non-renal manifestations of systemic lupus erythematosus: a systematic review. Scand J Rheumatol 2007;36(5):329–37.

136. Edge J, Outland J, Dempsey J, Callen J. Mycophenolate mofetil as an effective corticosteroid-sparing therapy for recalcitrant dermatomyositis. Arch Dermatol 2006;142(1):65–9.

137. Rouster Stevens KA, Pachman LM. Mycophenolate mofetil in juvenile dermatomyositis. Arthritis Rheum 2006;54:S680.
138. Riley P, Maillard S, Wedderburn L, Woo P, Murray K, Pilkington C. Intravenous cyclophosphamide pulse therapy in juvenile dermatomyositis. A review of efficacy and safety. Rheumatology (Oxford) 2004;43(4):491–6.
139. Olson N, Lindsley C. Adjunctive use of hydroxychloroquine in childhood dermatomyositis. J Rheumatol 1989;16:1545–7.
140. Salmon J, Roman M. Accelerated atherosclerosis in systemic lupus erythematosus: implications for patient management. Curr Opin Rheumatol 2001;13:341–4.
141. Huber A, Lang B, LeBlanc C, et al. Medium- and long-term functional outcomes in a multicenter cohort of children with juvenile dermatomyositis. Arthritis Rheum 2000; 43(3):541–9.
142. Collison C, Sinal S, Jorizzo J, Walker F, Monu J, Snyder J. Juvenile dermatomyositis and polymyositis: a follow-up study of long-term sequelae. South Med J 1998;91(1):17–22.
143. Huber A, Feldman B. Long-term outcomes in juvenile dermatomyositis: how did we get here and where are we going? Curr Rheumatol Rep 2005;7(6):441–6.
144. Lundberg I. The heart in dermatomyositis and polymyositis. Rheumatology (Oxford) 2006; 45(Suppl 4):iv18–21.
145. Eimer M, Young L, Abbott K, et al. Abnormal cardiovascular risk profile in adult patients with juvenile dermatomyositis. Arthritis Rheum 2006;54:S519.
146. Pachman L, Ramsey-Goldman R, Lipton R, et al. The NIAMS Juvenile Dermatomyositis Registry parent assessment of child's symptoms at 36 months after diagnosis. Arthritis Rheum 2002;46:S307.
147. Tse S, Lubelsky S, Gordon M, et al. The arthritis of inflammatory childhood myositis syndromes. J Rheumatol 2001;28(1):192–7.
148. Constantin T, Ponyi A, Orban I, et al. National registry of patients with juvenile idiopathic inflammatory myopathies in Hungary—clinical characteristics and disease course of 44 patients with juvenile dermatomyositis. Autoimmunity 2006;39(3):223–32.
149. Singh S, Bansal A. Twelve years experience of juvenile dermatomyositis in North India. Rheumatol Int 2006;26(6):510–5.

# Chapter 5
# Inclusion Body Myositis

Lawrence J. Kagen

**Abstract** Inclusion body myositis is an insidious, slowly progressive myopathy of middle-aged and older individuals. Because of these characteristics, diagnosis is often delayed. Affected muscle is marked by the presence of rimmed vacuoles, inclusions, and an inflammatory infiltrate largely made up of CD8 T lymphocytes and macrophages. The inclusions contain beta-amyloid and phosphorylated tau protein, as well as other components. Theories of the pathogenesis of this disorder of older individuals include those based on evidence of the unfolded protein response leading to endoplasmic reticulum stress, abnormalities of proteosomal degradative function, mitochondrial dysfunction, the immune response, and amyloid toxicity. There is no proven, reliably effective medication for this disorder.

**Keywords** Inclusion body myositis • Beta amyloid • Tau protein • Endoplasmic reticulum stress • Unfolded protein response • MHC-1 • CD8 T cells

## Introduction

The precise diagnosis of inclusion body myositis rests on biopsy findings, which have been recognized, over the last four decades, to be directly related to a distinct clinical syndrome. In 1965, Adams and coworkers (*1*) described the occurrence of nuclear and cytoplasmic inclusions in the muscle of a 20-year-old male student with a syndrome of progressive weakness of the extremities and trunk. Finger flexor strength was spared. Serum creatine kinase activity was mildly elevated. Biopsy of muscle demonstrated the presence of histiocytes and lymphocytes distributed perivascularly, interstitially, and around necrotic fibers. Of particular

L.J. Kagen
Department of Rheumatology, Weill Medical College of Cornell University,
Hospital for Special Surgery, New York Presbyterian Hospital, New York, NY, USA
e-mail: kagenl@verizon.net

L.J. Kagen (ed.), *The Inflammatory Myopathies*,
DOI 10.1007/978-1-60327-827-0_5,
© Humana Press. a part of Springer Science + Business Media, LLC 2009

interest in this report was the presence of eosinophilic inclusions in the cytoplasm of myofibers and in sarcolemmal nuclei.

Two years later, Chou (2) reported findings of intracytoplasmic and intranuclear inclusions in myofibers of a 60-year-old man with chronic polymyositis, manifested by generalized progressive weakness, dysphagia, and muscle atrophy. Electromyograms suggested myositis, although serum enzyme levels were not significantly elevated. A mononuclear cell infiltrate was found in muscle on biopsy.

In 1970, a third case was reported by Carpenter and colleagues (3) of a 39-year-old woman, who had suffered from a progressive myopathy for 10 years. The onset of her weakness, which affected both proximal and distal muscles, was insidious. Her forearm and hand muscles, however, were strong. Serum creatine kinase values were normal. Cytoplasmic and nuclear filamentous inclusions were found in muscle on biopsy. In addition, this report called attention to the presence of vacuoles within the cytoplasm of myofibers.

In 1971, Yunis and Samaha (4), describing biopsy findings in muscle of a 26-year-old woman, suggested the name *inclusion body myositis*. This patient had weakness of both upper and lower extremities that developed over the course of several years. Although there was severe wasting in multiple areas, the strength of the quadriceps in the lower extremities and of the muscles of the hands was preserved. Serum creatine kinase levels were normal. Biopsy of muscle revealed the "typical picture of chronic polymyositis." Again, nuclear and cytoplasmic inclusions were found with a "focal and mild diffuse round cell infiltration." In their discussion, these investigators cast doubt on the previously suggested viral etiology of the filamentous nuclear and cytoplasmic inclusions. These reports, in the latter half of the twentieth century, laid the basis for the recognition of inclusion body myositis as a distinct clinical entity.

The present description of the typical patient recognized with this disorder, however, would be somewhat different from that of two of the patients initially reported. Inclusion body myositis is now understood to affect older individuals, with an insidious progressive myopathy that does affect the quadriceps and finger flexors as well as other musculature (see clinical finding discussion). Another early major advance in the delineation of this syndrome was the finding of Mendell and colleagues (5) of the presence of amyloid in the filamentous inclusions.

## Clinical Findings

Inclusion body myositis is seen predominantly in middle-aged and older individuals, generally over age 50. However, it can occasionally occur in younger patients. It affects both sexes, although some series have noted a male preponderance. The disorder is marked by the insidious progression of painless weakness. Its slow progression may delay diagnosis and even its recognition by an affected individual. Many patients are seen late in the course of illness and are unaware that weakness is the result of disease rather than the natural consequence of aging. It is the occurrence of a fall, a misstep over a street curb, or the inability to negotiate a flight of stairs, which may bring the patient to seek medical attention. In many cases, it is a friend or relative who points out the progressive weakness that an affected individual has experienced and suggests medical examination.

The delay in diagnosis was demonstrated in a report of patients with inflammatory muscle disease. There were 15 patients with inclusion body myositis; in these individuals, there was an average time of 6.5 years from the onset of disease to diagnosis *(6)*. This was considerably longer than the delay noted for patients with dermatomyositis, which was 0.07 years on average. In this review, asymmetrical muscle weakness, with prominent wrist flexor, finger flexor, and knee extensor involvement were distinctive in comparison with the findings in those with dermatomyositis or polymyositis (Table 5.1).

Often on first meeting a patient with inclusion body myositis, the physician can note an unusually weak handshake, with the lack of firm finger grip, due to weakness of the flexors of the digits. Weakness of ankle dorsiflexors may have led to difficulty in walking, causing tripping or falling. This distal muscle involvement of both the upper and lower extremities is often a clue to diagnosis (Table 5.2).

In addition, however, many other muscle groups of the extremities and trunk and neck flexors also demonstrate weakness. Dysphagia is common late in the disease. Rarely, it may even be a presenting symptom *(7, 8)*. Laboratory evaluation demonstrates elevation of the levels of the serum enzymes creatine kinase (CK), lactate dehydrogenase (LDH), alanine aminotransferase (ALT), and aspartate aminotransferase (AST) and of the serum myoglobin, but as indicated, these values may be unexpectedly low or even in the normal range. Electromyography indicates myopathic involvement. At this point, support for the diagnosis then rests on the muscle biopsy (Table 5.3).

## Muscle Biopsy

Muscle biopsy findings are characteristic and diagnostic *(9)*. Inclusion body myositis is a vacuolar myopathy, with cytoplasmic vacuoles rimmed by basophilic granules. In addition, an inflammatory infiltrate composed largely of CD8 T lymphocytes

**Table 5.1** Clinical features

1. Age: Usually 50 or greater
2. Gender: Both sexes affected
3. Duration of illness: Over 6 months at presentation, often much longer

**Table 5.2** Physical findings: Muscle weakness

1. Distal: Finger and wrist flexors, ankle dorsiflexors
2. Proximal: Trunk and shoulder musculature, hip and leg flexors
3. Weakness: May be asymmetrical

**Table 5.3** Laboratory findings

1. Serum enzymes: CK, LDH, AST, ALT may all be elevated, CK most prominently, up to ten times normal, but may be lower and even within normal limits
2. Serum myoglobin: Moderately elevated

**Table 5.4**  Muscle biopsy findings

1. Rimmed cytoplasmic vacuoles
2. Cytoplasmic and nuclear inclusions
3. Presence of amyloid
4. Ragged red fibers
5. Variable fiber size, angulated fibers
6. Necrotic and regenerating fibers
7. Inflammatory infiltrate of lymphocytes and macrophages
8. Cytoplasmic and nuclear filamentous inclusions seen with electron microscopy (electron microscopy usually not necessary for diagnosis)

and macrophages is present. Filamentous inclusions in both the cytoplasm and nuclei of myofibers are seen on electron microscopy. These inclusions, which are eosinophilic, on light microscopy contain beta-amyloid and phosphorylated tau protein. There is a mitochondrial disorder marked by the presence of ragged red fibers and also manifested by increased numbers of myofibers that lack cytochrome oxidase. In this regard, electron microscopy reveals abnormal mitochondria, and genetic techniques have demonstrated an increase in the number of mitochondrial DNA deletions in affected patients. Muscle fiber size is variable; there are groups of angulated fibers and necrotic as well as occasional regenerating fibers. The findings of typical changes by light microscopy usually suffice for diagnosis, and electron microscopy, although providing powerful insight into disease morphology, is generally reserved for research and not employed in general practice. These findings, although characteristic, may be variably present in individual biopsy samples, and can, in certain samples, be difficult to discern (Table 5.4).

# Pathogenesis

Theories of pathogenesis take into account two major pathological features present in affected muscle: the degenerative component (the vacuoles and inclusions) and the inflammatory component (the lymphocytic and macrophagic infiltrate). These theories may be thought of as concentrating on toxic-metabolic factors and on the immune response.

## *Toxic-Metabolic Factors*

Askanas and Engel *(10)* pointed out that myofiber degeneration in this disorder is characterized by progressive fiber atrophy and vacuolization, with accumulation of multicomponent aggregates, the amyloid-containing inclusion bodies.

The amyloid inclusions are of two types, one of which contains amyloid beta and the other phosphorylated tau protein. In addition, both types of inclusions contain other proteins. These other proteins are thought to be subject to misfolding in the endoplasmic reticulum, leading to abnormalities in function of this intracellular organelle, a mechanism that can result in stress within the cell. This stress-producing process has been termed the *unfolded protein response*. Further evidence for the possible role of endoplasmic reticulum stress within affected myofibers is suggested by the presence of chaperone proteins in the inclusions. These proteins would otherwise assist in the folding of newly formed polypeptides. Their presence in inclusions has been taken to be an indication of the unfolded protein response and of endoplasmic reticulum stress. This stress-evoking process may set in motion a series of pathogenic events, including the induction of mystatin, a factor in muscle atrophy, and the expression of major histocompatibility complex (MHC) by myofibers. This last factor in turn may play a role in the elicitation of the immune response.

The presence of proteasomal components, and of ubiquitin and mutated ubiquitin in inclusions, indicates abnormalities in the cell's catabolic processes. Also present are alpha synuclein and presenilin 1, markers of oxidative stress, and heat shock proteins. These constituents of the inclusions are indicative of several coexisting abnormalities in the metabolism of affected muscle cells. The vacuoles represent autophagosomes filled with membranous debris, a sign of incomplete cellular processing or catabolism.

Askanas and Engel *(10)* emphasized the importance of amyloid beta precursor protein and of its metabolite, the proteolytic fragment amyloid beta, as toxic upstream factors in the cascade of degenerative processes, which results in the findings mentioned that are characteristic of inclusion body myositis.

Amyloid beta, in experimental studies, has been shown to act as a toxin on myofibers, leading to vacuolization, atrophy, and changes typical of those seen in inclusion body myositis. Moreover, there is evidence of increased transcription of amyloid beta precursor protein in muscle of patients with inclusion body myositis. Beta amyloid may accumulate as the result of abnormalities found in components that otherwise could process it. These include the secretase enzymes (which cleave amyloid beta), free cholesterol (which may influence amyloid beta deposition), cystatin C (a protease inhibitor), and transglutaminases 1a and 2 (which may allow cross-linking of amyloid beta molecules). All of the foregoing factors are thought to account for the accumulation of amyloid beta, a toxic material, in myofibers.

There is also evidence of oxidative stress and free-radical toxicity and of inhibition of normal proteasome function. The last abnormality is indicated by the presence of both ubiquitin and mutated ubiquitin in the inclusions. Inhibition of proteasomal function has also been suggested to be related to amyloid beta. Also, as indicated, significant mitochondrial abnormalities are present in affected muscle.

How these processes are linked, and the order of their appearance in the pathogenesis of inclusion body myositis, awaits further research. At present, the manifestations of this disorder are felt to be due to cascades of multifactorial, toxic, pathological events.

## *The Immune Response*

As reviewed by Dalakas *(11)*, in addition to the vacuoles and inclusions, muscle tissue in inclusion body myositis contains an inflammatory infiltrate made up in large part of macrophages and cytotoxic CD8 T lymphocytes, which can be seen invading intact myofibers. Other features of inclusion body myositis suggest its association with autoimmune disease.

In approximately 20–30% of patients, another disorder considered to be autoimmune may be present. Autoimmune disorders that have been observed include autoimmune thyroid disease, multiple sclerosis, rheumatoid arthritis, and Sjögren's syndrome. An increased frequency of genes associated with autoimmunity, such as human leukocyte antigen (HLA) DR3, has been found in up to 75% of patients. Moreover, a genetic factor in disease susceptibility is suggested by the rarely observed occurrence of inclusion body myositis in twins and in other family members of affected individuals *(12)*.

In his review, Dalakas *(11)* pointed out that there have been cases of inclusion body myositis associated with dysproteinemia, paraproteinemia, and immunodeficiency syndromes, again suggestive of a relation of disease susceptibility to altered immune mechanisms. Also, there have been reports of inclusion body myositis in patients infected with HIV and human T-lymphotrophic virus 1 (HTLV-1), both agents which may alter normal immune mechanisms.

Overexpression of MHC antigens occurs in muscle of patients with inclusion body myositis. Under normal circumstances, myofibers do not express detectable amounts of MHC. Along with the upregulation of MHC, T-cell activation is present, with expression of ICAM-1 (intercellular adhesion molecule-1), MHC-1, and ICOS (inducible costimulatory molecule). The activated, cytotoxic T cells, which invade myofibers, display perforin granules capable of inducing fiber necrosis. Moreover, there is evidence (based on T-cell receptor types) that the cytotoxic T-cell population has been specifically recruited to muscle and locally expanded there after exposure to antigen.

Taken together, these findings suggest that muscle fibers can act as antigen-presenting cells to CD8 lymphocytes. There is also evidence of upregulation of chemokines, cytokines, and metalloproteinase in muscle, all of which may contribute to myofiber damage. The presence of activated, cytotoxic, antigen-driven, T-cell populations in muscle of genetically susceptible individuals points to the likely importance of immune mechanisms in the disorder (Table 5.5).

**Table 5.5** Pathogenetic factors

| Toxic-metabolic factors | Immune-inflammatory factors |
| --- | --- |
| Amyloid beta | Invasion by activated, cytotoxic lymphocytes |
| Mitochondrial disorder | MHC expression on myofibers |
| Oxidative stress | Upregulation of cytokines, chemokines, and metalloproteinases |
| | |
| Proteasomal abnormality | |
| Endoplasmic reticulum stress | |

## Summary of Theories of Pathogenesis

Based on our present knowledge, in inclusion body myositis, it is likely that the two processes, those involving toxic-metabolic factors (related, at least in part, to amyloid beta) and immune-inflammatory mechanisms (related to cytotoxic T lymphocytes), may be acting concurrently. The stimulus or factor responsible for the initiation of these processes remains unknown, however. Whether one of these two processes is secondary to the other or whether they act synergistically in production of disease still remains to be determined. Further, intriguing hypotheses of a putative role of aging, genetics, or a possible, as yet unknown, infectious agent, remain open for investigation.

## Therapy

Presently, there is no therapy that has been reliably effective. A number of agents, including corticosteroids, cytotoxic-immunosuppressive agents, anti-TNF (tumor necrosis factor) agents, interferon beta, and intravenous gamma globulin, have been tried. In some cases, there have been modest gains, but overall there has been no dependably effective therapeutic approach to this disorder. However, it is possible that some patients who demonstrate marked signs of inflammation (such as markedly elevated enzymes or serum myoglobin and an exuberant infiltrate on biopsy) or those with rapidly progressive disease may obtain benefit from treatment. Many physicians, on initial diagnosis, will employ a course of therapy with careful ongoing assessment to determine whether there may be some benefit to be attained in individual cases.

The lack of success of measures designed to address autoimmunity has been suggested by some to indicate that immune mechanisms may not be central to disease initiation or perpetuation. This is an area requiring further investigation.

It is likely, however, that the presence of irreversible degenerative mechanisms, perhaps related at least in part to aging, as well as the late stage of illness at which many patients are first seen may be important factors in the poor response to therapy so characteristic of this disorder. This underscores the need for knowledge of the modifiable, pathological pathways in inclusion body myositis.

Beyond consideration of therapeutic measures aimed at pathogenetic mechanisms in this disorder, in the elderly patient attention should be paid to nutrition, physical therapy, and remediation of any existing comorbidities.

## Hereditary Inclusion Body Myopathy

Although inclusion body myositis may at times be familial, it should not be confused with hereditary inclusion body myopathy. This last name is applied to a number of different genetic disorders, which may be autosomal, recessive, or dominant and can appear in childhood or later in life. The biopsy findings, although similar, do not include an inflammatory infiltrate, and there is no upregulation of MHC markers in muscle tissue.

# References

1. Adams RD, Kakulas BA, Samaha FA. A myopathy with cellular inclusions. Trans Am Neurol Assoc 1965;90:213–6.
2. Chou SM. Myxovirus-like structures in a case of human chronic polymyositis. Science 1967;158:1453–5.
3. Carpenter S, Karpati G, Wolfe L. Virus-like filaments and phospholipid accumulation in skeletal muscle. Neurology 1970;20:889–903.
4. Yunis EJ, Samaha FJ. Inclusion body myositis. Lab Invest 1971;25:240–8.
5. Mendell JR, Sahenk Z, Gales T, Paul L. Amyloid filaments in inclusion body myositis. Arch Neurol 1991;48:1229–34.
6. Amato AA, Gronseth GS, Jackson CE, et al. Inclusion body myositis: clinical and pathological boundaries. Ann Neurol 1996;40:581–6.
7. Verma A, Bradley WG, Adesina AM, Sofferman R, Pendlebuty WW. Inclusion body myositis with cricopharyngeus muscle involvement and severe dysphagia. Muscle Nerve 1991;14:470–3.
8. Riminton DS, Chambers ST, Parkin PJ, Pollock M, Donaldson IM. Inclusion body myositis presenting solely as dysphagia. Neurology 1993;43:1241–3.
9. Dubowitz V, Sewry CA. Muscle biopsy: a practical approach. 3rd ed. Philadelphia: Saunders, 2007.
10. Askanas V, Engel WK. Inclusion-body myositis, a multifactorial muscle disease associated with aging: current concepts of pathogenesis. Curr Opin Rheum 2007;19:550–9.
11. Dalakas M. Inflammatory, immune, and viral aspects of inclusion-body myositis. Neurology 2006;66:Suppl:S33–8.
12. Needham M, Mastaglia FL. Inclusion body myositis: current pathogenetic concepts and diagnostic and therapeutic approaches. Lancet Neurol 2007;6:620–31.

# Chapter 6
# The Role of Muscle Biopsy in the Diagnosis of Inflammatory Myopathy

Sakir Humayun Gultekin

**Abstract** Muscle biopsies of patients with immune-mediated inflammatory myopathies are characterized by a combination of chronic inflammatory infiltrates and muscle fiber necrosis. In addition, there are typical histochemical, immunohistochemical, and ultrastructural findings of each type of inflammatory myopathy. Accurate classification of inflammatory myopathies is important because inclusion body myositis does not respond to immunosuppressive treatment, polymyositis is frequently part of an overlap syndrome, and dermatomyositis is associated with cancer in adults. Necrotizing myopathy without inflammation may be due to a partially treated inflammatory myopathy, a toxic myopathy, or a paraneoplastic myopathy. Metabolic myopathies and muscular dystrophies may clinically and rarely pathologically mimic inflammatory myopathy. Correct identification of these entities depends on better awareness of clinical similarities between metabolic myopathy and inflammatory myopathy; appropriate utilization of immunohistochemical, ultrastructural, biochemical, and genetic techniques on muscle samples in difficult cases; and maximizing communication between the clinician and the pathologist.

**Keywords** Mitochondrial myopathy • Glycogen storage disease • Inclusion body myositis • Muscular dystrophy • Limb-girdle • Dysferlin • Statin myopathy

## Classification of Idiopathic Inflammatory Myopathies

Over many decades after the publication of the Bohan and Peter criteria for the diagnosis of myositis *(1,2)*, clinicoserologic variants of polymyositis and dermatomyositis have been identified. In addition, inclusion body myositis (IBM) has been defined and identified as the most common idiopathic inflammatory myopathy (IIM) over the age of 50 *(3,4)*. The main subtypes of IIM are:

S.H. Gultekin
Department of Pathology, Division of Neuropathology, Oregon Health and Science University, Portland, OR, USA

L.J. Kagen (ed.), *The Inflammatory Myopathies*,
DOI 10.1007/978-1-60327-827-0_6,
© Humana Press. a part of Springer Science+Business Media, LLC 2009

- Pure polymyositis (PM)
- Pure dermatomyositis (DM)
- Juvenile dermatomyositis
- Overlap myositis
- Cancer-associated myositis
- Inclusion body myositis (IBM)
- Focal myositis
- Granulomatous myositis

## Histopathology of Inflammatory Myopathy

The pathologist looks for the following fundamental features for a diagnosis of IIM:

- Presence of chronic inflammatory infiltrates between individual muscle fibers (endomysial), around muscle fascicles (perimysial), and around blood vessels (Fig. 6.1a)
- Presence of myofiber necrosis and regeneration (Fig. 6.1b)

In addition, there are several histological, histochemical, immunohistochemical, and electron microscopic features that are helpful for a diagnosis of myositis and subclassification:

- Autoaggressive T cells: T cells that invade intact muscle fibers (PM and IBM)
- Connective tissue labeling with alkaline phosphatase histochemical stain (Fig. 6.1c)

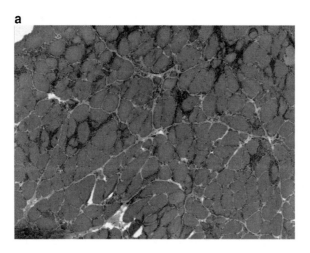

**Fig. 6.1** Inflammatory myopathy. (**a**) Lymphocytic infiltrates among muscle fibers. Hematoxylin and eosin stain ×100. (**b**) Myofiber necrosis. Hematoxylin and eosin stain ×400. (**c**) Connective tissue reactivity. Alkaline phosphatase ×200. (**d**) De novo expression of MHC-1 molecule in myofiber membranes. MHC-1 immunohistochemistry ×200

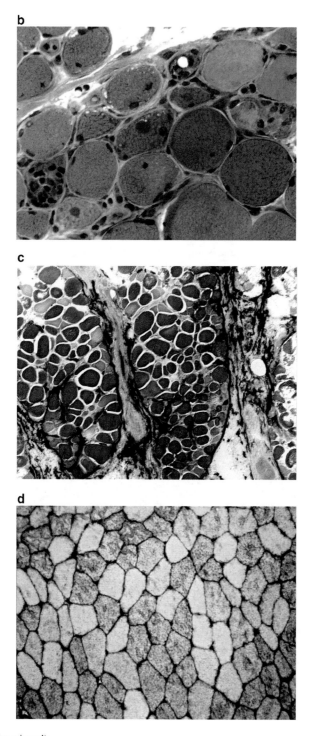

**Fig. 6.1** (continued)

- Diffuse de novo sarcolemmal expression of major histocompatibility complex 1 (MHC-1) molecule (Fig. 6.1d)
- Perifascicular atrophy/necrosis or perifascicular MHC-1 expression (DM)
- Membrane attack complex ($C^{5-9}$) deposits in capillaries (DM)
- Thickened capillaries and capillary depletion (DM)
- Tubuloreticular inclusions in endothelial cells (DM)
- Rimmed vacuoles (IBM)
- Fibrillary inclusion bodies (IBM)
- Amyloid deposits (IBM)

Not all features of a particular entity are found in every biopsy sample. Identification of muscle fiber necrosis and chronic inflammation remains essential for a probable diagnosis of myositis. The finding of perifascicular atrophy is diagnostic for dermatomyositis, even in the absence of inflammation (Fig.6.2). In cases for which corticosteroid treatment has been initiated prior to the biopsy, the inflammation may not be detected in the tissue sample. Those cases may be difficult to tell from any other necrotizing myopathy (toxic, drug induced, paraneoplastic, dystrophic). Additional histological findings and ancillary studies described may be helpful to arrive at a correct diagnosis *(5)*. Good communication between the clinician and the pathologist remains essential in this regard.

Statin myopathy is an important example of drug-induced myopathy with symptoms that both may mimic an IIM (myalgia, weakness, creatine kinase [CK] elevation, rhabdomyolysis) and reveal a necrotizing myopathy with or without inflammation on muscle biopsy *(6)*. Statin treatment may also may trigger an existing genetic myopathy to become clinically manifest. This possibility should be considered if the patient's muscle symptoms and CK levels are not gradually improving after cessation of statin treatment.

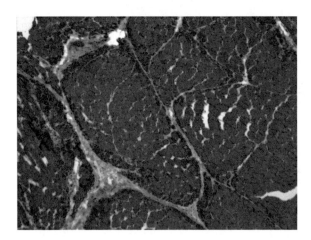

**Fig. 6.2** Dermatomyositis: perifascicular atrophy and myofiber necrosis. Hematoxylin and eosin stain ×100

Muscle biopsy may reveal the underlying cause of a "treatment-resistant myositis" *(7)*: Some pure dermatomyositis and polymyositis cases are inherently less responsive to treatment. The diagnosis may be a recognized treatment-resistant subtype of myositis.

## Inclusion Body Myositis

Inclusion body myositis *(8)* has been identified as the most common IIM in patients above the age of 50. It is twice as common in males and typically runs an indolent course. Combined proximal and distal weakness (finger extensors) is characteristic, and the quadriceps femoris muscle is frequently involved. Serum CK is elevated two to five times normal. Myositis-associated antibodies are not detected in patient sera. Histopathology is characterized by predominantly T-cell infiltrates that may have autoaggressive features, muscle fiber necrosis, atrophy, hypertrophy, fibrosis, frequent rimmed vacuoles, amyloid deposits in muscle fibers, and fibrillary inclusion bodies (Fig. 6.3). IBM patients do not respond to corticosteroid treatment. Diagnostic criteria that have been proposed for the diagnosis of IBM *(9)* are as follows:

*Definitive IBM*: Muscle biopsy shows autoaggressive inflammation, rimmed vacuoles, and amyloid deposits or ubiquitin (+)/SMI-31 (+) inclusions or demonstration of 15- to 18-nm paired helical filaments by electron microscopy.

*Probable IBM*: If the muscle biopsy shows only autoaggressive inflammation, then the diagnosis of probable IBM can be made if the following characteristic clinical and laboratory features are present:

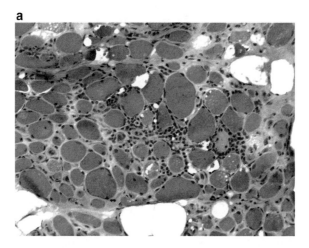

**Fig. 6.3** Inclusion body myositis. (**a**) Lymphocytic infiltrates among muscle fibers. Hematoxylin and eosin stain ×200. (**b**) Suppressor T cells invading intact muscle fibers (autoaggressive inflammation). CD8 immunohistochemistry ×400. (**c**) Multiple rimmed vacuoles within a muscle fiber. Hematoxylin and eosin stain ×400. (**d**) Ubiquitin deposits in muscle fibers. Ubiquitin immunohistochemistry ×200. (**e**) Fibrillary inclusion involving a myofiber nucleus. Electron microscopy

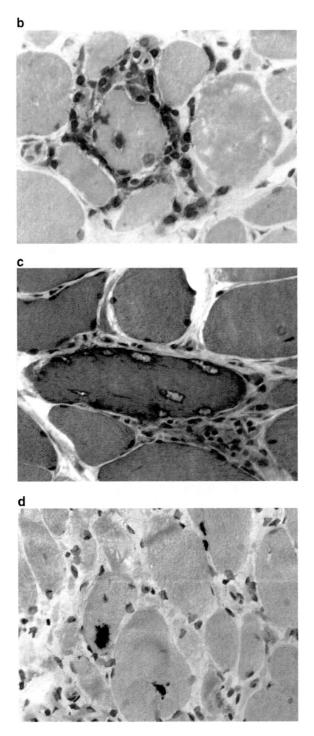

**Fig. 6.3** (continued)

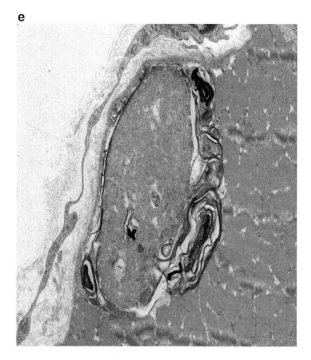

**Fig. 6.3** (continued)

- Duration of illness more than 6 months
- Onset over 30 years of age
- Weakness both proximal and distal and one of the following: finger flexor weakness, weaker wrist flexors than wrist extensors, quadriceps femoris weakness on the MRC scale of less than 4.
- Serum CK less than 12 times upper limit of normal.
- Electromyography consistent with IBM

Muscle biopsy and biochemical genetic testing may reveal another disease that clinically mimics myositis. Fatigue and muscle pain are also symptoms of a variety of other diseases, such as fibromyalgia and polymyalgia rheumatica. Symptoms of myositis, such as muscle pain, cramps, fatigue, weakness, and exercise-induced weakness are shared by patients with other primary diseases of the muscle. These diseases include:

- Endocrine myopathy
- Drug-induced myopathy
- Paraneoplastic myopathy
- Metabolic myopathy
- Muscular dystrophy
- Graft-versus-host disease
- HIV-associated myopathy
- Other viral diseases

Endocrine, drug-induced, HIV-associated, and other viral myopathies are generally suspected and investigated by clinical and laboratory methods other than biopsy. Paraneoplastic myopathy is a necrotizing myopathy with minimal or no inflammation on muscle biopsy and would lead to a search for an occult malignancy if the patient is not known to have cancer. Adult patients, especially above the age of 50, with polymyositis and dermatomyositis should also be screened for an underlying neoplasm *(10)*. Therefore, we look at metabolic myopathies and dystrophies more closely in this section as they have specific diagnostic features on muscle biopsy, or pathology findings can lead to a more specific biochemical/genetic test.

Muscular dystrophies can present during childhood or at any stage of adulthood. They usually have a progressive course, but the rate of progression depends on the type of dystrophy, among other factors. Most dystrophies can be specifically diagnosed by either immunohistochemical testing or Western blotting on muscle samples or with specific molecular testing for the underlying mutation. In some cases, both protein-level and DNA-level testing can be necessary to arrive at a definitive diagnosis.

Dystrophic histology is generally readily identifiable on muscle biopsies with chronic changes, such as fibrosis, muscle fiber loss, fatty infiltration, and a specific constellation of morphologic signs in a subset of disease entities. Subsequently, immunohistochemical testing can be performed to screen for specific entities, such as most limb-girdle dystrophies (LGMDs), and dystrophinopathies (Duchenne, Becker, symptomatic female careers of dystrophinopathy). However, in rare early cases of adult muscular dystrophy, in addition to muscle fiber necrosis, an inflammatory histology may emerge. This may lead to an erroneous diagnosis of a primary IIM. Dystrophies that may reveal an initial inflammatory phenotype on muscle biopsy are:

- Facioscapulohumeral (FSH) dystrophy
- Limb-girdle muscular dystrophies:
  - Dysferlinopathy (LGMD-2B)
  - Fukutinopathy (LGMD-2I)-pediatric
  - Eosinophilic myositis with Calpain-3 mutation *(9)*
- Emery-Dreifuss muscular dystrophy (mostly pediatric)
- Merosin (laminin alpha-2) deficiency (pediatric)

Facioscapulohumeral dystrophy is the third most common muscular dystrophy. It is characterized by a specific distribution of weakness involving facial, periscapular, and humeral muscles. It may progress to distal leg muscles. In unsuspected cases with atypical distribution of weakness and lack of family history, an "inflammatory" muscle biopsy result may be misleading *(12)*. A genetic test is available for identification of the genetic defect, a tandem repeat (D4Z4) on chromosome 4q.

Dysferlinopathy (LGMD-2B), which is autosomal recessive, may present as a predominantly limb-girdle syndrome or as a distal myopathy syndrome (Miyoshi type). In the limb-girdle form, the proximal weakness is present at the onset, usually in adolescence and early adulthood. Serum CK may be markedly elevated. Muscle biopsies may have inflammatory features *(13)* and sarcolemmal MHC-1 expression. Immunohistochemical and Western blot testing for dysferlin protein is important to distinguish these from IIM by histology alone (Fig. 6.4). Clinical history is the main distinguishing feature *(14)*.

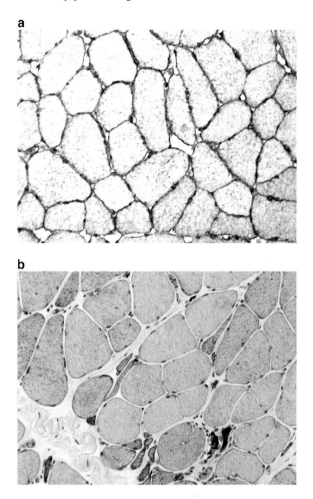

**Fig. 6.4** Dysferlinopathy. (**a**) Normal sarcolemmal distribution of dysferlin in adult muscle tissue. (**b**) Loss of dysferlin in muscle fibers in a patient with LGMD-2B. Dysferlin immunohistochemistry ×200

Metabolic myopathies can mimic myositis clinically *(15)*. Vague myalgias and occasional cramps are not uncommon complaints. Exercise-induced stiffness, weakness, cramps, and rhabdomyolysis (myoglobinuria) are typical dynamic symptoms. Fixed muscle weakness or very slowly progressive weakness may be a presenting feature. These myopathies are diagnosed by a variable combination of muscle pathology; biochemical tests, including enzyme measurements on various tissues and fibroblast cultures; human exercise laboratory tests; and genetic testing.

Mitochondrial myopathy may be a result of single or multiple mitochondrial or nuclear DNA mutations. Some are well-characterized syndromes, such as Kearns-Sayre, Leigh, MELAS, MERRF, for which a distinct constellation of signs and symptoms and multisystem involvement lead to an early suspicion of a mitochondrial cytopathy. Diagnostic difficulty arises when an adult patient without a family history presents with isolated muscle symptoms. Myalgias and CK elevation may lead to a clinical suspicion if IIM. Muscle biopsies may reveal classic findings of a mitochondrial myopathy, such as ragged red fibers due to abnormal accumulation of mitochondria in muscle fibers, similar abnormalities with mitochondria-specific succinyl dehydrogenase (SDH) histochemical stain, complete absence of cytochrome oxidase labeling in individual muscle fibers, or electron microscopic evidence of abnormal mitochondria (Fig. 6.5). When the muscle biopsy does not yield a diagnosis, biochemical and genetic testing are required when clinical suspicion of a primary mitochondrial disease remains high *(15)*.

Various enzyme defects in the glycolytic pathway give rise to glycogen storage disorders. Entities that affect primarily the skeletal muscle include myophosphorylase

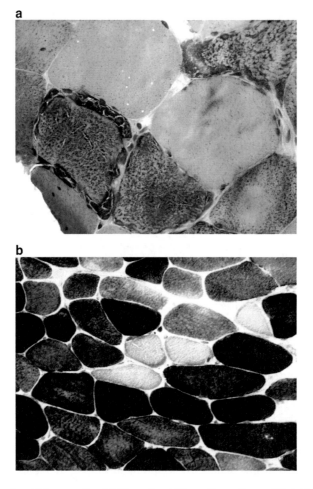

**Fig. 6.5** Mitochondrial myopathy. (**a**) Ragged red fibers. Gomori's modified trichrome ×400. (**b**) Total absence of cytochrome oxidase in scattered muscle fibers. COX stain ×400. (**c**) Ragged blue fibers with excess succinyl dehydrogenase activity. SDH stain ×400. (**d**) Mitochondria with paracrystalline inclusions in skeletal muscle. Electron microscopy

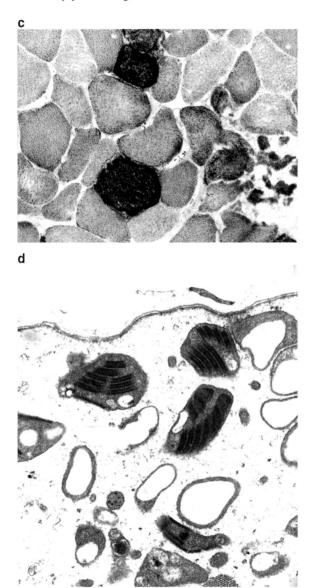

**Fig. 6.5** (continued)

deficiency, phosphorylase b kinase deficiency, phosphofructokinase deficiency, debrancher enzyme deficiency, Pompe's disease, and LAMP-2 deficiency, among others. While most present in childhood, some more common ones, like Pompe's and myophosphorylase deficiency, have adult onset forms that pose a diagnostic problem *(16)*.

Pompe's disease (glycogenosis type 2) is due to a deficit of lysosomal acid maltase (acid glucosidase). Adult form presents as a slowly progressive proximal weakness with pelvic girdle more involved than the shoulder. Respiratory muscle involvement is not uncommon. CK is variably elevated, and electromyography may show myotonic discharges in paraspinal muscles. Muscle biopsies may reveal typical vacuolar myopathy with abnormal glycogen deposits within lysosomes (Fig. 6.6). In adult form of Pompe's disease, muscle pathology may be entirely unremarkable. Direct enzyme measurement is available on leukocytes. Since specific enzyme replacement therapy has become available, a specific diagnosis is paramount for effective treatment *(17)*.

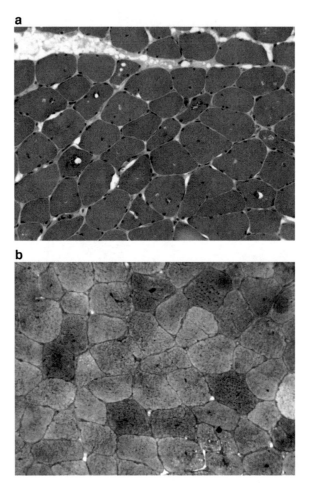

**Fig. 6.6** Acid maltase deficiency (Pompe's disease). (**a**) Vacuolar myopathy without inflammation. Hematoxylin and eosin stain ×100. (**b**) Small carbohydrate deposits in muscle fibers. PAS stain ×100. (**c**) Complete digestion of glycogen deposits. Diastase ×100. (**d**) Vacuoles labeled with lysosomal enzymes. Acid phosphatase ×100. (**e**) Glycogen pools in myofibers. PAS stain on plastic-embedded 1-m-thick section. (**f**) Free and lysosomal (membrane-bound) glycogen deposits in muscle. Electron microscopy

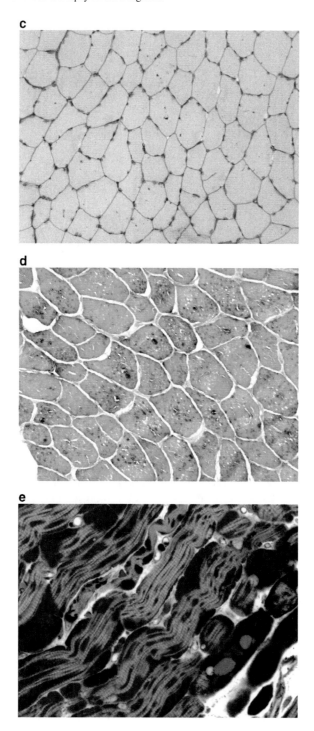

**Fig. 6.6** (continued)

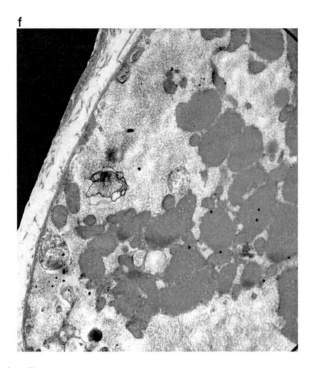

**Fig. 6.6** (continued)

Myophosphorylase deficiency (McArdle's disease, glycogenosis type V) is one of the most common inherited metabolic diseases. Adult onset is rare. Symptoms are identical to other metabolic myopathies. Serum CK is frequently elevated. Episodes of myoglobinuria are common, but electromyography may be normal between these episodes. A forearm ischemic exercise test may show abnormally low rise in venous lactate concentration. Muscle biopsies may show abnormal subsarcolemmal glycogen deposits, electron microscopic evidence of glycogen deposits, and the diagnostic absence of myophosphorylase reaction by histochemistry (Fig. 6.7). Rare cases mimicking IIM have been reported *(18,19)*.

Other metabolic disorders that may mimic myositis:

- *Myoadenylate deaminase (MAD) deficiency.* Although most patients with this autosomal recessive condition are asymptomatic, exercise-induced cramps, pain, early fatigue, cramps, and fibromyalgia-like complaints may occur. The defective enzyme is AMPD1 (muscle specific) on chromosome 1p. A secondary reduction in adenosine monophosphate (AMP) may be detected with another enzyme deficiency or dystrophy in some cases *(20)*. A histochemical stain for MAD on muscle biopsy specifically identifies the deficiency of this enzyme.
- *Carnitine palmitoyl transferase II (CPT II) Deficiency.* This "muscular" form of fatty acid oxidation defect is due to a defect in CPT II located on the inner mitochondrial membrane. Paroxysmal myoglobinuria and attacks of muscle stiffness, tightness, and pain are typical. Adolescent/young adult onset is typical, and evolution

a

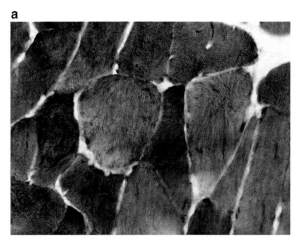

b

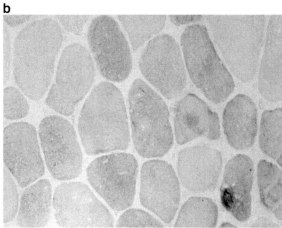

**Fig. 6.7** (a) Normal quantity and distribution of myophosphorylase in muscle by histochemical staining. ×200. (b) Absent myophosphorylase activity in skeletal muscle tissue of a patient with McArdle's disease. ×200

is slow. Heterozygous individuals may present with vague symptoms. Renal failure due to hemoglobinuria is a major risk. Electromyography and CK levels are not helpful between the episodes. Muscle biopsies are frequently normal, but enzyme analysis or mutation screening *(21)* will yield the specific diagnosis.

# References

1. Bohan A, Peter JB. Polymyositis and dermatomyositis (first of two parts). N Engl J Med 1975;292(7):344–7.
2. Bohan A, Peter JB. Polymyositis and dermatomyositis (second of two parts). N Engl J Med 1975;292(8):403–7.

3. Greenberg SA. Inflammatory myopathies: evaluation and management. Semin Neurol 2008;28(2):241–9.
4. Dalakas MC. Inflammatory disorders of muscle: progress in polymyositis, dermatomyositis and inclusion body myositis. Curr Opin Neurol 2004;17:561–77.
5. Sadeh M, Dabby R. Steroid-responsive myopathy: immune-mediated necrotizing myopathy or polymyositis without inflammation? J Clin Neuromuscul Dis 2008;9:341–4.
6. Needham M, Fabian V, Knezevic W, et al. Progressive myopathy with up-regulation of MHC-I associated with statin therapy. Neuromuscul Disord 2007;17:194–200.
7. Mastaglia FL. When the treatment does not work: polymyositis. Pract Neurol 2008;8(3):170–4.
8. Askanas V, Engel WK. Inclusion-body myositis, a multifactorial muscle disease associated with aging: current concepts of pathogenesis. Curr Opin Rheumatol 2007;19:550–9.
9. Mikol J, Engel AG. Inclusion body myositis. In: Engel AG, Franzini-Armstrong C, eds. Myology. 3rd ed. New York: McGraw Hill, 2004:1367–88.
10. Hill CL, Zhang Y, Sigurgeirsson B, et al. Frequency of specific cancer types in dermatomyositis and polymyositis: a population-based study. Lancet 2001;357:96–100.
11. Amato AA. Adults with eosinophilic myositis and calpain-3 mutations. Neurology 2008;70:730–1.
12. Fitzsimons RB. Facioscapulohumeral muscular dystrophy. Curr Opin Neurol 1999;12:501–11.
13. Fanin M, Angelini C. Muscle pathology in dysferlin deficiency. Neuropathol Appl Neurobiol 2002;28:461–70.
14. Dubowitz V, Sewry CA. Metabolic myopathies I: glycogenoses. In: Dubowitz V, Sewry CA, eds. Muscle biopsy: a practical approach. 3rd ed. Philadelphia: Saunders/Elsevier, 2007:453–68.
15. Wortmann RL, DiMauro S. Differentiating idiopathic inflammatory myopathies from metabolic myopathies. Rheum Dis Clin North Am 2002;28:759–78.
16. Benatar M. Metabolic myopathy. In: Benatar M, ed. Neuromuscular disease: evidence and analysis in clinical neurology. Totowa, NJ: Humana Press, 2006:397–419.
17. Katzin LW, Amato AA. Pompe disease: a review of the current diagnosis and treatment recommendations in the era of enzyme replacement therapy. J Clin Neuromuscul Dis 2008;9:421–31.
18. O'Brien T, Collins S, Dennett X, Byrne E, McKelvie P. McArdle's disease resembling an inflammatory myopathy. J Clin Neurosci 1998;5:210–2.
19. Horneff G, Paetzke I, Neuen-Jacob E. Glycogenosis type V (McArdle's disease) mimicking atypical myositis. Clin Rheumatol 2001;20:57–60.
20. Sabina RL. Myoadenylate deaminase deficiency. In: Karpati G, ed. Structural and molecular basis of skeletal muscle diseases. Basel: ISN Neuropath Press, 2002:214–5.
21. Deschauer M, Wieser T, Zierz S. Muscle carnitine palmitoyltransferase II deficiency: clinical and molecular genetic features and diagnostic aspects. Arch Neurol 2005;62:37–41.

# Chapter 7
# Electromyography

Hans L. Carlson

**Abstract** Electrodiagnostic studies are a routine component of the workup of myopathy and are fundamentally an extension of the physical examination. The examiner must be aware of factors that may influence the findings of a study. An understanding of neuromuscular anatomy and physiology, as well as the ability to recognize relevant patterns during the clinical evaluation, will guide the diagnostic evaluation. Specialized techniques may increase the diagnostic accuracy of these tests for the inflammatory myopathies.

**Keywords** Electrodiagnosis • Myopathy • Neuromuscular • Muscular weakness

## Introduction

Electrodiagnostic studies (nerve conduction studies and electromyography [EMG]) are a routine component of the workup of myopathy. The electrodiagnostic evaluation, combined with a careful history and physical examination, helps direct the diagnostic process. However, the results need to be considered carefully with respect to the clinical picture and other diagnostic tools. Electrodiagnostic studies are not as sensitive in evaluating myopathies as they are for many other neuromuscular conditions (*1*). To utilize the electrodiagnostic study effectively, an understanding of neuroanatomy and its relevance to the electrodiagnostic data is essential.

H.L. Carlson
Orthopaedics and Rehabilitation, Oregon Health and Science University, Portland, OR, USA

L.J. Kagen (ed.), *The Inflammatory Myopathies*,
DOI 10.1007/978-1-60327-827-0_7,
© Humana Press. a part of Springer Science + Business Media, LLC 2009

## Approach to the Patient with Weakness

When initially evaluating a patient who presents with weakness, the history and physical examination remain the single most important diagnostic tools. The etiology of weakness may represent central lesions, myelopathy, motor neuron disease, radiculopathy, plexopathy, mononeuropathy, polyneuropathy, neuromuscular junction disorders, or myopathy. Muscle weakness can be commonly confused with fatigue or asthenia (2). Characterizing the onset, location, nature, and frequency of the symptoms begins to narrow the differential diagnosis. It is important to note that electrodiagnostic studies are fundamentally an extension of the physical examination. A careful evaluation with respect to motor function, sensory abnormalities, reflexes, distribution of weakness (distal or proximal), and neurologic pattern of weakness (single or multiple myotomes or nerves) is required to put the electrodiagnostic data in the proper context (Table 7.1). In general, myopathies are distinguished by symmetric proximal weakness without sensory abnormalities, normal tone and normal or decreased muscle stretch reflexes, and no bowel or bladder dysfunction. Atrophy may or may not be present. This initial evaluation will effectively direct further workup, including the electrodiagnostic evaluation.

## Physiologic Basis of Electrodiagnostic Studies

Electrodiagnostic studies can be extremely useful in the evaluation of patients with weakness. While many factors can affect the electrodiagnostic results, the electrodiagnostic findings should correlate with the clinical evaluation. Just as imaging studies (X-rays, magnetic resonance imaging [MRI]) should be directly observed by the ordering practitioner in addition to reviewing the radiologist's report, inspection of the study should ensure the electrodiagnostic data support the electrodiagnostic conclusion. This is a useful practice for clinicians even if they do not perform electrodiagnostic studies.

Having a basic comprehension of the anatomy and physiology of the peripheral nervous system is the key to a more thorough understanding of the study. The electrodiagnostic study evaluates the peripheral nervous system, which consists of the peripheral nerves, the motor (anterior horn cell) and sensory (dorsal root ganglion) neurons, the neuromuscular junction, and the muscles. Localization of a peripheral nervous system lesion as well as characterization of the pathology (motor, sensory, axonal, demyelinating) and severity are possible.

Nerves transmit both motor and sensory data by chemical and electrical processes that result in an electrical impulse in the nerve (3). These impulses transmit sensory information from sensory receptors to the spinal cord/central nervous system to control muscle function. In motor nerves, these electrical impulses initiate acetylcholine release at the neuromuscular junction, which then binds to receptors on the muscle membrane. This results in depolarization of the muscle fiber and a subsequent muscle fiber electrical potential known as a *muscle fiber action potential (3)*.

**Table 7.1** Patterns of neurologic deficits

| | Motor weakness | Sensory loss | Reflexes | Limb distribution | Nerve distribution | Other |
|---|---|---|---|---|---|---|
| Myelopathy | Yes | Yes | Increased | Symmetric | Sensory and motor levels | No atrophy |
| Motor neuron disease | Yes | No | Increased | Symmetric, asymmetric, or cranial | Segmental | Fasciculations, atrophy |
| Radiculopathy | Yes | Yes | Decreased | Asymmetric | Single myotome, multiple nerves | Pain, polyradiculopathy |
| Plexopathy | Yes | Yes | Decreased | Asymmetric | Multiple myotomes and nerves | Viral (idiopathic), compressive, traumatic |
| Mononeuropathy | Yes | Yes | Decreased | Asymmetric | Multiple myotomes, single nerve distribution | Multiple mononeuropathies |
| Polyneuropathy | Yes | Yes | Decreased | Symmetric, distal | Multiple myotomes and nerves | Stocking/glove |
| Neuromuscular junction disorder | Yes | No | Decreased or no change | Symmetric, proximal, cranial | Multiple myotomes and nerves | Flexor weakness, ptosis, fatigue |
| Myopathy | Yes | No | Decreased or no change | Symmetric, proximal | Multiple myotomes and nerves | Extensor weakness, some distal |

Contributed by Nels L. Carlson

A motor unit consists of an anterior horn cell, axon, and all associated neuromuscular junctions and muscle fibers. When a motor unit is activated (depolarized), the subsequent electrical potentials of all of the associated muscle fibers are known as

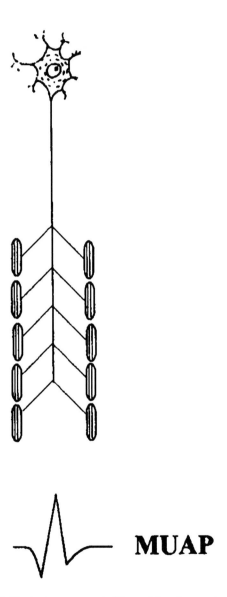

**MUAP**

**Fig. 7.1** The motor unit. The basic component of the peripheral nervous system is the motor unit, defined as an individual motor neuron, its axon, and associated neuromuscular junctions and muscle fibers. The extracellular needle electromyography recording of a motor unit is the motor unit action potential (MUAP). (From **Ref. 3**. Reprinted from Clinical-Electrophysiologic Correlations, copyright Butterworth-Heinemann. 1998. Reproduced with permission from copyright holder Butterworth-Heinemann/Elsevier)

a *motor unit action potential* (MUAP) (Fig. 7.1). Nerve conduction studies and EMG record these electrical potentials to quantify nerve or muscle abnormalities. Nerves may be myelinated or unmyelinated and vary in structure and diameter. Nerve conduction studies only record large myelinated fibers as small fiber neuropathies may have unremarkable routine nerve conduction studies *(3)*.

## Standard Electrodiagnostic Studies

### *Nerve Conduction Studies*

Nerve conduction studies and EMG compose an electrodiagnostic evaluation, each component having strengths and limitations. The test will often be referred to as EMG, a nerve conduction study, or a nerve conduction velocity (NCV). Except in cases with specific contraindications, both EMG and nerve conduction studies should be performed in a complete electrodiagnostic evaluation, which is more appropriately labeled as an electrodiagnostic study *(4)*.

Motor fibers, sensory fibers, or a combination (mixed nerve conduction studies) may be evaluated with nerve conduction studies. The resultant electrical potentials that are recorded for sensory nerve studies are known as sensory nerve action potentials (SNAPs) or compound motor action potentials (CMAPs) for motor nerve studies. It is possible to study a variety of nerves. Nerves of the extremity that are routinely studied include the median, peroneal, radial, sural, tibial, and ulnar. Other nerves may be evaluated, as indicated by the clinical question of interest. A nonroutine nerve conduction study may be limited by an examiner unfamiliar with the study and what is considered a normal response. A study of the symptomatic side should be compared to a study of the contralateral side *(1)*.

In addition to localizing a lesion, nerve conduction studies also assist in characterizing pathophysiology. Axonal loss lesions display decreased SNAP and CMAP amplitudes. These lesions may also prolong latency and slow conduction velocity but not below the normal physiologic range. Demyelinating lesions cause significantly prolonged latencies and reduced conduction velocities with CMAP and SNAP amplitudes that may be normal or decreased. Acquired demyelination may lead to conduction block, resulting in decreased CMAP amplitudes *(1)*.

### *Sensory Studies*

During sensory nerve conduction studies, a recording and reference electrode is placed over the nerve to be examined while it is stimulated, either proximally (antidromic) or distally (orthodromic). The recorded electrical potential (SNAP) is quantified by measuring the latency, amplitude, and conduction velocity (Fig. 7.2). A SNAP is stimulated and recorded over the nerve; therefore, conduction velocity

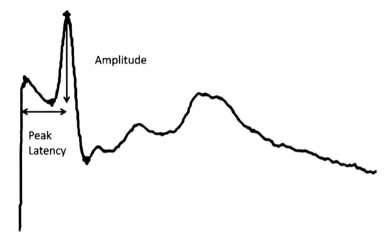

**Fig. 7.2** Sensory nerve action potential (SNAP)

may be calculated with a single stimulation site since neuromuscular junction and muscle depolarization time do not have to be accounted for *(1)*.

## Motor Studies

A recording electrode is placed over a muscle while the innervating nerve is stimulated to produce a motor nerve conduction study. An active electrode is placed over the motor end plate, and a reference electrode is placed distally over the tendon. Proximal and distal sites of the nerve are stimulated. The resultant electrical potential recorded over the muscle is the compound muscle action potential and is quantified in terms of latency, amplitude, and conduction velocity (Fig. 7.3). Neuromuscular junction and depolarization time are cancelled out using distal and proximal stimulation sites to produce accurate nerve conduction velocities *(1)*.

## Late Responses

Late responses are studies that reflect the electrophysiologic properties of the segments of the nerve both proximal and distal to the stimulation site. For most routine nerve conduction studies, stimulation of the limb is not more proximal than the knee or elbow. The late responses provide another electrodiagnostic tool for more comprehensive assessment of nerve function. There are two commonly assessed late responses: F waves and H reflexes. The F waves are thought to illustrate the "backfire" of a motor neuron *(5)* after the CMAP; they are not present on all motor nerve studies. The commonly performed F waves are of the ulnar, median, tibial, and peroneal nerves. This study assesses proximal nerve segments. However,

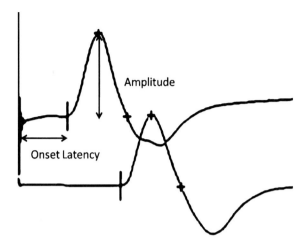

**Fig. 7.3** Compound motor action potentials (CMAPs)

a prolonged F wave does not necessarily localize the pathology to a proximal site. Because the F wave is routinely measured from a distal muscle, latency may be prolonged in distal entrapments *(1)*. The F wave is a test of the entire nerve circuit, not just proximal segments *(3)*. The H reflex assesses the S1 nerve root, an electrophysiologic equivalent of the ankle jerk reflex.

## *Electromyography*

Needle EMG examinations evaluate spontaneous and voluntary muscle fiber electrical potentials through an EMG needle that is placed in the muscle. The needle EMG examination is an integral piece of the electrodiagnostic study and is the most useful part of the evaluation of myopathies. The needles for routine EMG examination are either concentric or monopolar, and while they differ in their construct, their function is quite similar. The active and reference electrodes are both contained in the concentric needle, while the monopolar needle is used with a surface reference electrode on the skin. Disease states ranging from motor neuron disease to myopathy display abnormal activity. The value of needle EMG examination is not limited to determining the severity of the pathology but also the chronicity *(1)*. This examination is also important for evaluating proximal muscles not easily studied with nerve conduction studies. It is possible to examine multiple muscles innervated by multiple peripheral nerves.

Performing and interpreting needle EMG examinations are contingent on detailed knowledge of muscle location, innervations, and action. Muscles are evaluated at rest and with active contraction. The presence of abnormal spontaneous activity is assessed while the muscle is at rest. Active contraction of the muscle allows for the evaluation of motor unit action potential morphology and recruitment.

Spontaneous activity is evaluated by observing the EMG activity read from an EMG needle in a muscle at rest *(1)*. A normal muscle will be electrically silent at rest.

As the needle is moved through the muscle, fleeting muscle fiber depolarization may occur, and this is referred to as *normal insertional activity*. The duration of the insertional activity may be increased with both myopathies and neuropathies. The presence of increased insertional activity in the absence of other electrodiagnostic study abnormalities is not considered adequate electrophysiologic evidence to make a diagnosis. Spontaneous activity corresponds to the spontaneous depolarization of muscle fibers and may be generated at any location from the motor neuron to the muscle fiber. This abnormal activity represents instability of the muscle fiber membrane secondary to either nerve or muscle fiber injury *(6)*. The source of the spontaneous activity determines the characteristics of the abnormal waveforms that are generated. The abnormal waveforms may represent single muscle fibers (e.g., fibrillations, positive sharp waves [PSWs]) or multiple muscle fibers (e.g., complex repetitive discharges [CRDs]) or motor units (e.g., fasciculations). The common findings in acute denervation include fibrillation potentials or positive sharp waves that represent the spontaneous depolarization of a single muscle fiber.

Voluntary motor unit action potential activity is evaluated by asking the patient to contract the muscle being examined with the EMG needle. The resultant waveform is known as a motor unit action potential and represents the summated electrical activity of a motor unit. Morphology (amplitude, duration, polyphasia) and activation and recruitment patterns are determined from motor unit action potentials *(1)*. When assessing motor unit action potential morphology, the patient is asked to contract the muscle gently. This allows for the more detailed assessment of individual motor unit action potentials. Normally, the motor unit depolarization will result in the associated muscle fibers depolarizing at approximately the same time, resulting in a typical shape to the recorded potential. Characteristics of this waveform can be measured (amplitude, duration, phases). The presence of an abnormality of either the nerve or the muscle fibers will affect the synchrony or number of muscle fibers depolarizing, resulting in changes to the amplitude, duration, or phases of the motor unit action potential. Reinnervation will further affect the motor unit action potential morphology.

As a general rule, the initial motor unit action potentials that fire are smaller motor units with type I muscle fibers, such that motor unit action potential morphology tends to evaluate type I muscle fibers selectively *(3)*. In the next phase of the evaluation, the patient is asked to increase the power of the muscle contraction. During this contraction, type II and type I motor unit action potentials are generated. The waveforms will increase in frequency and number with multiple motor unit action potentials firing such that individual motor unit action potential morphology is not able to be analyzed. With the increased force of the muscle contraction, the activation, recruitment, and interference patterns of the motor unit action potential are evaluated. *Activation* refers to the capacity to increase the firing rate of the motor unit and is centrally mediated, while *recruitment* refers to the capacity to recruit more motor units as the firing rate increases, reflecting function of the peripheral nerve *(3)*. Abnormalities of the interference pattern are related to the activation or recruitment of motor unit action potentials.

Large-amplitude, long-duration, or polyphasic motor unit action potentials are displayed in general neuropathies with adequate time for reinnervation. Myopathies

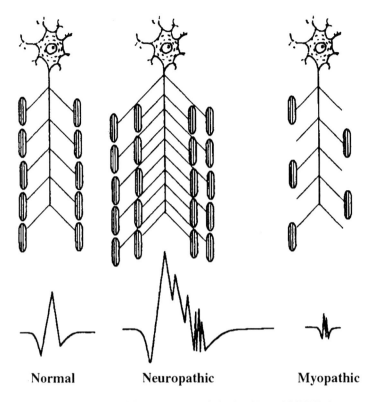

**Normal**          **Neuropathic**          **Myopathic**

**Fig. 7.4** Motor unit action potential (MUAP) morphologies. Normal MUAPs have two to four phases. In chronic neuropathic lesions that occur after reinnervation, the number of muscle fibers per motor unit increases, resulting in long-duration, high-amplitude, and polyphasic MUAPs. In myopathies or in neuromuscular junction disorders with block, the number of functional muscle fibers in the motor unit decreases. This leads to short-duration, small-amplitude, and polyphasic MUAPs. (From **Ref. 3**. Reprinted from Clinical-Electrophysiologic Correlations, copyright Butterworth-Heinemann. 1998. Reproduced with permission from copyright holder Butterworth-Heinemann/Elsevier)

can demonstrate decreased amplitude and duration, polyphasic motor unit action potentials (Fig. 7.4). Recruitment of motor unit action potentials is decreased with axonal loss or with demyelination and conduction block and may also be seen with severe myopathies *(1,3)*.

## Technical Issues

Numerous factors are capable of affecting nerve conduction studies, including age, height, temperature, anomalous innervations, onset of injury, and timing of the electrodiagnostic study *(1)*. While the physiologic reason for these factors is beyond the scope of this chapter, it is important to acknowledge these variables and patterns to avoid errors in diagnosis. With cool temperatures, studies will display slowed conduction velocities, prolonged latencies, and increased CMAP and SNAP amplitudes. During the electrodiagnostic examination, skin temperatures should be monitored and maintained between 33 and 34°C *(3)*. Advanced aging causes reduction in conduction velocities and amplitudes of CMAPs, and SNAPs *(7)*. Anomalous innervations and their subsequent nerve conduction study patterns can easily be mistaken for normal anatomic variants if knowledge of these innervations and patterns is not taken into account *(1)*.

## Special Electrodiagnostic Studies

Several special needle EMG studies can be performed to assist in making the diagnosis of individuals with suspected myopathy. These studies are time intensive, require special equipment, and generally are not part of the routine electrodiagnostic studies. Standard needle EMG records the electrical potential of a motor unit and some of its associated muscle fibers. This technique does not allow for analysis of single muscle fibers and is limited in that only a small area of the muscle is screened. Furthermore, the routine analysis of motor unit action potential morphology and recruitment may miss subtle abnormalities. Specialized techniques, including single-fiber EMG, macro-EMG, and quantitative motor unit action potential analysis, provide increased precision for the evaluation of patients with possible myopathy, specifically when customary electrodiagnostic studies are indistinct *(8)*.

Quantitative motor unit action potential analysis requires the recording of multiple motor units from a single muscle and involves several needle insertions in the examined muscle. Motor unit action potential characteristics such as mean duration and amplitude are calculated. These measurements can be compared to age-stratified normal values for specific muscles. Twenty to forty motor unit action potentials should be studied to increase the sensitivity of this test for myopathies *(9)*. Motor unit action potential duration is thought to be more sensitive than amplitude in identifying abnormalities *(5)*. Interference patterns of motor unit action potentials can also be evaluated. The turns-amplitude analysis of the interference pattern is the most commonly used and may be more sensitive in detecting myopathies than quantitative motor unit action potential analysis *(1,10)*. Other interference pattern analyses have also been described *(1)*.

Perhaps the most useful of the special needle EMG techniques is single-fiber EMG. The motor unit action potential has previously been described as the waveform that results when motor unit depolarization leads to the associated muscle fibers depolarizing at approximately the same time. The time between firing of the single muscle fibers within a motor unit is known as *jitter* and largely reflects the function of the neuromuscular junction. Abnormalities of the neuromuscular junction will prolong transmission time, resulting in increased deviation of adjacent muscle fiber depolarization, known as increased jitter. *Blocking* occurs when the delayed transmission is significant enough that the muscle fiber does not fire *(3)*. Routine needle EMG examination does not allow for this difference to be detected. A special needle is used for single-fiber EMG that facilitates the recording of adjacent muscle fibers from the same motor unit to measure jitter and blocking. Multiple pairs of adjacent muscle fibers are evaluated in the examined muscle, and the mean consecutive difference is calculated. Both increased jitter and blocking are indicative of neuromuscular junction disorders but can also be seen in myopathies as well as neuropathic disease *(3)*.

Another special EMG study is macro-EMG. This again requires a special EMG needle to record nearly all of the muscle fibers associated with a motor unit. In addition to motor unit action potential amplitude, muscle fiber density can be estimated. Once more, multiple motor unit action potentials from multiple sites are assessed, and the studies can be time intensive. Myopathies are characterized by small-amplitude motor unit action potentials with increased fiber density *(1)*.

Muscle fiber conduction velocity is another specialized technique influenced by muscle fiber properties that are affected by inflammatory myopathies. This technique, combined with EMG, increases the specificity and diagnostic accuracy with respect to inflammatory myopathies *(11)*.

## Inflammatory Myopathies

Electrodiagnostic studies used in conjunction with other diagnostic tests, such as muscle biopsy, are essential tools for the diagnosis and characterization of myopathic disorders *(1)*. Myopathies represent a wide and varied group of disorders, and for the most part, electrodiagnostic findings in the inflammatory myopathies are similar to metabolic and congenital myopathies and muscular dystrophies (Table 7.2). The electrodiagnostic study should not be relied on to differentiate the inflammatory myopathies from other myopathies. Myopathies classically present with symmetric proximal weakness involving the upper extremities, lower extremities, or both and may be either acquired or hereditary *(1)*. Weakness and functional impairments range from mild to severe, and sensation is not disturbed. Exceptions exist: Some myopathies may be asymmetric (i.e., inclusion body myositis [IBM], facioscapulohumeral muscular dystrophy), distal (i.e., myotonic dystrophy, IBM) *(3)*, or painful (dermatomyositis, polymyositis, toxic myopathies) *(12)*. Physical exam findings include proximal weakness and atrophy, spared sensation, and usually normal reflexes *(1)*.

Routine motor nerve conduction studies of upper and lower extremities (i.e., median, ulnar, tibial, peroneal) use recording electrodes over distal muscles and usually produce normal results because myopathies typically affect proximal muscles. Compound motor unit action potential amplitudes may be decreased in severe or distally involved myopathies *(1)*. Sensory nerve conduction studies are routinely normal, and although sensory neuropathies associated with inflammatory myopathies are rare, they have been described *(13)*. The F waves are usually normal as the

**Table 7.2** Electrodiagnostic findings in myopathies

| Parameter | Muscular dystrophy | Congenital | Mitochondrial | Metabolic | Inflammatory | Channelopathy |
|---|---|---|---|---|---|---|
| DL | Normal | Normal | Normal | Normal | Normal | Normal |
| NVC | Normal | Normal | Normal | Normal | Normal | Normal |
| H reflex | Normal or absent | Normal or absent | Normal | Normal | Normal or absent | Normal |
| SNAP amplitude | Normal | Normal | Normal | Normal | Normal | Normal |
| CMAP amplitude | Normal or decreased | Normal or decreased | Normal or decreased | Normal or decreased | Normal or decreased | Normal |
| MUAP duration | Decreased or increased | Decreased and/or normal | Decreased or normal | Decreased or normal | Decreased or increased (IBM) | Decreased or normal |
| MUAP amplitude | Decreased or increased | Decreased or normal | Decreased or normal | Decreased or normal | Decreased or increased (IBM) | Decreased or normal |
| Polyphasics | Increased | Increased or normal | Increased or normal | Increased or normal | Increased | Increased or normal |
| Recruitment | Increased | Increased or normal | Increased or normal | Increased or normal | Increased | Increased or normal |
| Fibrillations and PSWs | Yes | Centronuclear myopathy | No | Yes | Yes | Occasionally |
| CRDs | Yes | Centronuclear myopathy | No | Yes | Yes | Occasionally |
| Myotonic potentials | Myotonic dystrophy | Centronuclear myopathy | No | Acid maltase deficiency | No | Yes |
| Electrical silence | No | No | No | Contractures in McArdle's diseases | No | During attacks of paralysis |

*Source:* **Ref. (1)**. Reprinted from Physical Medicine and Rehabilitation: State of the Art Reviews, Clinical Electrophysiology. Used with permission from Hanley and Belfus/Elsevier

*DL* distal latency; *NCV* nerve conduction velocity; *SNAP* sensory nerve action potential; *CMAP* compound motor action potential; *MUAP* motor unit action potential; *PSWs* positive sharp waves; *CRD* complex repetitive discharge; *IBM* inclusion body myositis

recording electrodes are placed over distal muscles. A recommended nerve conduction workup for the patient with a suspected myopathy is one upper extremity and one lower extremity motor conduction, sensory conduction, and F wave (3). Disorders that present similarly to myopathies, such as motor neuron disease, motor neuropathies, and neuromuscular junction disorders, are evaluated with nerve conduction studies (3).

Needle EMG examination is the most important part of the electrodiagnostic study in the workup of myopathy (1). A recommended EMG evaluation consists of two distal and two proximal muscles from one upper and one lower extremity as well as paraspinal muscles. Muscle with weakness should be evaluated and may require more than one needle insertion as the muscle involvement may be irregular with respect to abnormalities (1,3). Paraspinal muscles are commonly involved in the inflammatory myopathies, and their evaluation is therefore recommended (3). It is fortunate that myopathies tend to be symmetric, so biopsies can be performed on the contralateral muscle with electrodiagnostic studies because trauma from the EMG needle can interfere with the accuracy of the needle biopsy (3).

## Polymyositis and Dermatomyositis

Spontaneous activity may be present in neuropathies or myopathies, and it is the distribution and pattern of the abnormal findings that help in narrowing the differential diagnosis. The muscles involved in polymyositis and dermatomyositis usually have abnormal spontaneous activity consisting of fibrillation potentials, positive sharp waves, or complex repetitive discharges. The degree of abnormal spontaneous activity may approximately correlate with the severity of the inflammatory myopathy (14). The abnormal fibrillation potentials can resolve with treatment as muscle strength improves, although relapses are not uncommon (3,15,16). Electrodiagnostic studies have limitations in assessing disease activity versus damage with respect to the inflammatory myopathies (17).

The classic finding when assessing voluntary activity of the myopathic muscle is small amplitude and duration, polyphasic motor unit action potentials secondary to muscle fiber dysfunction, or dropout (3). This type of motor unit action potential can be seen in a variety of disorders, however, including neuromuscular junction disorders, early reinnervation, and periodic paralysis (3). As these inflammatory myopathies become chronic, large-amplitude or long motor unit action potentials can develop and may be secondary to the increased density of the muscle fibers following the process of segmental necrosis and collateral regeneration, potentially leading to confusion with neuropathic processes (5). Duration, rather than amplitude, may be a more useful motor unit action potential characteristic to examine when evaluating myopathies, although long-duration motor unit potentials can be seen with dermatomyositis/polymyositis and may not correlate to the chronicity of the disease (5,18). Amplitude can increase with chronic myopathies and is also affected by technical factors associated with the EMG needle (5).

The analysis of motor unit action potential recruitment is helpful for both acute and chronic myopathies. Recruitment is assessed by the examiner resisting the force generated by the patient during active muscle contraction. Less force is generated than is generally observed for the same amount of motor unit action potentials being activated because the activated motor unit action potentials with the inflammatory myopathies have fewer muscle fibers (1). This phenomenon is referred to as *early recruitment*.

Chronic myopathies may be confused with neuropathies secondary to large-amplitude motor unit action potentials, but myopathies will have normal or early recruitment as opposed to decreased recruitment in neuropathies (3). When single-fiber EMG is performed with myopathy, increased jitter and blocking may be seen, which reflects the effect of denervation/reinnervation of the neuromuscular junction (3).

## Inclusion Body Myositis

Inclusion body myositis is more common than dermatomyositis/polymyositis in older adults (19). IBM has different clinical features than polymyositis/dermatomyositis, but the electrodiagnostic features are, for the most part, similar. With respect to the nerve conduction studies, sensory nerve conduction studies will be normal. Distal muscles are frequently involved with IBM, and compound motor unit action potential amplitudes may be decreased. IBM may have a tendency to involve certain muscles in the lower extremity, such as the Iliopsoas, quadriceps, and tibialis anterior, and the biceps, triceps, and flexor digitorum profundus in the upper extremity; thus, needle EMG should be performed accordingly (1,3,19). Abnormal spontaneous activity associated with IBM (fibrillation potentials, positive sharp waves, complex repetitive discharges) can be more common than that seen in polymyositis/dermatomyositis and may be expected in all examined muscles (20). The lack of abnormal spontaneous activity would call the diagnosis into question (5). IBM tends to be slowly progressive, and often the diagnosis is not made until the disease process is chronic. IBM motor unit action potential morphology may be myopathic (small, short motor unit action potentials with polyphasia), neuropathic (large, long motor unit action potentials with polyphasia), or both, which is consistent with the chronic nature of this myopathy (3). Some individuals with IBM may also have peripheral neuropathy (21). These findings can lead to further difficulties in pinpointing the diagnosis.

## Conclusion

Electrodiagnostic studies are useful diagnostic tools for localizing and characterizing neuropathology. Knowledge of the peripheral nervous system and functional anatomy are essential during the process of distinguishing myopathies from radiculopathies, plexopathies, polyneuropathies, or other lesions. Recognition of patterns of neuromuscular involvement (weakness, sensory abnormalities, or pain) during the initial clinical evaluation can help direct the electrodiagnostic evaluation. Relevant patterns include proximal versus distal, symmetric versus asymmetric, motor versus sensory, and so on *(1)*. It is important to remember that electrodiagnostic studies function as an extension of the history and physical examination. The electrodiagnostic workup is focused, with a thorough history and physical examination directed by a specific clinical question (or questions). Specialized techniques may increase the diagnostic accuracy of these tests for the inflammatory myopathies.

# References

1. Krivickas LS, Carlson NL. Myopathies. Phys Med Rehabil Clin N Am 1999;13:307–32.
2. Saguil A. Evaluation of the patient with muscle weakness. Am Fam Physician 2005; 71(7):1327–36.
3. Preston DC, Shapiro BE. Electromyography and neuromuscular disorders: clinical-electrophysiologic correlations. Newton, MA: Butterworth-Heinemann, 1998.
4. American Association of Neuromuscular and Electrodiagnostic Medicine (AANEM). Proper performance and interpretation of electrodiagnostic studies. Muscle Nerve 2006;33(3):436-9.
5. Dumitru D. Electrodiagnostic medicine. Philadelphia: Hanley and Belfus, 1995.
6. Daube JR. AAEM minimonograph #11: needle examination in clinical electromyography. Muscle Nerve 1991;14(8):685–700.
7. Kimura J. Electrodiagnosis in diseases of nerve and muscle: principles and practice. 3rd ed. New York: Oxford University Press, 2001.
8. Dorfman LJ, McGill KC. AAEE minimonograph #29: automatic quantitative electromyography. Muscle Nerve 1988;11(8):804–18.
9. Engstrom JW, Olney RK. Quantitative motor unit analysis: the effect of sample size. Muscle Nerve 1992;15(3):277–81.
10. Liguori R, Dahl K, Fuglsang-Frederiksen A, Trojaborg W. Turns-amplitude analysis of the electromyographic recruitment pattern disregarding force measurement. II. Findings in patients with neuromuscular disorders. Muscle Nerve 1992;15(12):1319–24.
11. Blijham PJ, Hengstman GJ, Ter Laak HJ, Van Engelen BG, Zwarts MJ. Muscle-fiber conduction velocity and electromyography as diagnostic tools in patients with suspected inflammatory myopathy: a prospective study. Muscle Nerve 2004;29(1):46–50.
12. Krivickas LS. Electrodiagnosis in neuromuscular disease. Phys Med Rehabil Clin N Am 1998;9(1):83–114.
13. Franca MC Jr, Faria AV, Queiroz LS, Nucci A. Myositis with sensory neuronopathy. Muscle Nerve 2007;36(5):721–5.
14. Streib EW, Wilbourn AJ, Mitsumoto H. Spontaneous electrical muscle fiber activity in polymyositis and dermatomyositis. Muscle Nerve 1979;2(1):14–8.
15. Sandstedt PE, Henriksson KG, Larrsson LE. Quantitative electromyography in polymyositis and dermatomyositis. Acta Neurol Scand 1982;65(2):110–21.
16. Agarwal SK, Monach PA, Docken WP, Coblyn JS. Characterization of relapses in adult idiopathic inflammatory myopathies. Clin Rheumatol 2006;25(4):476–81.
17. Dayal NA, Isenberg DA. Assessment of inflammatory myositis. Curr Opin Rheumatol 2001;13(6):488–92.
18. Blijham PJ, Hengstman GJ, Hama-Amin AD, Van Engelen BG, Zwarts MJ. Needle electromyographic findings in 98 patients with myositis. Eur Neurol 2006;55(4):183–8.
19. Jackson CE, Barohn RJ, Gronseth G, Pandya S, Herbelin L. Inclusion body myositis functional rating scale: a reliable and valid measure of disease severity. Muscle Nerve 2008;37(4):473–6.
20. Dumitru D, Newell-Eggert M. Inclusion body myositis. An electrophysiologic study. Am J Phys Med Rehabil 1990;69(1):2–5.
21. Rendt K. Inflammatory myopathies: narrowing the differential diagnosis. Cleve Clin J Med 2001;68(6):505–19.

# Chapter 8
# Magnetic Resonance Imaging of Myopathies and Myositis

Carolyn M. Sofka

**Abstract** Magnetic resonance imaging (MRI) has broad applications in evaluating the patient with a suspected myopathy. The superior soft tissue contrast and spatial resolution of MRI make it a useful tool in evaluating the anatomy, morphology, and potential functionality of muscles. Specifically, MRI is extremely sensitive for resolving areas of muscle edema, thus identifying areas of active involvement, detecting potential subclinical disease, and providing guidance for muscle biopsy. As MRI is a fairly reproducible examination, the longitudinal course and disease progression (or regression) of myopathies can be evaluated, with MRI providing potential prognostic information and evaluating response to treatment.

**Keywords** Magnetic resonance imaging • Myositis • Polymyositis • Dermato myositis • Pyomyositis • Myositis ossificans

## Introduction

The inflammatory myopathies encompass a broad range of abnormalities that often have a similar clinical presentation and symptoms. A definitive diagnosis is often only made after a muscle biopsy. Even after such an invasive procedure, the diagnosis can remain elusive if an affected muscle was not addressed for biopsy, often resulting in a false-negative diagnosis.

Most imaging studies are noncontributory in evaluating the patient with a presumed inflammatory myositis. Conventional radiographs are limited to identifying soft tissue calcifications in the setting of dermatomyositis or ossification in

C.M. Sofka
Department of Radiology and Imaging, Hospital for Special Surgery,
Weill Medical College of Cornell University, New York, NY, USA

L.J. Kagen (ed.), *The Inflammatory Myopathies*,
DOI 10.1007/978-1-60327-827-0_8,
© Humana Press. a part of Springer Science + Business Media, LLC 2009

suspected cases of myositis ossificans. They lack the resolution needed to evaluate the soft tissues and they do involve ionizing radiation. Computed tomography (CT) is exquisite at demonstrating cortical bone and therefore can detect small areas of calcification or ossification that X-rays might overlook, but it lacks the soft tissue contrast resolution needed to depict muscle morphology clearly.

Ultrasound has some utility in evaluating the patient with a suspected inflammatory myositis, demonstrating areas of both chronic changes with fatty atrophy as well as active disease with power Doppler. One of its main advantages is to provide guidance for muscle biopsy. The use of ultrasound is described in detail in another chapter.

Magnetic resonance imaging (MRI) with its superior soft tissue contrast and spatial resolution, is excellent for evaluating the soft tissue structures in the musculoskeletal system. Detailed anatomic and often functional information regarding muscle can be obtained from an MRI.

In addition to its detailed morphologic information, MRI can provide a large anatomic overview of a region of interest, including the evaluation of the contralateral limb for comparison and symmetry. MRI uses no ionizing radiation, so it is useful across a broad patient population. Last, and perhaps most important, MRI findings can help direct muscle biopsy by identifying areas of abnormal muscle that may have subclinical involvement. By accurately demonstrating distinct abnormal muscle groups, an appropriate site can be chosen for biopsy, thus avoiding a potential false-negative result.

In this chapter, the basic principles of MRI are discussed, including specific protocol recommendations for evaluating the inflammatory myopathies. The specific MR appearances of a variety of commonly encountered muscle abnormalities are also reviewed. This review received institutional review board approval

## MRI Technical Considerations

In contrast to imaging the small joints of the hand and foot, where a very small field of view is needed, the imaging of the myopathies generally necessitates a larger field of view with a more global anatomic overview, usually imaging the contralateral limb for comparison and symmetry at the same sitting. To that end, larger coils are usually used, such as those often employed in abdominal or body imaging.

Magnetic resonance imaging has the ability to provide exquisite anatomic images. In the case of muscle, this is usually done by performing T1-weighted imaging (Fig. 8.1). As muscle abnormalities may often be an unsuspected finding, however, other standard pulse sequences used in musculoskeletal imaging (proton density and T2, for example) can also provide anatomic information as well (Fig. 8.2).

In a T1-weighted image, there is a large contrast range between fat and skeletal muscle (Fig. 8.1) *(1)*. Skeletal muscle has higher signal intensity than water on a T1-weighted image, but the intensity is much lower than that of fat *(2)*. Normally, skeletal muscle is seen as a structure with intermediate to low signal intensity, usually with a few, very fine linear internal striations of fat on a T1-weighted image.

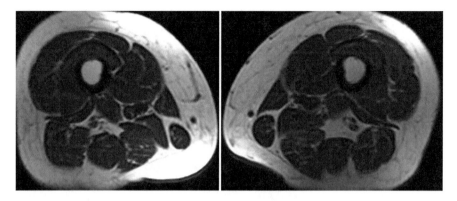

**Fig. 8.1** Axial T1-weighted image through the distal third of the thighs bilaterally demonstrating the normal appearance of skeletal muscle. The muscles are of uniform intermediate-to-low signal intensity bilaterally, symmetrically. There are only a few thin internal fatty septae. Muscle bulk is preserved and symmetric

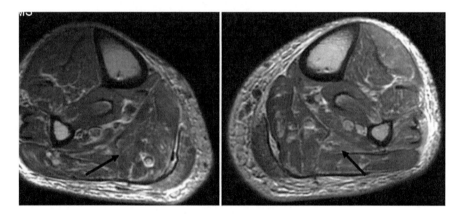

**Fig. 8.2** Axial proton density-weighted image through the legs demonstrates mild loss of muscle bulk and fatty infiltration (*arrows*)

A more "marbled" appearance or increased fatty infiltration of muscle, often associated with decreased muscle bulk, is indicative of chronic atrophy (Figs. 8.3–8.5).

Fat suppression sequences are invaluable in evaluating the myopathies. By rescaling fat and water contrast, such sequences accentuate areas of free mobile water within muscle, indicating abnormalities, such as potential inflammatory involvement or trauma. There are two main pulse sequences available to accomplish this with MRI: frequency-selective fat suppression and short tau inversion recovery (STIR). Frequency-selective fat suppression sequences are sensitive to local field inhomogeneities (e.g., in the presence of instrumentation, large fields of view);

**Fig. 8.3** Coronal
T1-weighted image through
the posterior aspect of the legs
demonstrates subselective
atrophy of the medial aspect
of the soleus on the right
(*arrow*)

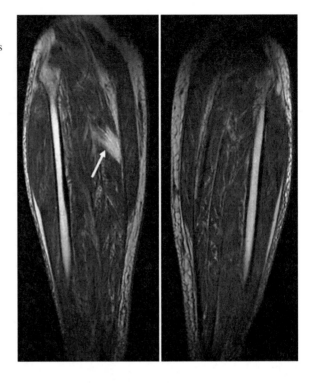

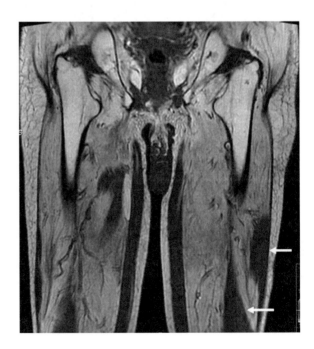

**Fig. 8.4** Coronal
T1-weighted image in a
patient with chronic
polymyositis demonstrating
severe marked atrophy of the
majority of the muscles of
the pelvis and thighs. Some
spared islands of uninvolved
skeletal muscle remain
(*arrows*)

a

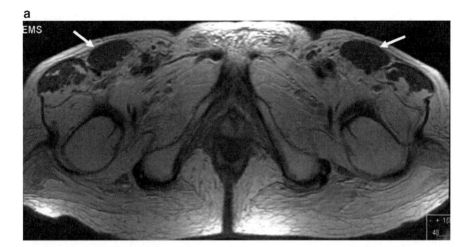

b

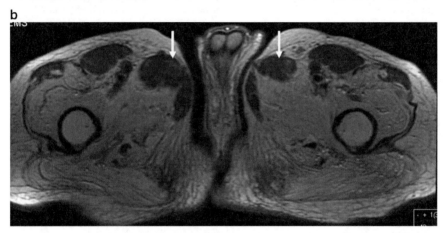

**Fig. 8.5** Axial proton density images through the low pelvis and proximal thighs in the same patient as Fig. 8.4 demonstrates the marked atrophy and loss of muscle bulk with relative sparing of the rectus femoris (*arrows*, **a**) and the adductor longus (*arrows*, **b**)

therefore, STIR sequences are generally employed when evaluating a patient with a suspected myopathy (Fig. 8.6).

The STIR sequence is extremely sensitive but largely nonspecific for muscle abnormalities. Muscle edema can be seen in a variety of disorders, such as polymyositis and dermatomyositis, injuries, infection, and denervation *(1,2)*. This sequence allows for a rapid general anatomic overview of large areas of the body, such as the pelvis and thighs, a common site of involvement by myositis (Fig. 8.7). Some authors have investigated the utility of large whole-body STIR imaging as a screening method for evaluating areas of subclinical involvement in myositis *(3)*. The STIR sequence is extremely sensitive in detecting areas of muscle edema,

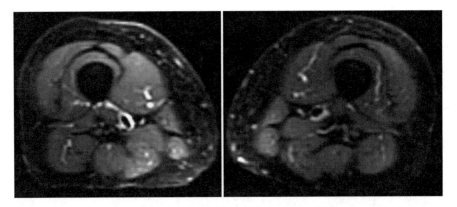

**Fig. 8.6** Axial inversion recovery through the distal third of thighs at the same level as Fig. 8.1. On inversion recovery, the signal from fat is suppressed and becomes closer in signal intensity to skeletal muscle. Faint areas of apparent increased signal at the posteromedial aspect of the thighs, right greater than left, are due to inhomogeneous fat suppression at the margins of the coil

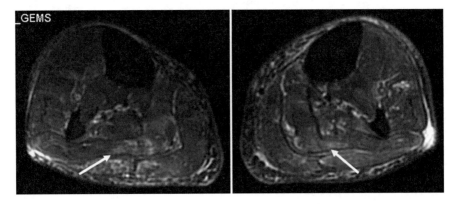

**Fig. 8.7** Axial inversion recovery images through both calves at the same level as Fig. 8.2 in a patient with lower extremity weakness. Nonspecific hyperintensity is seen in the deep muscles of the posterior compartments bilaterally (*arrows*)

thereby identifying areas of disease activity and potentially directing biopsy (Figs. 8.8–8.10) (*4–8*).

Choosing an appropriate site for biopsy is important to reduce the false-negative rate and therefore the incidence of repeat biopsies. By choosing an appropriate site prospectively, this can decrease delays in diagnosis, patient discomfort, and cost (*8*). While the cost of MRI is often higher than other cross-sectional imaging modalities, studies have shown an overall cost-effectiveness in getting premuscle biopsy MRI to guide for an appropriate site to sample, thus decreasing false-negative biopsy rates and the potential need to rebiopsy (*6,9*).

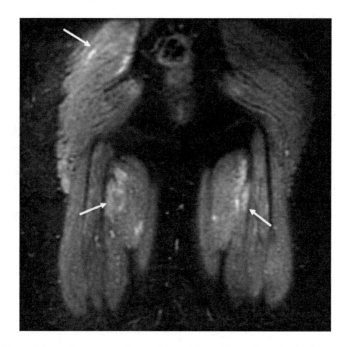

**Fig. 8.8** Coronal inversion recovery image in a patient with weakness in the lower extremities. There are subtle areas of hyperintensity in the semimembranosis muscles posteriorly (*arrows*) as well as the right gluteus maximus muscle (*superior arrow*)

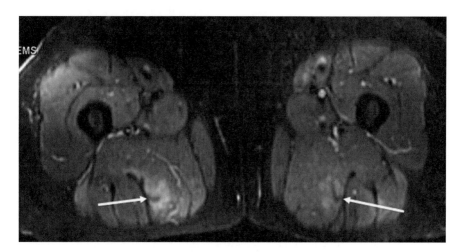

**Fig. 8.9** Axial inversion recovery image in the same patient as Fig. 8.8 demonstrates the subtle increased signal in the semimembranosis muscles (*arrows*)

Functional MRI, while not performed routinely in the clinical setting, can potentially provide even more detailed molecular analysis of muscle. Qi et al. *(10)* found diffusion-weighted imaging helpful in differentiating inflamed from normal

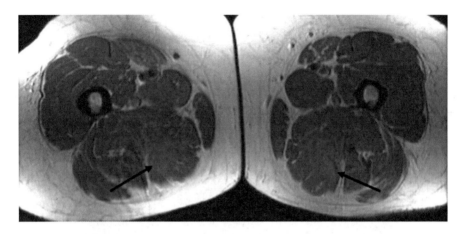

**Fig. 8.10** Axial proton density image through the thighs at the same level as Fig. 8.9 demonstrates faint increased signal in the muscles (*arrows*); however, the abnormality is not as conspicuous as on the inversion recovery sequences, which was used to suggest locations for muscle biopsy

muscles in dermatomyositis and polymyositis. With diffusion-weighted imaging, the amount of extracellular diffusion of water is measured, suggesting areas of abnormal pathology (inflammation, trauma). In their series, Qi et al. observed greater unrestricted motion of water due to infiltration of fluid in the extracellular space in cases of muscle inflammation.

## Dermatomyositis and Polymyositis

Dermatomyositis and polymyositis are both disorders of skeletal muscle. In dermatomyositis, both skin and muscle are involved, while in polymyositis only muscle is involved. Clinically, patients present with proximal muscle weakness, usually in the thighs and pelvic girdle, progressing to later involvement in the upper extremity, laryngeal, and pharyngeal muscles. Weakness is usually the more common clinical presentation rather than tenderness or pain.

The role of MRI is to identify the affected muscles, sometimes those with subclinical disease. While often the MRI findings are nonspecific, the pattern of involvement can suggest a specific disease entity, especially when the contralateral extremity is imaged for comparison and symmetry *(11)*.

Also, MRI can help to distinguish polymyositis from other processes, such as infection. For example, polymyositis is the most common muscular manifestation in patients with HIV infection and needs to be distinguished from infectious pyomyositis, which also is not uncommon in the same population, because the treatments are clearly different. MRI with intravenous contrast can help to distinguish the two because rim enhancement does not occur in polymyositis *(12)*.

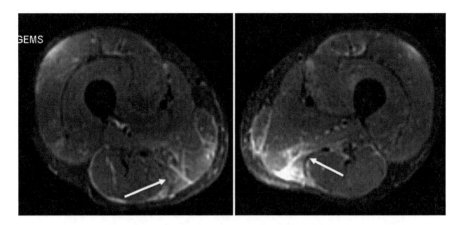

**Fig. 8.11** Axial inversion recovery image through both thighs in a patient with known dermatomyositis demonstrates infiltrative hyperintensity in the posterior muscle compartments bilaterally, left greater than right (*arrows*)

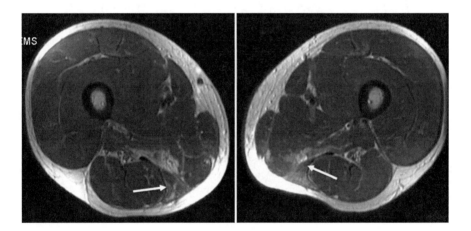

**Fig. 8.12** Axial proton density sequence through the same level as Fig. 8.11 demonstrates abnormal signal intensity in the same muscle groups (*arrows*)

Dermatomyositis involves both skeletal muscle and skin. It often has the same muscle distribution and involvement as polymyositis, with preferential involvement of the lower extremities; however, the clinical presentation (skin involvement) can help distinguish the two (Figs. 8.11–8.13). Of note, in the lower extremities, relative sparing of the rectus femoris and biceps femoris muscles has been inconsistently observed *(13)*.

By identifying areas of muscle involvement, MRI can also be used to direct muscle biopsy. In some cases, deciding clinically what muscle group to sample (most often the quadriceps due to its usual involvement) can be difficult. Biopsying

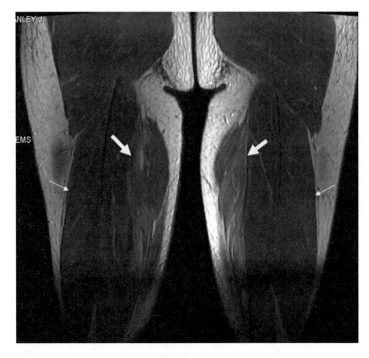

**Fig. 8.13** Coronal proton density image through the posterior legs further demonstrates the abnormal muscle inflammation (*short thick arrows*). Contrast the appearance of the abnormal muscle with adjacent normal muscle (*thin arrows*)

an unaffected muscle can result in a false-negative diagnosis. MRI with STIR imaging can clearly identify areas of abnormality and suggest areas to sample. MRI can also be used as an outcomes measure, evaluating long-term follow-up and assessment of ongoing disease activity or resolution *(14)*.

## Inclusion Body Myositis

Sporadic inclusion body myositis (IBM) is a chronic inflammatory myopathy presenting clinically as progressive, asymmetric proximal and distal weakness that typically initially involves the quadriceps and the flexor muscles of the forearm. Hereditary IBM occurs earlier in life (20–30 years of age) with a distinctly different pattern of involvement from sporadic IBM. In hereditary IBM, there is distal weakness of the lower limbs, with relative sparing of the quadriceps *(15)*.

Classically, MRI demonstrates a nonspecific appearance of fatty infiltration with increased T1 signal intensity in the affected muscles and atrophy *(15)*. As noted with respect to polymyositis and dermatomyositis, the MRI appearance can in and of itself be nonspecific, however; the clinical history and distribution of involvement can suggest the diagnosis.

Dion et al. *(11)* studied the MRI appearance of IBM and contrasted it to polymyositis. They found that in sporadic IBM, the muscles tended to be more atrophic and fatty replaced compared to those in polymyositis. Moreover, the pattern of involvement between the two diseases was found to be distinctly different. In sporadic IBM, asymmetrical involvement of the thighs was most often encountered, with a distal predominance in the anterior muscle group. This was in contrast to those lesions found in polymyositis, for which there was a symmetrical involvement most often involving the posterior muscle group.

Contrast is of limited utility in evaluating patients with IBM except when the clinical picture is nonspecific and other diagnoses are being entertained, such as pyomyositis. In IBM, the lesions typically do not enhance *(16)*.

## Focal Myositis

Focal myositis is a rare benign inflammatory pseudotumor of unknown origin *(17)*. Clinically, patients present with a painful mass in an extremity. On muscle biopsy, these lesions have similar histologic characteristics as polymyositis and occur most commonly in the thigh or lower extremity *(18)*. MRI can demonstrate an area of focal myositis as focal enlargement of a muscle, with a hypointense or isointense lesion on T1-weighted images with surrounding edema *(18,19)*. There may be relative sparing of some muscle fibers, resulting in a slightly heterogeneous appearance on MRI, corresponding histologically to a "checkerboard"-like pattern *(20)*. As with the other nonsuppurative myopathies, contrast administration is of limited utility. Contrast enhancement is variable *(19)*, although it can be intense *(2)*.

## Pyomyositis and Muscle Infarction

Pyomyositis is uncommon in temperate climates. When it does occur outside the tropics, there is usually a preexisting condition in adults. In children, however, there infrequently is a coexistent disease, and it can occur sporadically. In the series by Karmazyn et al. *(21)*, pyomyositis in children occurred either from direct extension from adjacent infection or from hematogenous spread.

In adults, coexistent diseases often include diabetes mellitus, HIV infections, connective tissue disorders, malignancies, chronic steroid use, or other immunocompromised states *(22)*. The most common organism implicated in skeletal muscle infection is staphylococcus, followed by mycobacteria, nocardia, streptococci, and *Cryptococcus (23)*.

Three clinical stages of pyomyositis are typically identified: invasive, in which the microorganism enters the muscle; purulent, in which a small collection of pus

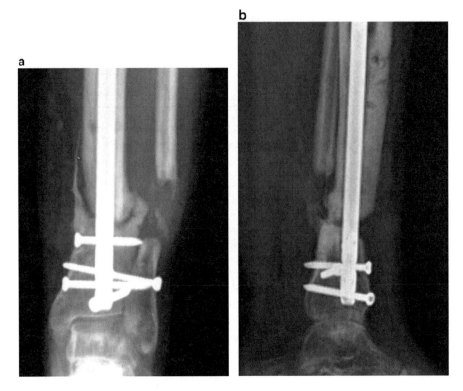

**Fig. 8.14** Anteroposterior (**a**) and lateral (**b**) radiographs of the distal leg in a patient with a chronic fracture deformity and osteomyelitis. The radiographs demonstrate nonspecific soft tissue swelling and the chronic ununited fracture deformity

is present; and late stage, in which there is a large abscess and patients are near septic shock *(22)*. The lower extremity is usually affected more than the upper limb, and the pelvic girdle is often involved *(23,24)*.

Magnetic resonance imaging is most useful in evaluating the location, extent, and distribution of disease involvement *(23)*, particularly patients in stages 1 and 2. In stage 1 (invasive), the clinical picture may be nonspecific. On MRI, focal or infiltrative areas of enhancement are identified on postcontrast T1-weighted images (Fig. 8.14–8.16) *(22)*. As normal muscle is replaced by inflammatory cells, the involved muscle becomes enlarged and demonstrates slightly increased signal intensity on T2- or STIR-weighted images *(24)*.

Given its tomographic abilities, MRI can identify small collections of pus (stage 2, purulent stage) that traditionally may have gone undetected (Figs. 8.17 and 8.18). The abscess is usually hypointense on T1-weighted images but can be isointense or hyperintense depending on the proteinaceous content of the fluid. There is characteristic rim enhancement of the abscess following the administration of intravenous gadolinium, with no enhancement of the central necrotic and purulent material *(24)*.

**Fig. 8.15**  Axial inversion recovery image demonstrates nonspecific multifocal signal abnormality in the muscles about the distal tibia in addition to abnormal signal within the tibia

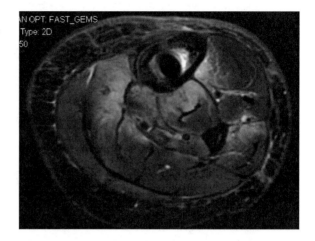

**Fig. 8.16**  Axial T1 fat-suppressed image postgadolinium administration demonstrates enhancement of the muscles that were of abnormal signal intensity on the STIR image at the same level as Fig. 8.15, consistent with infection (pyomyositis), as well as the tibia (osteomyelitis). No drainable abscess or focal fluid collection is present. Note that MRI can provide diagnostic images even in the setting of indwelling orthopedic devices and hardware

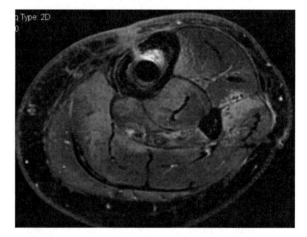

In patients with diabetes, in addition to being at risk for pyomyositis, they may sustain muscle infarctions. MRI is useful in evaluating these patients as it can potentially differentiate among infarction, abscess, and focal or nodular myositis. Diabetic muscle infarcts are usually isointense to muscle on T1-weighted images.

Of note, the internal architecture of muscle is usually preserved in the early setting, thus aiding in distinguishing this lesion from a neoplasm or focal myositis. The muscle is usually hyperintense on T2 or STIR images, and a focal abscess will not be present unless the muscle is superinfected. Intravenous contrast enhancement should demonstrate a heterogeneous mass with peripheral rim enhancement. Visualization of central linear nonenhancing fibers is indicative of necrosis, which may be seen sur-

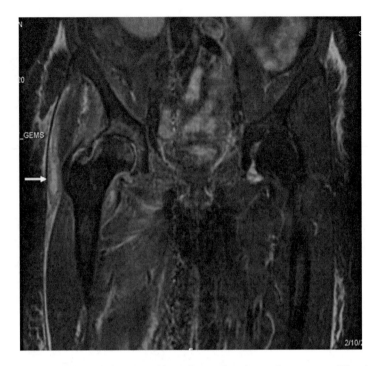

**Fig. 8.17** Axial large field of view coronal inversion recovery image demonstrates diffuse increased signal intensity in all the muscles about the hip as well as a focal fluid collection laterally (*arrow*)

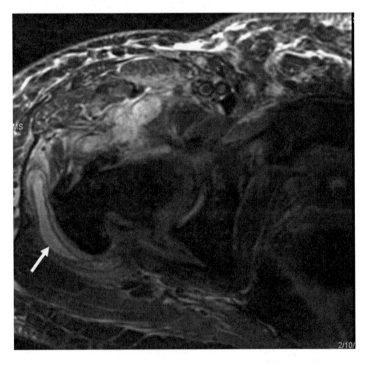

**Fig. 8.18** Axial inversion recovery image in the same patient as Fig. 8.17 further demonstrates the multifocal abnormal muscle signal as well as the fluid collection (*arrow*) in this patient with pyomyositis

rounded by normal muscle fibers, or those demonstrating streaky enhancement, indicative of inflammation *(16)*.

## Trauma and Myositis Ossificans

In the setting of trauma, MRI can identify not only the extent, location, and degree of injury to the involved muscle but also complications such as hematoma or seroma formation as well as myositis ossificans *(25)*.

With a mild muscle injury such as a contusion, the muscle is usually slightly increased in size, although the muscle fibers remain in continuity with increased signal intensity on T2- or STIR-weighted images (Fig. 8.19) *(26)*. Hematomas are of variable signal intensity on MRI and can be complex, depending on the age and stage of evolution of the hematoma.

While not a true inflammatory process ("myositis" being somewhat of a misnomer), in myositis ossificans there is damage to muscle with proliferation of connective tissue that ultimately differentiates into mature bone *(27)*. MR images demonstrate increased signal intensity within the muscle shortly after the injury, progressing to a more focal

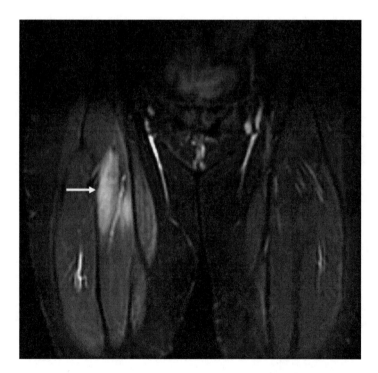

**Fig. 8.19** Coronal inversion recovery image through the anterior aspect of both thighs demonstrating asymmetric focal increased signal intensity in the right rectus femoris muscle, consistent with mild strain (*arrow*)

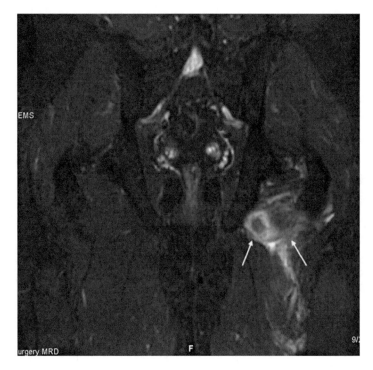

**Fig. 8.20** Coronal inversion recovery image through the posterior aspect of the hip in a patient with hip pain following trauma demonstrates diffuse increased abnormal signal intensity in the quadratus femoris, superior gemellus, and obturator internus muscles (*arrows*)

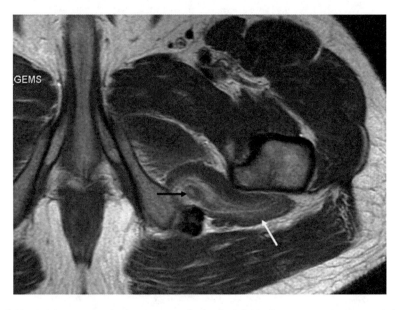

**Fig. 8.21** Axial proton density image centered over the left hip demonstrates the abnormal signal in the quadratus femoris muscle (*white arrow*). There is a more focal area of nodular hyperintensity in the more medial aspect of the muscle (*black arrow*) as seen in the setting of developing myositis ossificans

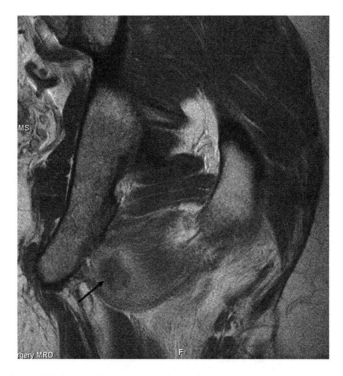

**Fig. 8.22** Coronal high-resolution proton density-weighted sequence centered over the left hip illustrates the focal nodular area of abnormal signal intensity consistent with a developing focus of myositis ossificans (*black arrow*)

mass several days to weeks after the injury (Figs. 8.20–8.22) *(2)*. It is during this time that the lesions may present a confusing clinical picture as they can look aggressive on MRI, and the patient may not recall a specific traumatic event, making the diagnosis of an underlying neoplasm often difficult to exclude. Following patients with plain film radiographs will demonstrate development and maturation of ossification following the weeks after injury in the setting of myositis ossificans. If repeat MRI examination is obtained, bone (seen as peripherally low-signal-intensity foci containing fat and trabeculae) will be observed in the setting of evolving myositis ossificans.

## Miscellaneous (Compartment Syndrome, Muscle Denervation)

A devastating complication of extremity injury is compartment syndrome. Compartment syndrome usually involves the muscles of the calf, often following blunt trauma or fracture *(28)*. Bleeding and edema within the muscle result in increased pressure in the affected muscle compartment, which leads to vascular insufficiency and infarction to the muscles and nerves *(26)*. While the gold standard for diagnosing compartment syndrome remains direct pressure measurements, MRI can be useful in suggesting the diagnosis in the proper clinical setting, with areas

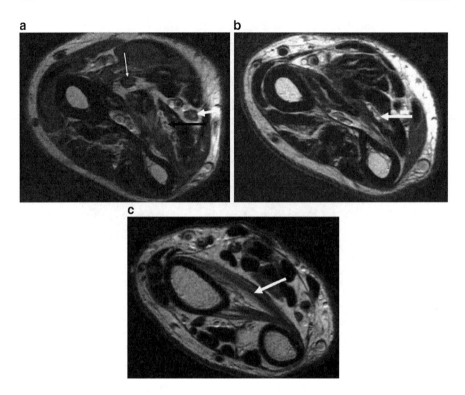

**Fig. 8.23** Axial proton density sequences through the proximal (**a**), mid- (**b**), and distal (**c**) forearm in a patient with chronic compartment syndrome. In (**a**), note the diffuse atrophy and loss of muscle bulk in the flexor digitorum profundus (FDP) muscle (*black arrow*) as well as the hypertrophy of the median (*long, thin white arrow*) and ulnar (*short, thick white arrow*) nerves. At the level of the mid-forearm (**b**), atrophy of both the FDP and the pronator quadratus is observed (*white arrow*), with the atrophy of the pronator quadratus extending to the level of the wrist (*arrow*, **c**)

of increased signal intensity within the affected muscle compartment. MRI also can be used to evaluate the morphology of the muscles and nerves in chronic compartment syndrome and serves as a prognostic indicator (Fig. 8.23).

Magnetic resonance imaging can identify muscle denervation several days to weeks after the initial insult, whether the denervation is due to a primary underlying neuropathy or trauma. In subacute denervation (2–4 weeks after the initial insult), MRI demonstrates nonspecific edema throughout the involved muscle, with some MRI changes reported as early as 2–4 days after the initial event *(2,29,30)*. The MRI appearance likely relates to shifting of water from intracellular to extracellular spaces *(30)*. The MRI appearance of muscle can return to normal if the innervation is restored; however, if it is not restored, chronic fatty infiltration and atrophy of the muscle will occur over the subsequent few months *(2,29)*.

# Conclusions

Magnetic resonance imaging has broad applications in evaluating the patient with a suspected myopathy. The superior soft tissue contrast and spatial resolution of MRI make it a useful tool in evaluating the morphology of muscles. The ability to image both extremities at the same time allows for determination of the pattern of involvement, often helpful in establishing a diagnosis (asymmetric, anterior compartment involvement in sporadic IBM versus symmetric, posterior compartment involvement in polymyositis, for example). MRI is exquisitely sensitive in detecting areas of muscle edema and abnormality, thus identifying areas of potential subclinical disease, as well as providing guidance for muscle biopsy. The longitudinal course and disease progression or regression of myopathies can also be evaluated, such as abscess collections in pyomyositis, muscle atrophy in end-stage myositis, or chronic compartment syndrome, or changes from denervation, thus providing potential prognostic information.

# References

1. Kuo GP, Carrino JA. Skeletal muscle imaging and inflammatory myopathies. Curr Opin Rheumatol 2007;19:530–5.
2. May DA, Disler DG, Jones EA, et al. Abnormal signal intensity in skeletal muscle at MR imaging: patterns, pearls and pitfalls. Radiographics 2000;20:S295–315.
3. Cantwell C, Ryan M, O'Connell M, et al. A comparison of inflammatory myopathies at whole-body turbo STIR MRI. Clin Radiol 2005;60:261–7.
4. Wong EH, Hui ACF, Griffith JF, et al. MRI in biopsy-negative dermatomyositis. Neurology 2005;64:750.
5. Adams EM, Chow CK, Premkumar A, et al. The idiopathic inflammatory myopathies: spectrum of MR imaging findings. Radiographics 1995;15:563–74.
6. Schweitzer ME, Fort J. Cost-effectiveness of MR imaging in evaluating polymyositis. AJR Am J Roentgenol 1995;165:1469–71.
7. Lampa J, Nennesmo I, Einarsdottir H, et al. MRI guided muscle biopsy confirmed polymyositis diagnosis in a patient with interstitial lung disease. Ann Rheum Dis 2001;60:423–6.
8. Connor A, Stebbings S, Hung NA, et al. STIR MRI to direct muscle biopsy in suspected idiopathic inflammatory myopathy. J Clin Rheumatol 2007;13:341–5.
9. Scott DL, Kingsley GH. Use of imaging to assess patients with muscle disease. Curr Opin Rheumatol 2004;6:678–83.
10. Qi J, Olsen NJ, Price RR, et al. Diffusion-weighted imaging of inflammatory myopathies: polymyositis and dermatomyositis. J Magn Reson Imaging 2008;27:212–7.
11. Dion E, Cherin P, Payan C, et al. Magnetic resonance imaging criteria for distinguishing between inclusion body myositis and polymyositis. J Rheumatol 2002;29:1897–906.
12. Restrepo CS, Lemos DF, Gordillo H, et al. Imaging findings in musculoskeletal complications of AIDS. Radiographics 2004;24:1029–49.
13. Park JH, Vansant JP, Kumar NG, et al. Dermatomyositis: correlative MR imaging and P-31 MR spectroscopy for quantitative characterization of inflammatory disease. Radiology 1990;177:473–9.
14. Studynkova JT, Charvat F, Jarosova K, et al. The role of MRI in the assessment of polymyositis and dermatomyositis. Rheumatology 2007;46:1174–9.

15. Ranque-Francois B, Maisonobe T, Dion E, et al. Familial inflammatory inclusion body myositis. Ann Rheum Dis 2005;64:634–7.
16. Donmez FY, Feldman F. Muscle compromise in diabetes. Acta Radiol 2008;6:673–9.
17. Garcia J. MRI in inflammatory myopathies. Skeletal Radiol 2000;29:425–538.
18. Llauger J, Bague S, Palmer J, et al. Focal myositis of the thigh: unusual MR pattern. Skeletal Radiol 2002;31:307–10.
19. Mulier S, Stas M, Delabie J, et al. Proliferative myositis in a child. Skeletal Radiol 1999;28:703–9.
20. Pagpnidis K, Raissaki M, Gourtsoyiannis N. Proliferative myositis: value of imaging. J Comput Assist Tomogr 2005;29(1):108–11.
21. Karmazyn B, Kleiman MB, Buckwalter K, et al. Acute pyomyositis of the pelvis: the spectrum of clinical presentations and MR findings. Pediatr Radiol 2006;36:338–43.
22. Yu CW, Hsiao JK, Hsu CY, et al. Bacterial pyomyositis: MRI and clinical correlation. Magn Reson Imaging 2004;22:1233–41.
23. Lalam RK, Cassar-Pullicino VN, Tins BJ. Magnetic resonance imaging of appendicular musculoskeletal infection. Top Magn Reson Imaging 2007;18:177–91.
24. Theodorou SJ, Theodorou DJ, Resnick D. MR imaging findings of pyogenic bacterial myositis (pyomyositis) in patients with local muscle trauma: illustrative cases. Emerg Radiol 2007;14:89–96.
25. Elsayes KM, Lammle M, Shariff A, et al. Value of magnetic resonance imaging in muscle trauma. Curr Probl Diagn Radiol 2006;35(5):206–12.
26. Armfeld DR, Kim DHM, Towers JD, et al. Sports-related muscle injury in the lower extremity. Clin Sports Med 2006;25:803–12.
27. Hendifar AE, Johnson D, Arkfeld DG. Myositis ossificans: a case report. Arthritis Rheum 2005;53(5):793–5.
28. Verrall GM, Slavotinek JP, Barnes PG, et al. Diagnostic and prognostic value of clinical findings in 83 athletes with posterior thigh injury: comparison of clinical findings with magnetic resonance imaging documentation of hamstring muscle strain. Am J Sports Med 2003;31:969–73.
29. Fleckenstein JL, Watumull D, Conner KE, et al. Denervated human skeletal muscle: MR imaging evaluation. Radiology 1993;187:213–8.
30. West GA, Haynor DR, Goodkin R, et al. Magnetic resonance imaging signal changes in denervated muscles after peripheral nerve injury. Neurosurgery 1994;35:1077–85.

# Chapter 9
# Ultrasound in the Evaluation of the Inflammatory Myopathies

**Ronald S. Adler and Giovanna Garofalo**

**Abstract** Imaging plays an important role in the assessment of disease activity and measuring the effectiveness in patients with inflammatory myopathies. Ultrasound is a noninvasive, relatively inexpensive, and simple examination to perform serially and has found increasing application in the diagnosis of muscle diseases, including polymyositis, dermatomyositis, and pyomyositis. The roles of newer applications of ultrasound, such as power Doppler sonography, contrast-enhanced ultrasound, and sonoelastography, have yet to be defined but show some promising results in further characterizing normal and pathological states. Technical developments and improvements in ultrasound image processing, including extended field of view, compound imaging, and harmonic imaging, enhance the ability to display changes in muscle morphology.

**Keywords** Muscle ultrasound • Power Doppler • Sonoelastography

## Introduction

The lack of precise measures of disease activity may complicate the care of patients with inflammatory myopathies (IMs) *(1)*. Assessment of disease activity is an important factor in measuring the effectiveness of therapy and the course of illness. The techniques currently available to physicians in practice rely on measurement of function, strength, laboratory indices, muscle biopsy, and imaging techniques.

R.S. Adler (✉) and G. Garofalo
Division of Ultrasound and Body Imaging, Hospital for Special Surgery,
Weill Medical College of Cornell University, New York, NY, USA

L.J. Kagen (ed.), *The Inflammatory Myopathies*,
DOI 10.1007/978-1-60327-827-0_9,
© Humana Press, a part of Springer Science + Business Media, LLC 2009

Several scales for assessing muscle function have been developed that rely on patient reporting of ability to perform activities of daily living but may prove unreliable in individuals who are either extremely weak or who, conversely, are doing well. Quantification of muscle strength with manual muscle strength testing, timed function tests, and biomechanical techniques depends on the ability of the patient to cooperate, may not be applicable to profoundly weak patients, and may be affected by interobserver variability *(2)*. Serial biopsy or electromyography, while definitive, are limited because of cost and invasiveness.

Many studies have documented the diagnostic sensitivity and specificity of magnetic resonance imaging (MRI) in IMs *(3–7)*. However, MRI is expensive, difficult for some patients to tolerate, and contraindicated in those with pacemakers, aneurysm clips, and other ferromagnetic biomedical implants. Ultrasonography (US) represents an alternative approach to the examination of the muscular system. It is a noninvasive, relatively inexpensive, and simple examination to perform serially. Traditional gray-scale US has found increasing application in the diagnosis of muscle diseases, including polymyositis and dermatomyositis, pyomyositis, Lyme myositis, sarcoid myositis, and myositis secondary to polyarteritis nodosa *(8–10)*.

The roles of newer applications of ultrasound, such as power Doppler sonography (PDS), contrast-enhanced ultrasound, and sonoelastography have yet to be defined but show some promising results in further characterizing normal and pathological states *(11–13)*. Technical developments and improvements in ultrasound image processing, including extended field of view (EFOV), compound imaging, and harmonic imaging, enhance ability to display changes in muscle morphology *(14–16)*.

Ultrasound has previously been shown to be useful in assessing disease duration and activity in a cohort of patients with chronic myopathies. Meng et al. *(17)* demonstrated that muscle echogenicity strongly correlates with disease duration and muscle atrophy, while power Doppler appears to better reflect disease activity. A study by Reimers et al. *(8)* reported findings correlating gray-scale US with concurrent histology in 70 patients with myositis. Chronic myositis presented with higher echo intensities and more atrophy than acute disease. The sensitivity of muscle US in detecting histologically proven disease was 82.9% with a specificity of 97.1%.

In this chapter, we review the sonographic appearances of normal and pathologic muscle conditions, with an emphasis on IMs. This includes a discussion of technical factors that should be remembered when performing musculoskeletal US. Included is a brief discussion of newer techniques that are becoming available and may enhance the diagnostic capabilities of US as well as the use of ultrasound in providing guidance for biopsy.

## Technical Factors and New Developments

Musculoskeletal ultrasound is generally best performed using a broadband linear phased-array transducer. For most applications, such as in the thighs or arms, an intermediate-frequency range from approximately 5 to 10 MHz will suffice.

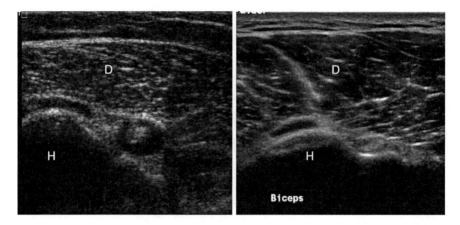

**Fig. 9.1** Transverse gray-scale ultrasound images over the anterior deltoid muscle in two patients. Both images display the anterior deltoid (D), humerus (H), and portions of the biceps tendon. The image on the *left* is a conventional gray scale without tissue compounding. In addition to the normal anatomical structures, low-level echoes are present throughout the image, appearing as relatively uniform white dots. The image on the *right* has had tissue compounding applied. Apart from the perimysial connective tissue (curvilinear echogenic lines) in the muscle, the background has a much more homogeneous appearance. The specular surfaces that give rise to the cortical surface of the humerus, overlying fascia, and fibroadipose septa appear less fragmented. The humerus (H) is labeled

The choice of frequency is generally governed by the depth of the tissue of interest, although the highest possible frequency for a particular application will afford the best axial resolution. Likewise, Doppler sensitivity may be affected by the choice of transducer center frequency. While a higher center frequency results in a larger Doppler shift, it may be necessary to scan at a lower center frequency to detect a Doppler signal.

*Speckle* refers to the inherent structured noise apparent in gray-scale ultrasound imaging *(18)*. A number of vendors have introduced schemes to reduce noise in ultrasound images, most notably using image compounding *(15)*. Spatial compounding employs multiple look directions to form a composite image, averaging over the contributions from each direction and retaining the dominant stationary echoes that arise from tissue interfaces. The resultant image has better contrast definition, enabling improved depiction of internal muscle morphology as well as muscle boundaries (Fig. 9.1).

The same inherent noise can be employed to construct an EFOV image, using in-plane speckle tracking, thereby producing an image with as much as 60 cm of information, as opposed to a small field-of-view image (Fig. 9.2) *(14)*. This technology has been less successful in producing volumetric images, largely due to poor out-of-plane resolution. It is sometimes of value, however, to display data as

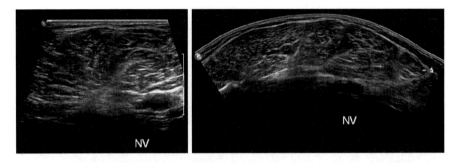

**Fig. 9.2** Small field-of-view transverse ultrasound image (*left*) and extended field-of-view (EFOV) image (*right*) obtained over the posterior thigh in a female patient with suspected hamstring injury. Only a portion of the hamstring complex is visualized in the image on the *left*. In the EFOV image of the posterior thigh (*right*), the full extent of the hamstring complex is displayed on a single image. Normal relationships among muscle groups can be more readily assessed in this manner. Because of the high in-plane resolution, these images are spatially registered and so can be used both to determine the nature and to quantify the extent of muscle abnormality. The neurovascular (NV) structures are evident at the *bottom* of the image

a rendered volume or in another plane (i.e., reconstructed image plane) to assess extent of disease. The production of a true volumetric image is expected to become possible in the near future as two-dimensional arrays become available.

Sonoelastography takes advantage of differences in relative hardness of soft tissues when an external force is applied to a tissue boundary *(13,19)*. Traditionally, it has been applied to characterizing hard nodules in a more deformable medium. The image produced reflects the translation of the tissue in response to a small surface deformation (Fig. 9.3). Because changes in internal muscle composition may occur in IMs, as well as in other pathologic conditions, muscle sonoelastography may provide a sensitive measure of atrophy, fatty infiltration, or other infiltrative processes. Investigation of the applications of this type of imaging is at an early phase, and the role of elasticity imaging as an adjunct to gray-scale imaging has yet to be defined.

Conventional color Doppler imaging, which provides an estimate of mean Doppler shift encoded in color, is useful for detecting the velocity distribution in high-flow vessels, but is limited for evaluating regional tissue perfusion. PDS is angle independent and is not subject to sampling artifact (aliasing) *(11, 20, 21)*. In power mode, low-amplitude noise in the color flow image can be eliminated, thereby extending the dynamic range over that of conventional color Doppler imaging. The angle independence, as well as the increased sensitivity, results in an angiographic display of color flow information (Fig. 9.4). PDS is not capable of detecting capillary flow, and it cannot differentiate between arterial and venous flow. PDS pixel intensity does relate, however, to the number of moving scatterers within the insonated volume and therefore provides a noninvasive quantifiable estimate of vascular volume *(21)*.

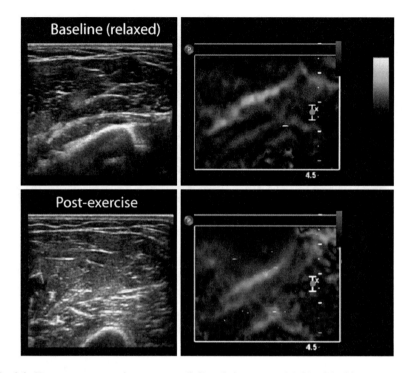

**Fig. 9.3** Transverse gray-scale sonograms (*left*) and elastograms (*right*) of the biceps at rest and following two sets of curls with 15-pound weight. Relative to the baseline gray-scale image (*top left*), the corresponding postexercise gray-scale image (*bottom left*) demonstrates the biceps to be enlarged and of increased echogenicity (muscle edema pattern). The elastograms (*right*) display strain images resulting from a small uniform surface deformation. Increasing levels of tissue softness (tissue that undergoes compression rather than translation) is represented by lighter hues of *red* (see *inset, right upper corner*). In this case, increased vascular engorgement results in a softer, more compressible (albeit enlarged), muscle mass, which is reflected by a broader distribution of the *lighter color hues*. (Image provided by iU22 [Philips Ultrasound, Bothell, WA] with prototype elastography software [Philips Research, Briarcliff, NY])

Improved sensitivity in estimating muscle blood flow requires the use of ultrasound contrast agents, of which a variety exists. Ultrasound contrast agents provide two to three orders of magnitude improvement in the detection of blood flow and have been shown to serve as capillary imaging agents. These agents consist of encapsulated microbubbles, 2–3 μm in size, which are metabolized and have variable biologic half-lives, depending on their composition. Whether the agent is imaged using power Doppler mode or gray scale, contrast agents provide a measure of both perfusion and vascular volume *(22)*.

*Phase aberration* refers to loss of internal coherence in the ultrasound beam and occurs whenever the beam insonates tissue of internally varying speed of sound *(23)*.

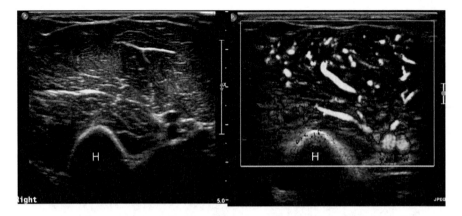

**Fig. 9.4** Postexercise vascular recruitment: Gray-scale (*left*) and power Doppler (*right*) images of the biceps muscle in an asymptomatic volunteer following two sets of ten repetitions with a 10-pound weight. Muscle enlargement and increased echogenicity are a consequence of increased blood volume. Following exercise, numerous vessels (*color*) are evident in multiple different orientations. The appearance has an angiographic quality without dropout of flow due to vessel orientation and no artifact due to undersampling of the Doppler shift (aliasing). Pixel intensity (*color hue*) in this representation directly represents the number of moving blood cells that produce a detectable Doppler shift. The humerus (H) is labeled

A consequence of phase aberration is the loss of cortical margins of bone, deep to an area of heterogeneous soft tissue. The most common example of phase aberration occurs when assessing organs, such as the liver or pancreas, through abdominal pannus. This phenomenon likely has implications in patients with underlying muscle infiltration due to the nature of the infiltrating material (i.e., fat, fibrosis), which tends to alter muscle speed of sound. Currently, no general phase aberration correction exists, although several vendors have instituted some early forms of correction.

## Normal Sonographic Appearances

Muscle fascicles normally appear hypoechoic on ultrasound, separated by echogenic fibroadipose or perimysial connective tissue (Fig. 9.5) (*24*). When seen in cross section, the perimysium appears as scattered, irregular, and sometimes punctuate echogenic foci in a hypoechoic background. In long axis, these appear more organized, typically assuming a multipenate appearance. The obliquely oriented muscle fascicles can be observed converging onto a central tendon or fascial plane. This ordered arrangement of muscle fascicles can produce an anisotropic effect similar to that noted in tendons, albeit less pronounced.

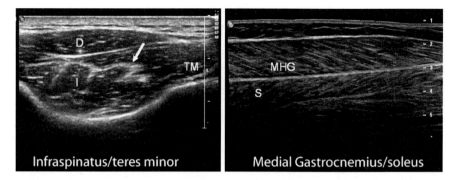

**Fig. 9.5** Normal muscle. *Left*: transverse image depicting portions of the infraspinatus (I), teres minor (TM), and deltoid muscles (D). A central echogenic area (*arrow*) within the infraspinatus corresponds to the myotendinous junction and can be distinguished from the remaining scattered short echogenic segments of perimysial connective tissue. A linear echogenic line represents the fascial plane separating the infraspinatus from the posterior deltoid. The remaining normal muscle is hypoechoic. *Right*: in contradistinction to the sonographic appearance of muscle seen in cross section, muscle fascicles assume a more ordered linear arrangement when seen longitudinally. Typically, a multipenate appearance is evident when viewed at the level of either a myofascial attachment as shown here, at the junction of the medial head of the gastrocnemius (MHG) and soleus muscles (S), or a myotendinous attachment

Vascularity within muscle appears in close relation to the intervening connective tissue. Alterations in muscle echogenicity or vascularity may be seen in normal muscle, simply reflecting the state of activity (see Fig. 9.4). Patchy areas of increased echogenicity likely relate to increases in the numbers of scattering interfaces in the insonated volume, thereby producing increased acoustic backscatter. Newman et al. *(11)* performed PDS in the biceps muscles of healthy volunteers to evaluate exercise-induced changes in muscle blood volume. Using a subjective scoring system as well as a semiquantitative vascularity measure, they demonstrated significant increases in intramuscular vascularity after exercise, reflecting increases in muscle perfusion.

## Muscle Edema Pattern

Apart from the intrinsic perimysial connective tissue, muscle normally appears hypoechoic, largely due to the uniformity presented by the muscle fascicles. Increased muscle echogenicity and size associated with a postexercise state provide the simplest example of a transient muscle edema pattern (see Figs. 9.3 and 9.4). Infiltrative disorders will in general result in increased muscle echogenicity,

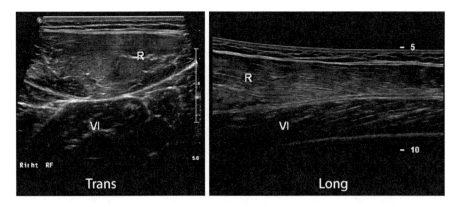

**Fig. 9.6** Transverse (*left*) and longitudinal (EFOV) gray-scale image of the quadriceps compartment in a professional athlete following a strain injury. The rectus femoris (R) is slightly enlarged and displays patchy areas of increased echogenicity (compare to vastus intermedius [VI] below). Internal muscle morphology is preserved. Notice that the underlying fascicular and multipenate morphology is maintained

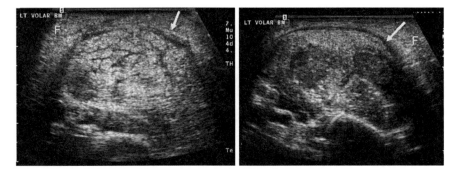

**Fig. 9.7** A 24-year-old female with history of septic arthritis and secondary involvement of the biceps due to *Staphylococcus aureus*. Transverse images of the biceps at two different levels demonstrate a muscle edema pattern that has a segmental distribution, resulting in a mosaic pattern of involvement in an enlarged biceps muscle. Helpful features here are thickening of the muscle fascia (*arrow*) as well as edema in the overlying subcutaneous fat (F). In our experience, this pattern is more indicative of an infectious process

reflecting increased acoustic backscatter. The etiology is nonspecific, and a variety of causative factors can produce increases in muscle echogenicity and size (Figs. 9.6–9.8). These include posttraumatic, inflammatory, or infectious etiologies (*9, 24*). Likewise, alterations in the composition of muscle, due to infiltration by

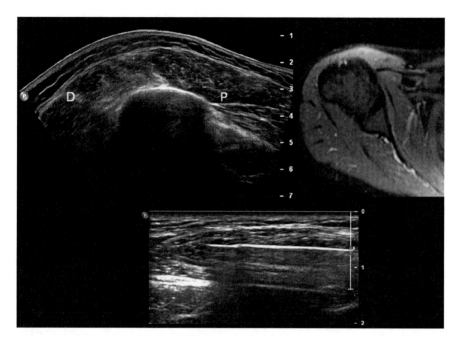

**Fig. 9.8** Patient with right upper extremity weakness and elevated muscle enzymes. EFOV transverse image of the right shoulder (*left*) demonstrates a muscle edema pattern in the anterior head of the deltoid muscle (D), affecting primarily the deep surface of the muscle. The adjacent pectoralis (P) muscle maintains normal echogenicity and morphology. Axial fat-suppressed T2-weighted fast spin echo (FSE) image of the right shoulder (*right*) shows increased signal intensity within the anterior head of the deltoid muscle. A 12-gauge biopsy gun (*bottom*) is deployed within the anterior deltoid while observing in real time to ensure specimen location. The biopsy confirmed this as a newly diagnosed inflammatory myopathy consistent with dermatomyositis

fat or fibrosis, can produce increases in muscle echogenicity (Figs. 9.9 and 9.10). In the latter case, the ultrasound beam may become incoherent (undergo phase aberration), distorting the appearance of the deeper tissues or cortical surface of underlying bone. The patterns of muscle involvement may be focal, diffuse, patchy, or uniform, with considerable overlap among different entities.

## Muscle Atrophy

In contradistinction to the so-called edema pattern, increased muscle echogenicity can also be seen in cases of atrophy (Fig. 9.11) *(9)*. Again, increased acoustic backscatter can be associated with a concomitant increase in the density of scattering interfaces in the insonated volume. In this case, however, the increased density of

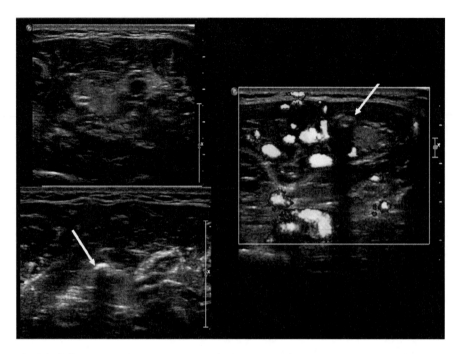

**Fig. 9.9** Infiltrative masses may present a similar pattern of abnormality to the muscle edema pattern. This patient had swelling involving the flexor compartment of the forearm. The gray-scale appearance (*left two images*) shows the flexor compartment muscles to be enlarged with areas of increased echogenicity. Corresponding power Doppler on the *right* shows numerous prominent blood vessels of varying size. In this case, a large hemangioma consisting of abnormal blood vessels and fat infiltrates the muscle, giving the appearance of muscle edema. The *arrows* depict focal calcifications, most likely phleboliths, within the mass. On ultrasound, calcifications appear echogenic with a relatively well-defined posterior acoustic shadows (hypoechoic band) deep to the calcific focus (*arrow*)

scatterers reflects diminished muscle fascicular size. Muscle atrophy is therefore characterized by increases in echogenicity and diminished volume. Most assessments of atrophy are subjective, with the only controls being unaffected muscles in the same individual or the extent to which one differentiates the perimysial septa from the normally hypoechoic fascicles. Using techniques similar to those employed to assess enhancement following administration of contrast, it is possible to make these determinations quantitatively (Fig. 9.12) *(25)*. Likewise, reports exist for normal muscle dimensions in limited case series; however, the assessment of muscle volume is variable, depending on a variety of factors, including age, gender, and level of training *(26, 27)*. While atrophy is commonly seen as a sequela of long-standing inflammatory myositis, it can also occur in neuromuscular

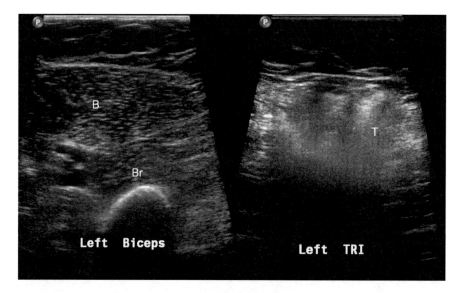

**Fig. 9.10** Patient with history of dermatomyositis and upper extremity weakness. Transverse ultrasound images of the left biceps/brachialis (*left image*) and left triceps (*right image*) in a patient shows varying levels of involvement with mild increased echogenicity in the biceps (B), where the muscle appears somewhat heterogeneous but maintains internal morphology. The brachialis (BR) appears to demonstrate more confluent areas of increased echogenicity, such that muscle fascicles are no longer distinguishable. The triceps (TRI) is diffusely echogenic and attenuating, typically seen in the setting of extensive fibrofatty infiltration. No discernible tissue organization is present, in part due to a loss of coherence in the ultrasound beam itself, also known as phase aberration

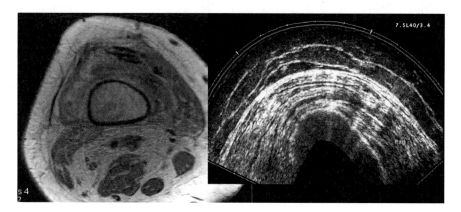

**Fig. 9.11** Axial FSE proton density MRI (*left*) and corresponding EFOV transverse image (*right*) of the thigh in a patient with disuse muscle atrophy. On MRI, the quadriceps muscles are of decreased volume and infiltrated with fat. Fatty infiltration displays signal characteristics similar to subcutaneous fat. On the corresponding ultrasound image (*right*), the subcutaneous fat appears hypoechoic relative to the muscle. The former is of a more uniform consistency with fewer scattering interfaces relative to the muscle. The increased density of scattering interfaces within muscle therefore manifests as increased, rather than decreased, echogenicity

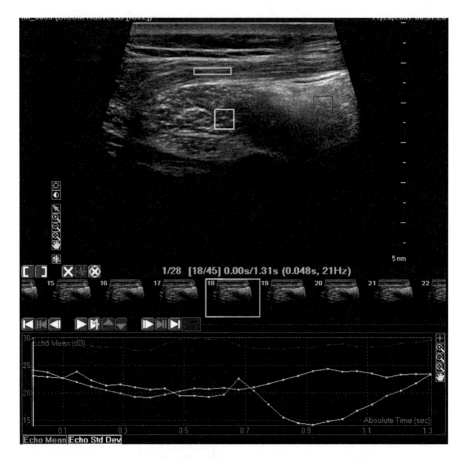

**Fig. 9.12** Patient with disuse muscle atrophy due to a chronic infraspinatus tendon tear and disuse. Current schemes for evaluation of muscle echogenicity rely on subjective assessment with respect to an internal control. Quantitative measures of mean gray value are available with mean intensities measured in decibels (dB). The curves depict mean gray-value intensity obtained during a volumetric sweep through the infraspinatus, teres minor, and deltoid muscles. Regions of interest (ROIs) are positioned in three different locations, with each point along the abscissa represented a single 2-D plane within the muscle. The average intensity within each *box* (dB/mm²) is depicted for different points within the muscle during a continuous sweep. The *red box* is placed with the echogenic infraspinatus muscle belly, while the remaining two ROIs are placed in the teres minor (*yellow*) and posterior deltoid (*green*). During a continuous sweep, a consistent difference of approximately 10 dB/mm² is evident between preserved and atrophic muscle

disease and denervation or due to disuse (Fig. 9.13) *(28,29)*. In our experience, muscle atrophy is more often uniform or segmental and tends not to present a patchy distribution of increased echogenicity.

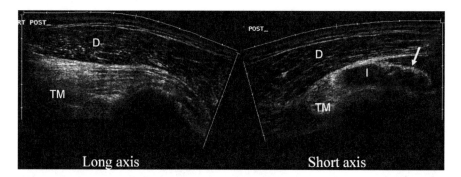

**Fig. 9.13** Denervation atrophy: long-axis (*left*) and short-axis (*right*) EFOV images of the posterior shoulder in a patient with a history of a stretch injury of the arm resulting in an axillary nerve injury within the quadrilateral space. The image on the *left* depicts the teres minor (TM) in long axis, which is diffusely echogenic. The overlying deltoid muscle (D) is normal in echogenicity and displays normal morphology. The image on the *right* shows portions of the teres minor and infraspinatus (I) in short axis, with the overlying deltoid in long axis. The central echogenic myotendinous junction (*arrow*) of the infraspinatus is apparent. Again, the teres minor displays increased echogenicity relative to the adjacent muscles due to selective atrophy resulting from a denervation injury to a branch of the axillary nerve

## Calcification

Calcification is generally not associated with adult forms of IMs, but it can be seen in both perifascial and intramuscular distributions in children with juvenile dermatomyositis *(9)*. It can also occur following trauma with hemorrhage, inflammation, or infection. Ultrasound is the most sensitive method to detect soft tissue calcification, more so than conventional radiographs or computed tomography. Calcification appears as echogenic foci with posterior acoustic shadowing (see Fig. 9.9). Posttraumatic calcification is usually peripheral (in the case of an intramuscular hematoma) or is linear, paralleling the adjacent bone *(30)*. Areas of cystic necrosis within muscle can undergo peripheral calcification *(31)*. Central calcification within abnormal intramuscular soft tissue should raise the possibility of neoplasm.

## Specific Disease Patterns

The IMs will typically present a mixed picture consisting of chronic disease with superimposed acute exacerbations. Consequently, no single pattern is unique to this disorder, but rather an admixture of muscle edema and atrophy patterns exists (see Fig. 9.10). This is complicated by the fact that a variety of other etiologies,

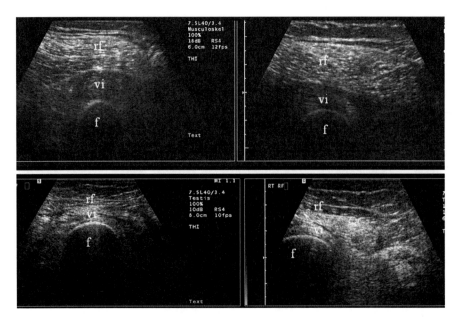

**Fig. 9.14** Transverse scans of the quadriceps compartment in three patients affected by polymyositis showing relationship to disease duration. The rectus femoris and vastus intermedius are depicted. *Upper left image*: transverse scan of the quadriceps compartment in a 36-year-old male patient affected by PM, diagnosed on biopsy, with moderate atrophy and disease duration of 3 years. The patient complained of weakness of neck flexors and of muscles of proximal compartment of upper and lower limbs. *Upper right image*: transverse scan of the quadriceps compartment in a 28-year-old female patient affected by PM, diagnosed on biopsy, with disease duration of 6 years. The patient complained of weakness of neck muscle flexors and weakness of proximal muscle compartment of upper and lower limb weakness. *Bottom images*: transverse scans of both quadriceps compartments in a 58-year-old male patient affected by PM, diagnosed on biopsy, with severe atrophy of both limbs, with disease duration of 10 years. The patient complained of generalized severe muscle weakness and was wheelchair bound. With increasing duration of disease, there are concomitant increases in muscle echogenicity and volume loss. *rf* rectus femoris; *vi* vastus intermedius; *f* femur

such as steroid-induced myopathy, infection, posttraumatic change, and denervation, may present similar sonographic features. What appears to be true, however, is that IMs present with certain characteristic anatomic distributions and patterns of muscle involvement, which can suggest a diagnosis *(9)*. Polymyositis, for instance, has a predilection for symmetric bilateral proximal muscle involvement, particularly of the quadriceps musculature (Fig. 9.14). Dermatomyositis often tends to affect the upper extremities (see Figs. 9.8 and 9.10). Hereditary inclusion body myositis (HIBM), alternatively, is quadriceps sparing and has been suggested to present unique patterns of muscle involvement (Fig. 9.15) *(32)*. The presence of linear

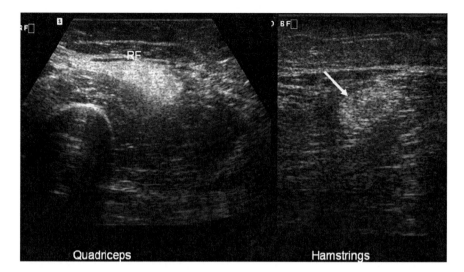

**Fig. 9.15** Transverse scan of the quadriceps compartment (*left*) and hamstrings (*right*) in a 41-year-old female affected by hereditary inclusion body myositis (HIBM), diagnosed on biopsy, with 10-year disease duration. Patient presented a lordotic Trendelenburg gait. Profound atrophy of the rectus femoris is seen as a hyperechoic area (RF) with relative sparing of the remaining quadriceps muscles. Image of the hamstring compartment (*right*) demonstrates central atrophy within the semitendinosus muscle. Isolated rectus atrophy and central atrophy (*white arrow*) with peripheral muscle is evident

calcification suggests the diagnosis of juvenile dermatomyositis and is not generally seen in adults. Further, once the diagnosis of IM is established, ultrasound can play a role in following disease progression. Likewise, ultrasound can serve as a useful adjunct to MRI by providing guidance for biopsy (see Fig. 9.8) *(33)*.

A study by Reimers et al. *(8)* reported findings correlating gray-scale US with concurrent histology in 70 patients with IM. Chronic IM presented with higher echogenicity and more atrophy than acute disease. Acute IM often presented with lower echogenicity and a muscle edema pattern. The sensitivity of muscle US in detecting histologically proven disease was 82.9% with a specificity of 97.1%. The only longitudinal study published to date looked at a small group of 12 patients with juvenile dermatomyositis and polymyositis; these patients had a mean duration of symptoms of 10 years. They found increased echogenicity in at least one muscle group in 60% of the patients and at least one residual finding on physical examination in 58% *(34)*.

Meng et al. *(17)* studied 37 patients with IM (27 with poly- or dermatomyositis and 10 with inclusion body myositis) and compared them to a control group. In this cohort, both upper and lower extremities were examined, including quadriceps, biceps, and triceps brachii. Gray-scale and PDS images were graded using a semi-quantitative scoring system, which was demonstrated to correlate with clinical scores, distinguishing between disease and control subjects. The differences between IM and control subjects on PDS were not as great as those on gray scale. None of the control subjects had abnormal gray-scale findings. Thus, the appearance of increased vascularity on PDS in the setting of abnormal gray-scale findings was indicative of myopathy. Increasing levels of echogenicity on gray-scale US, indicating muscle atrophy, were associated with disease of longer duration. In contrast, PDS findings of increased vascularity appeared to detect disease of shorter duration. Nine patients who were followed serially over approximately 6 months showed no significant differences in gray-scale findings, while alterations in PDS values appeared to reflect changes in clinical status. Combining these techniques may therefore help guide the clinician to assess acute exacerbations of disease. Interestingly, in the study by Meng et al. it was peak vascularity that best reflected the status of the muscle. In general, vascularity alone was not a good predictor of disease. This may in part reflect the poor sensitivity of PDS in detecting abnormal vascularity. The use of ultrasound contrast agents will likely be necessary to achieve the necessary sensitivity to demonstrate abnormal vascularity in patients with IM *(12)*.

## Conclusion

Patients with IM pose important challenges to the clinician. Disease flares can be confused with changes due to steroid myopathy, chronic atrophy, or other comorbid conditions. Imaging plays an important role in detecting and localizing disease and provides guidance for biopsy. While MRI is currently the gold standard for assessing patients with suspected IM, US may offer a reasonable alternative, and certainly it can offer a cost-effective means to follow these patients once the diagnosis is established. New developments in ultrasound technology may allow greater sensitivity in detecting early disease. Furthermore, software now exists to enable quantitative assessment of both muscle echogenicity and vascularity. US is unique in its real-time capabilities, providing a method to monitor and optimally direct muscle biopsy. It is reasonable to anticipate that ultrasound will continue to play an increasingly important role in assessing patients with IM.

## References

1. Mader R, Keystone E. Inflammatory myopathy—do we have adequate measures of the treatment response? J Rheumatol 1993;20:1105–7.
2. Stoll T, Bruhlmann P, Stucki G, Burkhardt S, Michel B. Muscle strength assessment in polymyositis and dermatomyositis evaluation of the reliability and clinical use of a new quantitative, easily applicable method. J Rheumatol 1995;22:473–7.
3. Kaufman L, Gruber B, Gerstman D, Kaell A. Preliminary observations on role of magnetic resonance imaging for polymyositis and dermatomyositis. Ann Rheum Dis 1987;46:569–72.
4. Fraser D, Frank J, Dalakas M, et al. Magnetic resonance imaging in the idiopathic inflammatory myopathies. J Rheumatol 1991;18(11):1693–700.

5. Barlett M, Ginn L, Beitz L, et al. Quantitative assessment of myositis in thigh muscles using magnetic resonance imaging. Magn Reson Imaging 1999;17(2):183–91.

6. Par J, Vansant J, Kumar N, et al. Dermatomyositis: correlative MR imaging and p-31 MR spectroscopy for quantitative characterization of inflammatory disease. Radiology 1990; 177(2):473–9.

7. Stonecipher M, Jorizzo J, Monu J, Walker F, Sutej P. Dermatomyositis with normal muscle enzyme concentrations: a single-blind study of the diagnostic value of magnetic resonance imaging and ultrasound. Arch Dermatol 1994;130(10):1294–9.

8. Reimers C, Fleckenstein J, Witt T, Muller-Felber W, Pongratz D. Muscular ultrasound in idiopathic inflammatory myopathies of adults. J Neurol Sci 1993;116:82–92.

9. Fleckenstein J, Reimers C. Inflammatory myopathies, a radiologic evaluation. Radiol Clin North Am 1996;34(2):427–39.

10. Collison C, Sinal S, Jorizzo J, Walker F, Monu J, Synder J. Juvenile dermatomyositis and polymyositis: a follow-up study of long-term sequelae. South Med J 1988;91:17–22.

11. Newman J, Adler R, Rubin J. Power Doppler sonography: use in measuring alterations in muscle blood volume after exercise. Am J Roentgenol 1997;168:1525–30.

12. Weber MA, Krix M, Jappa U, et al. Pathologic skeletal muscle perfusion in patients with myositis: detection with quantitative contrast-enhanced US—initial results. Radiology 2006;238(2):640–9.

13. Gennisson JL, Cornu C, Catheline S, Fink M, Portero P. Human muscle hardness during incremental isometric contraction using transient elastography. J Biomech 2005;38:1543–50.

14. Weng L, Tirumalai AP, Lowery CM, et al. Extended field-of-view imaging technology. Radiology 1997;203:877–80.

15. Lin DC, Nazarian LN, O'Kane PL, McShane JM, Parker L, Merritt CR. Advantages of real-time spatial compound sonography of the musculoskeletal system versus conventional sonography. Am J Roentgenol 2002;179(6):1629–31.

16. Desser TS, Jeffrey RB. Tissue harmonic imaging techniques: physical principles and clinical applications. Semin Ultrasound CT MR 2001;22(1):1–10.

17. Meng C, Adler RS, Peterson M, Kagen L. Combined use of power Doppler and gray scale sonography: a new technique for the assessment of inflammatory myopathy. J Rheumatol 2001;28(6):1271–82.

18. Wagner RF, Insana MF, Brown DG. Statistical properties of radio-frequency and envelope-detected signals with application to medical ultrasound. J Opt Soc Am A 1987;4:910–22.

19. Levinson SP, Shinagawa M, Sato T. Sonoelastic determination of human skeletal muscle elasticity. J Biomech 1995;28:1145–54.

20. Rubin JM, Bude RO, Carson PL, Bree RL, Adler RS. Power Doppler US: a potentially useful alternative to mean frequency-based color Doppler US. Radiology 1994;290:853–6.

21. Rubin JM, Adler RS, Fowlkes JB, et al. Fractional moving blood volume: estimation using power Doppler US. Radiology 1995;197:183–90.

22. Averkious M, Powers J, Skyba D, Bruce M, Jenson S. Ultrasound contrast imaging research. Ultrasound Q 2003;19(1):27–37.

23. O'Donnell M, Flax SW. Phase aberration measurements in medical ultrasound: human studies. Ultrason Imaging 1988;10(1):1–11.

24. Campbell S, Adler RS, Sofka C. Ultrasound of muscle abnormalities. Ultrasound Q 2005; 21(2):87–94.

25. Bohan A, Peter J, Bowman R, Pearson C. Computer-assisted analysis of 153 patients with polymyositis and dermatomyositis. Medicine 1977;56:255–86.

26. Young A, Stokes M, Crowe M. The size and strength of the quadriceps muscles of old and young men. Clin Physiol 1985;5(2):145–54.

27. Kawakami Y, Abe T, Kanehisa H, Fukunaga T. Human skeletal muscle size and architecture: variability and interdependence. Am J Hum Biol 2006;18(6):845–8.

28. Pillen A, Art IM, Zwarts MJ. Muscle ultrasound in neuromuscular disorders. Muscle Nerve 2008;37(6):679–93.

29. Sofka CM, Haddad AK, Adler RS. Detection of muscle abnormalities on routine ultrasound of the shoulder. J Ultrasound Med 2004;23(8):1031–4.
30. Fornage BD, Eftekkhari F. Sonographic diagnosis of myositis ossificans. J Ultrasound Med 1989;8(8):463–6.
31. Sofka C, Batz R, Adler RS, Mintz D. Ultrasound evaluation and treatment of calcific myonecrosis in the leg. Skeletal Radiol 2005;5:1–4.
32. Adler RS, Garolfalo G, Paget S, Kagen L. Muscle sonography in six patients with hereditary inclusion body myopathy. Skeletal Radiol 2008;37(1):43–8.
33. O'Sullivan PJ, Gorman GM, Hardiman OM, Farrell MJ, Logan PM. Sonographically guided percutaneous muscle biopsy in diagnosis of neuromuscular disease: a useful alternative to open surgical biopsy. J Ultrasound Med 2006;25(1):1–6.
34. Collison C, Sinal S, Jorizzo J, Walker F, Monu J, Synder J. Juvenile dermatomyositis and polymyositis: a follow-up study of long-term sequelae. South Med J 1988;91:17–22.

# Chapter 10
# Serological Findings

Ira N. Targoff

**Abstract** Patients with polymyositis and dermatomyositis (DM) have a high frequency of autoantibodies to cytoplasmic and nuclear cellular antigens. No single autoantibody is present in the majority of patients, but a group of these autoantibodies is relatively specific for myositis (myositis-specific autoantibodies [MSAs]). The MSAs tend to be mutually exclusive and have distinctive clinical associations, resulting in autoantibody-defined disease subgroups. Anti-Jo-1 and other ant synthetases are associated with several extramuscular features as well as myositis, including interstitial lung disease (ILD), arthritis, and other features that together constitute an "antisynthetase syndrome." Anti-signal recognition particle (anti-SRP) is associated with a clinically and histologically distinctive myopathy that is often severe and sometimes rapidly progressive and relatively refractory, while anti-Mi-2 is associated with DM. Several recently identified autoantibodies also have relative myositis specificity and are associated predominantly with DM. Anti-p155/140 and anti-MJ are associated with juvenile DM, which has a low frequency of established MSAs. Anti-p155/140 has been increased in myositis with malignancy in adults. Anti-caDM-140 has been associated with clinically amyopathic DM (anti-caDM-140), often with ILD. These and additional new autoantibodies are increasing the proportion of myositis patients for whom specific autoantibodies can be identified. The MSAs can be helpful for diagnosis in patients with myositis and for patient characterization and classification. They also continue to provide insights into disease mechanisms. The new autoantibodies will improve the utility of the autoantibodies for these purposes.

**Keywords** Autoantibodies • Dermatomyositis • Polymyositis • Myositis diagnosis • Immunoprecipitation • Anti-Jo-1 • Anti-Mi-2 • Anti-PM-Scl • Anti-p155/140

I.N. Targoff
Department of Veterans Affairs Medical Center, Oklahoma City;
Department of Medicine, University of Oklahoma Health Sciences Center;
and Oklahoma Medical Research Foundation, Oklahoma City, OK, USA

L.J. Kagen (ed.), *The Inflammatory Myopathies*,
DOI 10.1007/978-1-60327-827-0_10,

Serological findings have become increasingly important in the evaluation of patients for myositis for diagnosis and patient classification. Myositis autoantibodies also are important in research regarding disease mechanisms. It has been long known that patients with myositis have a high frequency of autoantibodies to cellular constituents, with evidence of autoantibodies even by general screening methods such as immunodiffusion and indirect immunofluorescence in close to 90% of patients *(1)*. At the time, only a fraction of these autoantibodies could be specifically identified, particularly in the clinical setting. In recent years, however, new autoantibodies have continued to be identified, and techniques for detection have improved and become more widely available. Thus, while in 2001 Brouwer et al. *(2)* found defined autoantibodies in 56% of myositis patients using various sophisticated techniques, in 2007 Koenig et al. *(3)*, using a combination of techniques, found that 80% of polymyositis (PM) and dermatomyositis (DM) patients had identifiable autoantibodies, often showing multiple autoantibodies. Koenig et al. did not include all the newer autoantibodies that have recently been described, suggesting that the proportion of patients with clinically identifiable autoantibodies is likely to grow. This chapter reviews the serological findings and their clinical significance in patients with myositis.

# Overview

## *Antinuclear Antibodies*

Using indirect immunofluorescence, antinuclear antibodies (ANAs) are found in over half of patients with PM and DM *(4)*, ranging up to 80% of patients *(1)*, but ANAs are usually not found as frequently in myositis as in systemic lupus erythematosus (SLE) or systemic sclerosis (SSc). Most patients with connective tissue disease overlap syndromes involving myositis have positive ANAs, for example 77% in the study of Love et al. *(4)*, while ANAs are infrequent in inclusion body myositis (IBM) (23%) and have not been associated with other forms of myositis. They would also not be expected in other myopathies and therefore have some diagnostic value by themselves, particularly in higher titer. The frequency of ANAs using more recently introduced ELISA (enzyme-linked immunosorbent assay)-based, automated ANAs is not well studied, and the wide diversity of autoantibodies found in myositis could be a cause for concern regarding these assays.

Consistent with the many different antibodies seen in myositis *(3)*, the ANA patterns are varied. Although the most common pattern is nuclear speckled, some of the myositis autoantibodies, including the antisynthetases and anti-signal recognition particle (anti-SRP) antibodies, are directed at cytoplasmic antigens and typically give cytoplasmic staining patterns by indirect immunofluorescence. Some patients with these antibodies, particularly those with antisynthetases, can have additional autoantibodies that lead to nuclear staining. However, approximately

10–15% of myositis patients show only cytoplasmic staining, which often is considered negative on the ANA test. Cytoplasmic immunofluorescence can be a clue to the presence of a myositis autoantibody, which can be particularly important in patients who present with extramuscular features.

## Myositis-Specific Autoantibodies and Myositis-Associated Autoantibodies

The identified and defined autoantibodies found in myositis have been divided into the myositis-specific autoantibodies (MSAs) and the myositis-associated autoantibodies (MAAs) (Table 10.1). This was originally based on the observation that MSAs appeared to have a primary association with myositis, with most patients with the antibodies having myositis even if they had other manifestations of their condition. In contrast, MAAs could be found in some patients with myositis but often had a primary association with other conditions. Most patients with the MSA, anti-Jo-1 for example, have myositis, which is often a significant clinical problem, but most with anti-Ro/SSA, considered an MAA, do not have myositis, although anti-Ro/SSA can be seen in some myositis patients SSA. Supporting this concept is that MSAs, in general, tend to be mutually exclusive; patients generally do not have more than one of the MSAs. Even different antisynthetases do not usually occur together. MAAs, however, often occur in combination with an MSA or other MAAs. For example, anti-Ro/SSA is more likely to occur in association with an MSA (5), and anti-Ro52 in particular occurs more commonly in association with antisynthetases (6) than in others with myositis. Also, MAAs are more likely to occur in patients with myositis in overlap syndromes.

While this separation can be useful, it should be emphasized that these are relative considerations, and all have exceptions. The MSAs should not be considered absolutely specific for myositis. Some patients with antisynthetases, for example, have other features of the antisynthetase syndrome without myositis, and certain of the antisynthetases are more strongly associated with interstitial lung disease (ILD) than with myositis (7,8). Antibody is considered to be an MAA, but the majority of patients with the antibody have myositis, and it has relative mutual exclusion with the MSAs (9). In addition, a few patients have been reported who have more than one MSA or more than one antisynthetase (2,10). Such cases remain unusual but may be significant in understanding the relationship of the antibodies to the disease.

## Disease Associations

Although, as noted, defined autoantibodies can be found in at least 50% of PM-DM patients and with multiple sensitive techniques this percentage can reach 80%, there

**Table 10.1** Autoantibodies in polymyositis and dermatomyositis

**Established myositis-specific autoantibodies**

*Antisynthetase autoantibodies*

| Name | Antigen | MW | Tests | IIF | Freq (%) | Clinical | Comments | Ref |
|---|---|---|---|---|---|---|---|---|
| Jo-1 | (a) Histidyl-tRNA synthetase (b) Transfer-RNA^his (direct reaction) | 50 | ID; IPP; WB; EIA | Cyto | (a) 18-20 (b) 6 | Antisynthetase syndrome: Myo (95%); ILD (80%); arthritis (60%); RP (60%); mechanic's hands (70%); fever | (1) PM > DM in some studies (2) Adult > juvenile (3) Titer may vary with disease activity (4) anti-tRNA always with anti-enzyme | *(4,28,41,50)* |
| PL-7 | Threonyl-tRNA synthetase | 80 | ID; IPP; EIA | Cyto | <5 | Similar to anti-Jo-1 | More DM than with anti-Jo-1 | *(44,103)* |
| PL-12 | (a) Alanyl-tRNA synthetase (b) Transfer RNA^ala | 110 | ID; IPP; EIA; IPP | Cyto | (a) <5 (b) <5 | Similar to anti-Jo-1, but lower freq Myo | Anti-tRNA usually with anti-enzyme | *(45,49)* |
| OJ | (a) Isoleucyl-tRNA synthetase (b) Multienzyme complex | 150 170, 130, 75 | IPP WB | Cyto | (a) <3 (b) <1 | Similar to anti-Jo-1, but lower freq Myo | Ile-RS usual main antigen; leu-RS, lys-RS can be seen with ile-RS | *(8,32,48)* |
| EJ | Glycyl-tRNA synthetase | 75 | IPP; WB | Cyto | <3 | Similar to anti-Jo-1 | More DM than with anti-Jo-1 | *(25,32)* |
| KS | Asparaginyl-tRNA synthetase | 65 (63) | IPP | Cyto | <2 | Similar to anti-Jo-1 but lower freq Myo | | *(7,46)* |
| Ha | Tyrosyl-tRNA synthetase | 62 (59) | IPP | Cyto (neg) | <1 | Similar to anti-Jo-1 | Preliminary report | *(104)* |
| Zo | Phenylalanyl-tRNA synthetase | 60 + 70 (57 + 66) | IPP | Cyto | <5 | Similar to anti-Jo-1 | 2 Strong bands by IPP; weak tRNA | *(47)* |

*Other myositis-specific autoantibodies*

| | | | | | | | | |
|---|---|---|---|---|---|---|---|---|
| SRP | Signal recognition particle | 54, 72 | IPP; WB | Cyto | 4–5 | (1) Most have PM (2) Severe weakness (3) May be rapidly developing (4) Sometimes resistant | Biopsy often shows little or no inflammation | (38,39) |
| Mi-2 | *NuRD helicases:* (a) Mi-2α (CHD3) (b) Mi-2β (CHD4) | 240 (a) 208–226 (b) 218 | ID; IPP; WB; EIA | NS | 5–14 | Most have DM PM | (1) Sera react with both forms by IPP (2) Freq varies geographically (3) Less DM specific by EIA,WB | (24,36,74, 75,77) |

**New dermatomyositis autoantibodies**

| | | | | | | | | |
|---|---|---|---|---|---|---|---|---|
| p155/140 (p155; 155/140) | Nuclear proteins 155 and 140 | 155, 140 | IPP; IPP-WB | NS | 20 (29 of JDM) | (1) Most have DM (2) JDM; CAM; caDM | (1) Increased risk of cancer in adults (2) Prominent rash | (16,17,21,23) |
| MJ | Nuclear protein | 140 | IPP; IPP-WB | NS (or neg) | 17.5 | JDM | Increased calcinosis | (18,22) |
| caDM-140 | Cyto protein | 140 | IPP | Cyto | 19 | (1) caDM (2) More ILD | Thus for reported only from Japan | (20) |
| SAE | Small ubiquitin-like modifier-activating enzyme | 90, 40 | IPP | NS | 8.4 of DM | (1) DM (2) Rash may precede myositis | | (19,98) |

**Myositis-associated autoantibodies**
*Overlap syndrome-associated autoantibodies*

| | | | | | | | | |
|---|---|---|---|---|---|---|---|---|
| PM-Scl | *Exosome proteins:* | 100, 75, other | ID; IPP; WB; EIA | NS/NO | (a) 5–10 (b) 3–5 | PM or DM (75); SSc (75); arthritis | (a) Myo may be more responsive (b) SSc usually limited-cutaneous | (9,105,106) |
| U1RNP | U1 small nuclear ribonucleoprotein | 70, 32A, C25 | ID; IPP; WB; EIA | NS | 5–10 | Myo; SSc; SLE | | |

(continued)

**Table 10.1** (continued)

| Name | Antigen | MW | Tests | IIF | Freq (%) | Clinical | Comments | Ref |
|---|---|---|---|---|---|---|---|---|
| NonU1-snRNPs | (a) U2RNP (b) U5RNP (c) U4/6RNP | (a) A', B (b) 200 (c) 150 | IPP; WB | NS | (a) Rare (b) Rare (c) Rare | (a) Myo; SSc (b) Myo; SSc (c) SSc; Myo | | (91,92,107) |
| U3RNP | Fibrillarin | 34 kDa | IPP; EIA | NO | <3; 14 | SSc overlap | Higher freq for EIA, WB | (3) |
| Ku | DNA-binding complex | 70, 80 | ID; IPP; WB | NS | <3; 23 | SSc; SLE; Myo | Higher freq for EIA, WB | (3) |

*Other myositis-associated autoantibodies*

| Name | Antigen | MW | Tests | IIF | Freq (%) | Clinical | Comments | Ref |
|---|---|---|---|---|---|---|---|---|
| Ro/SSA | (a) Ro60 (b) Ro52 | 60 52 | ID; IPP; EIA; WB EIA; WB | Nu | (a) 10 (b) 25 | Sjögren's; SLE | (a) Anti-La can also be seen (b) Both forms associated with antisynthetases | (2,6,94) |
| PMS1 related | DNA mismatch repair enzymes: PMS1 PMS2 MLH1 | 120 | IPP | Nu | 7.5 4 4 | Limited information | Different antienzymes can occur together or separately | (96) |
| 56 kDa | Ribonucleoprotein component | 56 | WB | Nu | 62–87 | All forms; More in JDM | | (108) |
| Fer | Elongation factor 1α | 48 | IPP | Cyto | <1 | Possibly Myo | | (109) |
| Mas | tRNA^ser and protein | 45 | IPP | Cyto | <2 | Myo; hepatitis | | (4) |
| KJ | Translation factor | 120 | ID; WB | Cyto | <1 | Myo; ILD | | (110) |
| Nucleoporins | Nuclear porins | 200, 130 | IIF | Rim | <=3 | Myo | | (3,111) |

Adapted from **Ref. 104**: Antibody names are derived from prototype patients or laboratory codes (PL - precipitin line) expect for those related to the antigen structure (SRP, p155/150, SAE, RNP (ribonucleoprotein), PMS1, 56 kDa) or disease association (caDM-140, PM-Scl, SSA (Sjögren's syndrome A).

*Abbreviations:* *caDM* clinically amyopathic dermatomyositis; *CAM* cancer-associated myositis; *cyto* cytoplasmic pattern; *DM* dermatomyositis; *EIA* enzyme immunoassay; *Freq* frequency; *ID* immunodiffusion; *IIF* indirect immunofluorescence; *ILD* interstitial lung disease; *IPP* immunoprecipitation; *JDM* juvenile DM; *MW* molecular weight in kilodaltons (for complexes, antigen subunit MW shown); *Myo* myositis; *NO* nucleolar pattern; *NS* nuclear speckled pattern; *Nu* nuclear pattern; *Ref* reference; *RP* Raynaud's phenomenon; *SLE* systemic lupus erythematosus; *SSc* systemic sclerosis; *WB* Western immunoblotting

is no currently detectable single autoantibody specificity that occurs in the majority of patients. The most common MSA, anti-Jo-1, is usually found in only approximately 20% of myositis patients overall (18-23%) *(2,4,5,11)*. This may relate to the heterogeneity of the condition. PM and DM are felt to be different in pathogenesis, and additional significant clinical heterogeneity is seen with regard to the myositis and the extramuscular features (as discussed elsewhere in this book). The diversity of antibodies, the mutual exclusion of MSAs, and the significant clinical associations seen with each MSA and some MAAs make them useful tools for defining disease subgroups in a way that is complementary to the classification based on clinical criteria *(4)*. Combining clinical and autoantibody criteria for classification can provide additional insights *(12)*.

The MSAs and MAAs are found in PM and DM, but MSAs rarely, if ever, occur in typical IBM *(4,13)*. A small number have had anti-Ro/SSA *(4)*. MSAs have been reported in a few IBM cases *(2,14)*, but the clinical details have not been described for most of these. Of interest was one case in which a patient with a diagnosis of IBM was found to have anti-Jo-1, and the patient responded well to treatment with corticosteroids, as might be expected with anti-Jo-1-associated myositis rather than IBM *(15)*. In other reports, the techniques for detection of some of the antibodies that were found differed from those that had previously established the disease specificity of the antibodies *(2)*. Clinically, the finding of an MSA, or even an MAA, in a patient with a diagnosis of IBM should raise questions regarding the diagnosis.

Traditional MSAs and most MAAs have been more common in PM than in DM *(5)* and more common in adults than in children and are usually not found in myositis with malignancy *(4,16)*. However, studies have identified new autoantibodies with relative specificity for DM *(17–20)*, some of which have been found at least as frequently in juvenile-onset myositis as in adults *(17,18,21,22)*, and one of these antibodies, anti-p155/140 (anti-155/140, anti-p155) has been associated with malignancy in adult patients *(23)*. While some MSAs and MAAs are found almost exclusively in PM (anti-SRP) or almost exclusively in DM (*(24)*, anti-p155/140 *(17)*), antisynthetases can be found in both PM and DM *(4,11)*. This is of interest in view of the apparent pathogenetic differences between PM and DM and further emphasizes that antibody-defined subgroups do not necessarily fit within clinically defined classes.

Patients who have MSAs and MAAs usually have them from the time of their initial presentation. The antibodies can sometimes be seen prior to the onset of myositis in patients who present with extramuscular features *(25,26)*. The antibodies usually persist throughout the patient's course, despite treatment, even if the condition is controlled or goes into sustained remission. Occasionally, an MSA can become undetectable, which is usually associated with disease remission or improvement *(27)*. There has also been previous suggestion of variation of antibody level with disease activity *(27)*, but this was more clearly shown in a recent study of anti-Jo-1 *(28)*. The amount of serum anti-Jo-1 antibody by ELISA varied with disease activity, not only for the myositis activity, as measured by strength, creatine phosphokinase (CPK), and function, but also for other antisynthetase manifestations.

## Autoantibody Testing

Most of the established MSAs and newer DM antibodies were first described using double immunodiffusion (DID) (anti-Jo-1 *(29)*, anti-Mi-2 *(30)*, anti-PM-Scl *(31)*) or protein A-assisted immunoprecipitation (IPP) (non-Jo-1 antisynthetases *(32)*, anti-SRP *(33)*, anti-p155/140 *(17,23)*, anti-SAE (small ubiquitin-like modifier-activating enzyme) *(19)*). Most of the clinical associations of these autoantibodies were determined in studies using these techniques to identify the autoantibodies. Since then, ELISA tests have been developed for anti-Jo-1 *(34)*, anti-Mi-2 *(2,35,36)*, and anti-PM-Scl *(3,37)*, some of which are widely available.

Other techniques based on recombinant antigens are also in use, such as line immunoassays for anti-Mi-2 and anti-PM-Scl *(3)*. At this time, anti-SRP, several non-Jo-1 antisynthetases, and the newer DM antibodies are detected only by IPP-based techniques *(7,8,38,39)* for clinical and investigational purposes, sometimes with modifications *(2)*. ELISA and IPP tests are intrinsically more sensitive techniques than DID and will sometimes detect antibody that cannot be detected by DID for quantitative reasons. In general, IPP with electrophoretic analysis of the antigen tends to be a more specific test for the antibody than ELISA. However, significant differences in the clinical associations of anti-Mi-2 that are unrelated to titer have been reported between antibody measured by different techniques (recombinant ELISA or line immunoassay versus IPP or DID) *(3,36)*. These different clinical associations may relate to differences in the predominant epitopes recognized by the different methods. The IPP and DID methods use antigen that is likely to be more native in configuration than the tests such as ELISA using recombinant antigen. The native antigen preserves some epitopes and hides others. Some studies have also suggested differences in the clinical associations for other MSAs when measured by different methods *(2)*. While IPP is sensitive and specific for detection of MSAs and some MAAs, IPP is considerably less sensitive for detection of certain of the MAAs than direct-binding methods such as ELISA or blotting, particularly for anti-Ku, anti-U3RNP (U3 ribonucleo-protein), and anti-Ro52 *(3)*. At least for, this difference appears to relate to epitopes since IPP can very sensitively detect antibody in certain patients, while in other sera, IPP does not detect antibody that can be seen by other techniques. The clinical associations of the subset of anti-Ku-positive patients who are IPP positive *(40)*, compared to those who are ELISA or blot positive, have not been well studied in myositis. Thus, the method of detection should be taken into account when assessing the clinical significance of antibody testing results.

## Established MSAs

### Antisynthetases

Anti-Jo-1 was the first well-defined MSA *(29)* and the first demonstrated to be an antisynthetase *(41)*. It is present in about 20% of all patients *(42)*, by far the most common antisynthetase in most studies *(11,12)*, usually more than others combined.

Most other populations have had a similar, relatively high frequency of anti-Jo-1 *(5)*, but the frequency was lower in some studies. For example, in a group of Mesoamerican Mestizos with myositis, only 5% had any antisynthetase. This might have been related to the higher-than-usual proportion with DM (69%) in this group and the higher frequency of anti-Mi-2 (30%) *(43)*.

The Jo-1 antigen, histidyl-tRNA synthetase, catalyzes the binding of histidine to its transfer RNA (tRNA$^{his}$). The other antisynthetases in myositis react with other aminoacyl-tRNA synthetases. There is a separate aminoacyl-tRNA synthetase enzyme for each amino acid, which must be able to specifically recognize the amino acid and the cognate tRNAs. It is thus not surprising that each enzyme is immunologically distinct; individuals usually have antibody to only one synthetase, with no cross-reaction of the antibody with other synthetases.

The antigen was identified originally by the finding that anti-Jo-1 autoantibodies specifically immunoprecipitated a tRNA for histidine and specifically inhibited the in vitro activity of histidyl-tRNA synthetase *(41)* without inhibiting other aminoacyl-tRNA synthetases. Anti-PL-7 (directed at threonyl-tRNA synthetase) *(44)*, anti-PL-12 (alanyl) *(45)*, anti-EJ (glycyl), anti-OJ (isoleucyl) *(32)*, and anti-KS (asparaginyl) *(46)* were identified as other antisynthetases by the observation that they also immunoprecipitated specific tRNAs, which could be distinguished from those seen with anti-Jo-1. Inhibition testing in each case demonstrated that they specifically inhibited the enzymatic activity of the antigenic enzyme. The report of anti-Zo, an antibody that reacts with phenylalanyl-tRNA synthetase, was unique in that the antigen was identified solely by mass spectrometry, with only a weak tRNA band *(47)*.

Each of these antibodies also immunoprecipitated a protein of the expected molecular weight for the enzyme. Thus, combining IPP for protein analysis and nucleic acid analysis can sensitively and specifically detect the antibodies (Figs. 10.1 and 10.2). Anti-OJ, directed at isoleucyl-tRNA synthetase, immunoprecipitates a multienzyme complex that contains the synthetase activities for nine amino acids *(48)*. Most anti-OJ sera can be demonstrated to react with the isoleucyl-tRNA synthetase component by enzyme inhibition studies and precipitate a similar tRNA that appears to be a tRNA for isoleucine. However, some have evidence of reactivity with other components of the multienzyme complex, either by inhibition or immunoblotting studies *(48)*. With this exception, which may represent intermolecular epitope spreading, it is unusual to find autoantibodies to more than one antisynthetase in the same serum, although this has been occasionally observed.

All patient sera with antisynthetases react with the synthetase enzyme, but some also react with the tRNA itself. This has been found for most anti-PL-12 (anti-alanyl-tRNA synthetase) sera *(45,49)* but can also occur with some sera with anti-Jo-1 *(50)*. There have not yet been any clinical associations with having antibodies that directly react with the tRNA. The precipitation of tRNA by other antisynthetases that do not react with the tRNA directly has been attributed to affinity of the enzyme for its substrate tRNA, although anti-OJ precipitates predominantly the tRNA for isoleucine, even though the other aminoacyl-tRNA synthetases in the multienzyme complex are precipitated.

Some studies have found anti-Jo-1 to be more common in PM than in DM in adults. For example, Arnett et al. *(5)* found anti-Jo-1 in 27% of PM versus 7% of DM.

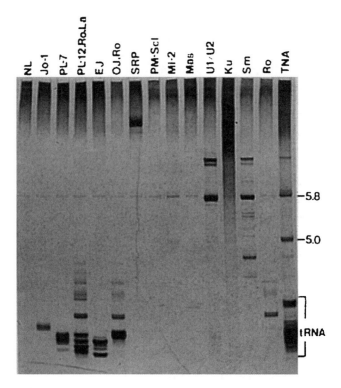

**Fig. 10.1** Immunoprecipitation with myositis autoantibodies. Immunoprecipitation for nucleic acid analysis. Immunoprecipitates were formed using protein A sepharose coated with patient antibody and incubated with HeLa cell extract. The immunoprecipitates were phenol extracted to remove proteins, and nucleic acids associated with the immunoprecipitated antigens were separated by urea–polyacrylamide gel electrophoresis, which was silver stained. The serum used in each *lane* is shown across the *top* (*NL* normal human serum; *TNA* total nucleic acid). The 5.8S and 5.0S small ribosomal RNAs seen in the TNA *lane* are labeled on the *right*, along with the transfer RNAs. Each antisynthetase antibody precipitates a distinctive set of transfer RNAs that are specific for the amino acid of the antigenic enzyme and can therefore be differentiated by electrophoresis. In contrast, anti-SRP antibody immunoprecipitates a larger, unique 7S RNA (7SL) that migrates more slowly and is easily distinguished. The PM-Scl and Mi-2 antigens do not have specific associated RNAs, and these antibodies cannot be identified by nucleic acid analysis. They each immunoprecipitate a distinctive set of proteins that can be identified by immunoprecipitation for protein analysis (as shown in Fig. 10.3). Anti-Mas antibody precipitates a weak RNA (see Table 10.1). "U1/U2" shows the U1 and U2 RNAs precipitated by a serum with specific anti-U2RNP and specific anti-U1RNP. Anti-Sm immunoprecipitates these same RNAs, along with U4, U5, and U6 RNAs. Anti-Ku precipitates heterogeneous DNA, but specific identification of the antibody requires other methods. (From **Ref. 103**. Reprinted from *Rheumatic Disease Clinics of North America*. Used with permission from Elsevier)

Fathi et al. *(51)* found that all six of their anti-Jo-1 patients had PM. Stone et al. *(28)* found that only 16 of 81 anti-Jo-1 patients had a diagnosis of DM. Others, however, found little or no difference in frequency of anti-Jo-1 between PM and DM *(11)*. This may relate to the populations studied or the criteria for a DM diagnosis.

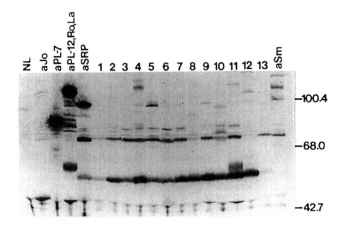

**Fig. 10.2** Immunoprecipitation with anti-SRP autoantibodies. Immunoprecipitation for protein analysis. Immunoprecipitates were formed using protein A sepharose coated with patient antibody and incubated with extract of S35-labeled HeLa cells. The immunoprecipitates were analyzed by 10% sodium dodecyl sulfate (SDS)–polyacrylamide gel electrophoresis. Sera 1 through 13 have anti-SRP; each sample showed the 7SL RNA by nucleic acid immunoprecipitation (see Fig. 10.1). The signal recognition particle includes six proteins. The major bands by immunoprecipitation are those of 54 and 72 kDa. Patients may differ in the relative strength of these bands (compare sample 12 to sample 13; see also **Ref. *38*)**. The anti-SRP reference serum immunoprecipitates an additional strong protein band of approximately 100 kDa because of a coexistent autoantibody. Immunoprecipitation with anti-Jo-1, anti-PL-7, and anti-PL12 shows strong proteins (the antigenic synthetases) that are easily distinguished. The position of molecular weight markers in kilodaltons is shown at the *right*. (From **Ref. *39***. Copyright © 1990 American College of Rheumatology. Reprinted with permission of Wiley-Liss, Inc., a subsidiary of Wiley)

However, DM may be more frequent with non-Jo-1 antisynthetases. DM was found in five of six with anti-EJ, for example *(25)*. The relative frequency of different antisynthetases may vary in different populations. For example, in the study of Arnett et al. *(5)*, anti-PL-12 was the most common non-Jo-1 antisynthetase, while Furuya et al. *(52)* found that anti-EJ was most common. Anti-EJ may be more common in Asian populations in general, although one study found an increase in anti-PL-7 *(53)*.

Among other clinical subgroups of the Bohan and Peter classification, anti-Jo-1 and other antisynthetases can occur in juvenile myositis *(54)*, with associated antisynthetase syndrome, but they are much less common than in adults and are not the most common MSA. Anti-Mi-2 *(55)*, anti-PM-Scl *(56)*, anti-p155/140 *(17,21)*, and anti-MJ *(56)* are more common than antisynthetases in children. The group that would be classified as connective tissue disease-associated myositis by Bohan and Peter, with diagnosed coexistent conditions, has a low frequency of antisynthetases *(4)*. However, Troyanov et al. *(12)* considered the connective tissue disease features that are part of the antisynthetase syndrome to represent an overlap syndrome and suggested classifying antisynthetase patients as having overlap myositis. Patients with myositis with malignancy usually do not have antisynthetases *(4,16)*, but several cases have been reported *(57,58)*, although coincidental unrelated cancer cannot be excluded.

The myositis seen in patients with anti-Jo-1 is generally similar clinically to that seen in patients without the antibody. However, some differences have been noted. Although it usually responds to treatment with corticosteroids and immunosuppressive agents, it may be more likely to recur as treatment is reduced compared to recurrence in other myositis patients (60% vs. 20% *(4)*). There also may be fever accompanying exacerbations more frequently *(4)*. Mozaffar et al. *(59)* found differences in the muscle histology of anti-Jo-1 patients compared to other myositis. All 11 anti-Jo-1 biopsies showed perifascicular atrophy and perimysial inflammation, findings usually associated with DM. However, the vasculopathy that is seen with DM, usually manifested by complement deposition and capillary loss (measured by reduced capillary index) was not seen in the anti-Jo-1 muscle. Anti-Jo-1 muscle did show perimysial connective tissue fragmentation suggesting fasciitis.

Patients with antisynthetases have an increased frequency of several additional features often seen in connective tissue diseases, including ILD, arthritis, and Raynaud's phenomenon. They may also show "mechanic's hands," lines of hyperkeratosis and splitting on the edges of the fingers. This constellation of features in a patient with an antisynthetase has been referred to as the *antisynthetase syndrome*. Patients with antisynthetases generally have one or more of these features but not necessarily all. While most patients with anti-Jo-1 have myositis, patients with antisynthetases may have one or more other antisynthetase features without myositis. This is most commonly ILD but can sometimes be arthritis. They may present with ILD or arthritis and develop myositis later or may not develop myositis over their course. Patients with certain antisynthetases are more likely to have this picture (they are more closely associated with ILD than with myositis). This has been most frequently observed with anti-PL-12 *(60)* but also appears to be true of anti-OJ *(8,48)* and anti-KS *(7)*.

The ILD is potentially the most significant extraarticular manifestation in view of effects on prognosis. It most often resembles nonspecific interstitial pneumonia *(61)*, but other histologic and clinical patterns can be seen *(60,62,63)*. The polyarthritis is very common *(4)* and can be deforming *(64)*, but usually not erosive. When the arthritis is the presenting feature, it may be diagnosed as rheumatoid arthritis before other features appear *(60)*. The syndrome associated with antisynthetases is described in greater detail in Chap. 11.

## *Anti-Signal Recognition Particle*

The SRP is a highly conserved complex of an RNA (the 7SL RNA) with six proteins (72, 68, 54, 19, 14, and 9 kDa). It binds to the signal sequence on nascent proteins that are destined for secretion or membrane expression and targets them to the endoplasmic reticulum for translocation by binding to docking proteins. Patient antibodies to the SRP 54-kDa protein block translocation in vitro *(65)*.

The 54- and 72-kDa proteins are recognized as antigens, and some patients react predominantly with one or the other of these proteins (Fig. 10.2) *(38,39)*. Thus far, no clinical association has been established for this difference between anti-SRP-positive patients. Most patients with anti-SRP react with the SRP proteins, and the RNA is precipitated indirectly through binding to the SRP proteins. However, anti-SRP patients with antibodies to the 7SL RNA have been reported; Satoh et al. *(66)* found them in 50% of Japanese patients but only 5% of North American patients.

Sera with anti-SRP autoantibody usually give a cytoplasmic pattern by ANA testing, although this may not be visible with weak sera and is not specific for this antibody. The antibody is usually detected by IPP with electrophoretic analysis of both RNA and protein *(33,38,39)* (see Figs. 10.1 and 10.2), but some studies have utilized a dot blot to analyze the immunoprecipitated RNA *(2)* and have found differences in clinical associations.

Anti-SRP is rare in DM. Most patients with the antibody have had a diagnosis of PM, although it is often atypical, as noted in this section. In the study of Satoh et al. *(66)*, among 32 anti-SRP patients, only 2 had DM, and both were among the 5 Japanese patients with anti-7SL RNA. Anti-SRP was also found in DM (5 of 20 anti-SRP patients), as well as a in patient with IBM, by Brouwer et al. *(2)* and by Hengstman et al. (3 of 23 patients) *(67)*, both using the dot-blot technique. Some studies had no DM *(39,68)*. Occasional patients have been reported with anti-SRP who have not had myositis *(38)*.

Anti-SRP patients are distinctive in most studies by the severity of their muscle weakness *(38,67,68)*. Miller et al. *(68)* noted that five of seven patients had a manual muscle testing score of 0 of 5 in their weakest muscles. Weakness often develops relatively rapidly and can be associated with relatively high CPKs (up to 25,000 in the study of Miller et al.). Some patients with this antibody have been relatively refractory to treatment, with often incomplete responses, recurrences, and an increased requirement for immunosuppressives *(39,69)*. Some patients are more responsive, however *(67,68)*. One study found an increase in cardiac involvement *(39)*, but this has not been seen in most other studies *(67)*. A poor prognosis has also been reported *(4,39)*, which has not been universally found. Patients with anti-SRP do not usually have the features of the antisynthetase syndrome, although these may be seen in a proportion similar to that in others with myositis *(39,67)*.

The muscle involvement seen with anti-SRP is distinctive in its histology. Often, a necrotizing myopathy is seen, which may be active and severe but with little or no inflammation *(67,68,70)*. The muscle biopsy may not be read as showing PM or other inflammatory myopathy. This suggests a distinctive pathogenesis. Supporting this impression was the finding that anti-SRP patients had a vasculopathy with some features resembling that of DM, including deposition of the membrane attack complex of complement and sometimes capillary loss *(68)*. However, unlike DM, perifascicular atrophy was not seen. The complement deposition has not been universally noted *(67)*. Further suggesting a difference in this myopathy from that of antisynthetases was the finding of a seasonal difference in the time of onset of weakness between anti-SRP patients (usually around November) and anti-Jo-1 patients (more in the spring) *(71)*. Others have also noted differences in season of onset *(66,68)*. Although most patients receive a diagnosis of PM and anti-SRP myopathy is considered among the inflammatory myopathies, this antibody might be marking a unique group of patients or a group with more in common with other necrotizing myopathies.

## Anti-Mi-2

Anti-Mi-2 autoantibodies immunoprecipitate a complex of proteins (240, 200, 150, 75, 65, 63, 34 kDa) *(72)* (Fig. 10.3), of which the major antigens, migrating in the 200- to 240-kDa range, are two closely related proteins (75% identity) that have been called Mi-2α and Mi-2β *(73–75)*. Most anti-Mi-2 patient sera react with both proteins. These are DNA-helicases, which are involved in transcriptional regulation on the chromatin level, controlling chromatin remodeling and thereby access to DNA. Studies of Mi-2β showed it to be part of a complex that also contains histone deacetylases, which have a related function, that has been referred to as nucleosome-remodeling deacetylase (NuRD) *(76–79)*. The proteins are formally labeled

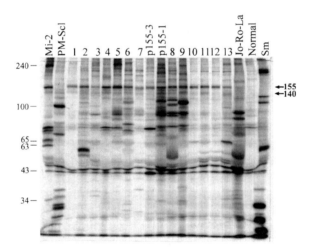

**Fig. 10.3** Immunoprecipitation with anti-p155/140 autoantibodies. Immunoprecipitation for protein analysis using S35-labeled HeLa cells as in Fig. 10.2. Samples p155-1 and p155-3 were used as reference sera for anti-p155/140 in the original study. Samples 1 through 13 have anti-p155/140 that was confirmed by immunoprecipitation blotting. Each shows a band of 155 kDa, usually accompanied by a weaker band of 140 kDa (positions indicated at the *right*). Although in this study the 155-kDa band was predominant, in other studies the bands were of equal strength *(23)*. Immunoprecipitation with anti-Mi-2 and anti-PM-Scl is also shown, each showing a distinctive set of multiple protein bands. They each react with components of a multiprotein complex. The position of molecular weight markers in kilodaltons is shown at the *left*; 65 and 63 are the positions of the indicated bands of Mi-2. (From **Ref. *17*.** Copyright © 2006 American College of Rheumatology. Reprinted with permission of Wiley-Liss, Inc., a subsidiary of Wiley)

CHD3 (Mi-2α) and CHD4 (Mi-2β) based on sequence domains, including chromo (chromatin organization modifier), helicase, and DNA binding.

Studies of anti-Mi-2 using immunodiffusion or IPP have shown high specificity for myositis (98%) and a strong association with DM (90-95%) *(4,5,24,30)*. Anti-Mi-2 is found in both adult and juvenile DM, although it may be more common in adults *(54)*. Occasional cases associated with malignancy have been reported. Most patients have typical DM with Gottron's and heliotrope signs, and the "V" and "shawl" signs (involvement of the base of the neck and upper back). The rash may be prominent. Overlap syndromes are usually not seen.

Anti-Mi-2 was observed to vary in frequency between populations, with a low frequency in some populations *(80)* and a higher frequency in others *(43)*. The high frequency of anti-Mi-2 in Mestizos noted seemed to be associated with both genetic and environmental factors *(43)*. In a further study of anti-Mi-2 in 15 cities around the world, Okada et al. *(81)* found that the frequency of anti-Mi-2 varied with differences in the frequency of DM and ranged from 60% in Guatemala City (associated with 83.3% DM) to 3.2% (with 48.4% DM) in Montreal. It had been noted that southern European regions had more DM *(2)*, and the DM rash is known to be photosensitive, and Okada et al. *(81)*, after examining a variety of possible geographic environmental influences, found that DM was most correlated with surface ultraviolet (UV) radiation, and that anti-Mi-2 was most correlated with UV radiation.

As noted, the frequency and clinical associations of anti-Mi-2 may be affected by the assay used for detection. An ELISA derived from overlapping fragments of the sequence of Mi-2β found a weaker association with DM *(2,36)* and lower specificity for myositis, although myositis specificity improved when confirmed by immunoblotting *(35)*. Initial studies suggested that this may have been related to reaction with different fragments, but subsequent studies found no fragment that could be used to reproduce the DM specificity seen with DID and IPP *(36)*, methods that involved native antigen. This may relate to the findings of Ge et al. *(74)*, using a recombinant fragment of Mi-2α, which suggested the importance of a conformational epitope.

# Overlap Antibodies

## *Anti-PM-Scl (Polymyositis-Scleroderma)*

Anti-PM-Scl autoantibodies usually give a characteristic nuclear and nucleolar staining pattern by indirect immunofluorescence, differing from the pure nucleolar patterns seen with and anti-U3RNP. Anti-PM-Scl autoantibodies immunoprecipitate a complex of at least 11 proteins, including major proteins of apparent molecular weights of 100, 70-75, 36, 35, 32, 31, 26, 24, 20 kDa and others *(9)* (see Fig. 10.3). Several studies found that the PM-Scl-100- and PM-Scl-75-kDa proteins are the major antigenic components of PM-Scl, but that some sera also react with other proteins *(82)*.

The majority of sera with anti-PM-Scl by IPP react with the 100-kDa protein by immunoblot *(83)*. Reaction with the 70- to 75-kDa protein was initially found in about 50% of anti-PM-Scl sera *(83,84)*, but a study using ELISA with an elongated recombinant form of this protein found a frequency of reactivity similar to that with the 100-kDa PM-Scl protein, including additional patients *(85)*, suggesting that PM-Scl-75 may be the major antigen. PM-Scl has been identified as the human exosome, the components of which are exoribonucleases that function in RNA processing *(82)*. A study found that another protein associated with the exosome, CID, is a frequent target of autoantibodies in patients with PM-scleroderma overlap syndrome, including some patients who do not have other evidence of anti-PM-Scl activity *(86)*. An ELISA has also been developed based on a helical peptide of a major epitope of the PM-Scl-100-kDa protein that may facilitate detection *(37)*.

Anti-PM-Scl is most commonly associated with an overlap syndrome with features of myositis and scleroderma *(9)*, but patients may have myositis or scleroderma alone. Occasionally, patients have had other diagnoses *(87)*, but the antibody is relatively specific for this syndrome, and there is relative mutual exclusion with MSAs (and with scleroderma antibodies). Many of the patients with myositis have DM, some with typical DM rashes *(3)*, and even mechanic's hands can be seen. The antibody also occurs in juvenile DM. The scleroderma is usually limited cutaneous. Patients may have other scleroderma-associated features such as Raynaud's or ILD. Arthritis may also be significant *(88)*. The myositis may be easier to treat than that of other myositis patients, responding to lower doses of steroids *(89)*. Anti-PM-Scl is strongly associated with human leukocyte antigen (HLA) DR3 and is rare among Japanese myositis patients.

## *Anti-U-snRNPs (small nuclear ribonucleoproteins)*

Arnett et al. *(5)* found anti-U1RNP in 16% of myositis patients, more in African Americans (26%) than in Caucasians (4%). It is common (60%) among patients with lupus-myositis overlap. Although it may occur in association with MSAs, it is more frequent among MSA-negative patients. The frequency of myositis in patients with anti-U1RNP is variable in different studies. Myositis is frequently seen in anti-U1RNP patients with mixed connective tissue disease (MCTD). Patients with MCTD and ILD, Raynaud's phenomenon, and arthritis may resemble those with antisynthetases. Although it has been suggested that the myositis may be milder *(89)*, and monophasic *(3)*, more severe or persistent myositis may occur.

Anti-Smith (Sm) can be seen in a small percentage of myositis patients, usually in association with anti-U1RNP. In addition, occasional patients have been found to have specific antibodies to particular small nuclear RNPs (snRNPs), without having anti-Sm. Antibodies to U2RNP *(90)*, U4/U6 RNP *(91)*, and U5RNP *(92)* have been reported. These antibodies react with proteins that are specific for these snRNPs, rather than the shared snRNP proteins targeted by anti-Sm. Most of these patients have had overlap syndromes involving myositis.

## *Anti-Ku*

The Ku antigen includes proteins of 72 and 86 kDa that bind to DNA ends and are involved in DNA repair. As noted, a much higher frequency of the antibody is seen with immunoblotting and line immunoassays than with DID or IPP *(3)*. Koenig et al. *(3)* found anti-Ku in 23% of French-Canadian myositis patients with line immunoassay but only in 3% by IPP. It is generally less common in Caucasians in other studies and most common in Japanese patients.

## *Other MAAs*

Koenig et al. *(3)* also found antifibrillarin antibodies in 14% of myositis patients; they used an addressable laser bead immunoassay and confirmed the finding by reaction with a transcription–translation product. There was an association with scleroderma overlap. This is usually considered a scleroderma-specific autoantibody, but other studies have noted more frequent occurrence of myositis in scleroderma patients with this antibody *(93)*.

Several studies have found an association of anti-Ro/SSA with myositis, with a higher frequency of anti-Ro52 (about 25%) than anti-Ro60 *(2,3,6)*. Anti-Ro52 was particularly common with anti-Jo-1 (58%) *(6)*, as well as with other antisynthetases *(94)*, anti-SRP or anti-PM-Scl. Anti-Ro52 in other settings is usually associated with anti-Ro60, but occurred without anti-Ro60 more frequently in myositis than usual. This frequency suggests that it may be useful in myositis diagnosis *(95)*, and the occurrence without anti-Ro60 could also have potential clinical significance, but it is not disease specific and tends to occur in association with other autoantibodies that are more disease specific.

Anti-PMS1 is directed at the DNA mismatch repair enzyme "postmeiotic segregation 1". It was found in 4 of 53 myositis patient sera (7.5%) and none of 94 with other rheumatic disease and 39 normal controls in one study *(96)*. It was often associated with other autoantibodies, including anti-Mi-2 in one patient. A small number of sera also reacted with other mismatch repair enzymes in the same enzyme family. Additional MAAs have also been reported, including those listed on Table 10.1.

## New DM Autoantibodies

## *Anti-p155/140*

An autoantibody that immunoprecipitates proteins of 155 and 140 kDa has been studied in several populations (see Fig. 10.3). Kaji et al. *(23)* found an antibody using IPP, labeled anti-155/140 in 7 of 52 DM patients but not in 9 PM, 50 normal, or 192 sera from other autoimmune disease. There were more cutaneous manifestations in the antibody-positive group, including a significant increase in flagellate erythema. Of particular note was an increase in malignancy (five of seven antibody-positive patients (71%) versus 11% of DM without the antibody) and a decrease in ILD (0% vs. 64%). Targoff et al. *(17)* studied an antibody labeled anti-p155 (since the 155 kDa was stronger than the 140 kDa in this study) by IPP with IPP blotting for confirmation (see Fig. 10.3). The antibody was found in 21% of myositis patients and only 1 of 138 controls. It was found in 29% of juvenile DM and 21% of adult DM but none with pure PM, although it was seen in a small number with connective tissue disease-associated PM. The antibody was found in six of eight with cancer-associated myositis, and 37.5% of those with the antibody had cancer. Chinoy et al. *(16)* found a similar antibody in 19 of their 103 with DM and none of the 109 with PM or 70 with overlap. Eight of the 19 had cancer-associated myositis (42%) versus 9% of other DM. There was also a lower-than-average frequency of other myositis antibodies in the patients with cancer. When these associations (anti-p155/140 and lack of other myositis antibodies) were combined, they were more useful than either alone in predicting malignancy risk, with a negative predictive value of 99.2%.

Gunawardena et al. *(21)* also found a high frequency of anti-p155/140 (23%) in juvenile DM. There were more ulcerations and skin disease in those with the antibody. The finding of the antibody in a significant proportion of children with juvenile DM was significant because of the lower frequency of MSAs in this group.

## Anti-MJ

Another autoantibody identified by IPP, labeled anti-MJ, has been associated with DM *(18,56)*. It showed a 140-kDa protein that was different from that seen with anti-p155/140 *(17)*. The antibody was found in 17.5% of 80 myositis patients, most of whom had DM (13 of 14), including more with juvenile than adult DM *(18)*. In a preliminary report in 156 patients with juvenile DM, anti-p140 (which appeared to be the same antibody) was found in 21% *(22)*. The group with the antibody had significantly more calcinosis than antibody-negative patients (52% vs. 13%), an association also noted by Oddis et al. *(18)*, who found calcinosis in 8 of 14 patients.

## Anti-caDM-140

Patients with clinically amyopathic DM (caDM), who have cutaneous DM without muscle involvement, appear to have a lower frequency of established MSAs than classical PM or DM *(20,97)*. However, Sato et al. *(20)* identified a new autoantibody in 8 of 15 caDM patients but not in control patients with myositis or other conditions. Those with the antibody had a higher frequency of ILD. Anti-caDM-140 showed a single 140-kDa band by IPP that was different from that of anti-MJ. Anti-p155/140 has also been found in caDM *(21,97)*.

## *Anti-Small Ubiquitin-like Modifier-Activating Enzyme*

One additional autoantibody, also identified by IPP, has been specifically associated with DM *(19)*. Protein bands of apparent molecular weight of 90 and 40 kDa by polyacrylamide gel electrophoresis were seen with this antibody, which were found to be subunits of the SAE using mass spectrometry. A preliminary report found the antibody in 11 of 266 myositis patients and none of 240 sera from rheumatic disease patients or normal controls *(98)*. All 11 had DM (8.4% of DM), including 2 with nonspecific interstitial pneumonia and 2 with cancer. In nine cases, the skin involvement preceded the clinical muscle involvement, although all developed myositis.

## Significance of the Myositis Autoantibodies

The main clinical role for the myositis autoantibodies has been to assist with diagnosis. The MSAs in particular have relative disease specificity that can be helpful in establishing the diagnosis when used in combination with other clinical information. For example, antisynthetases have relatively high specificity for PM or DM compared to other connective tissue diseases. However, most of the patients with antisynthetases who do not have myositis have other features of the antisynthetase syndrome *(26,60,99)*; therefore, the specificity is even higher in comparison to other myopathies *(35)*. Thus, in patients with evidence of myopathy by enzymes, electromyography, or magnetic resonance imaging, the confirmed presence of an antisynthetase would be strong evidence for PM or DM, particularly if other common predispositions to myopathy are excluded, such as hypothyroidism, medications, or alcoholism. It is unlikely that a muscle biopsy would change the initial treatment plan in this context. The case noted of a patient with a biopsy consistent with IBM whose response to treatment was more consistent with the anti-Jo-1 found in the serum is illustrative in this regard *(15)*.

The MAAs have less specificity for myositis and are therefore less useful for diagnosis. However, this also is generally in comparison to other connective tissue diseases, and they would be expected to have a low frequency in other myopathies. Thus, they also would have a relatively high positive predictive value in a group of patients with undiagnosed myopathy.

The antibodies also have diagnostic utility in patients who present with extramuscular features of PM or DM or myositis overlap syndromes. They can be helpful in identifying patients with ILD or arthritis whose condition is actually part of an antisynthetase syndrome. Sometimes, mild myositis can be identified in such patients that was not previously appreciated. However, the antibody is not itself evidence of clinical myositis.

As discussed in Chap. 2, the antibodies can also be useful for patient classification *(4,12)*. They can help in patient characterization, possibly in predicting responsiveness and risk of recurrent disease, and in predicting areas of concern, such as the potential for ILD in antisynthetase patients, which could possibly affect treatment choices. Patients with anti-SRP who have evidence of a rapidly progressive course may be candidates for earlier or more aggressive treatment *(4)*, although this is not always the case *(38)*, and characteristics of the individual case must be considered. Despite the typical clinical associations of the antibodies that have been discussed, individual presentations are generally not specific for particular antibodies.

Studies have also suggested potential new roles for the antibodies, as noted. For example, the demonstration that the titer of anti-Jo-1 varies with disease activity suggests a role for the antibody in assessing disease activity. This would be most helpful for longitudinal assessment of individual patients. For example, an increase in titer may help distinguish a flare of disease from other causes of recurrent symptoms. However, the clinical utility or optimal use of this finding has not yet been specifically studied. Similarly, the finding of an association of anti-p155/140 with malignancy in myositis suggests a possible role in identifying myositis patients who might benefit from a more thorough or repeated search for occult malignancy.

Finally, the antibodies have been used as tools for research in pathogenesis and disease mechanisms. One interesting study demonstrated that mice immunized with histidyl-tRNA synthetase (Jo-1 antigen), particularly the murine form leading to an autoimmune response, developed inflammation in the muscle and lung that resembled the antisynthetase syndrome *(100)*. Other studies have suggested that myositis autoantigens, as in other conditions, tend to be ones that can be cleaved by granzyme B, which could be important in directing immune response to these antigens *(101)*, and that there may be increased expression of myositis antigens in myositis muscle compared to normal muscle *(102)*. In addition, a form of histidyl-tRNA synthetase that was more susceptible to granzyme B cleavage was most prominent in the lung, suggesting a possible mechanism by which autoimmunity to synthetases could lead to the associated clinical picture. Such studies are likely to continue to provide insights into these conditions.

# References

1. Reichlin M, Arnett FC. Multiplicity of antibodies in myositis sera. Arthritis Rheum 1984;27:1150–6.
2. Brouwer R, Hengstman GJ, Vree Egberts W, et al. Autoantibody profiles in the sera of European patients with myositis. Ann Rheum Dis 2001;60(2):116–23.
3. Koenig M, Fritzler MJ, Targoff IN, Troyanov Y, Senecal JL. Heterogeneity of autoantibodies in 100 patients with autoimmune myositis: insights into clinical features and outcomes. Arthritis Res Ther 2007;9(4):R78.

4. Love LA, Leff RL, Fraser DD, et al. A new approach to the classification of idiopathic inflammatory myopathy: myositis-specific autoantibodies define useful homogeneous patient groups. Medicine 1991;70:360–74.
5. Arnett FC, Targoff IN, Mimori T, Goldstein R, Warner NB, Reveille JD. Interrelationship of major histocompatibility complex class II alleles and autoantibodies in four ethnic groups with various forms of myositis. Arthritis Rheum 1996;39:1507–18.
6. Rutjes SA, Vree Egberts WT, Jongen P, Van Den Hoogen F, Pruijn GJ, van Venrooij WJ. Anti-Ro52 antibodies frequently co-occur with anti-Jo-1 antibodies in sera from patients with idiopathic inflammatory myopathy. Clin Exp Immunol 1997;109:32–40.
7. Hirakata M, Suwa A, Takada T, et al. Clinical and immunogenetic features of patients with autoantibodies to asparaginyl-transfer RNA synthetase. Arthritis Rheum 2007;56(4):1295–303.
8. Sato S, Kuwana M, Hirakata M. Clinical characteristics of Japanese patients with anti-OJ (anti-isoleucyl-tRNA synthetase) autoantibodies. Rheumatology 2007;46(5):842–5.
9. Oddis CV, Okano Y, Rudert WA, Trucco M, Duquesnoy RJ, Medsger TA Jr. Serum autoantibody to the nucleolar antigen PM-Scl: clinical and immunogenetic associations. Arthritis Rheum 1992;35:1211–7.
10. Gelpi C, Kanterewicz E, Gratacos J, Targoff IN, Rodriguez-Sanchez JL. Coexistence of two antisynthetases in a patient with the antisynthetase syndrome. Arthritis Rheum 1996;39:692–7.
11. Chinoy H, Salway F, Fertig N, et al. In adult onset myositis, the presence of interstitial lung disease and myositis specific/associated antibodies are governed by HLA class II haplotype, rather than by myositis subtype. Arthritis Res Ther 2006;8(1):R13.
12. Troyanov Y, Targoff IN, Tremblay JL, Goulet JR, Raymond Y, Senecal JL. Novel classification of idiopathic inflammatory myopathies based on overlap syndrome features and autoantibodies: analysis of 100 French Canadian patients. Medicine 2005;84(4):231–49.
13. Hengstman GJ, van Engelen BG, Badrising UA, van den Hoogen FH, van Venrooij WJ. Presence of the anti-Jo-1 autoantibody excludes inclusion body myositis. Ann Neurol 1998;44:423.
14. Koffman BM, Rugiero M, Dalakas MC. Immune-mediated conditions and antibodies associated with sporadic inclusion body myositis. Muscle Nerve 1998;21:115–7.
15. Hengstman GJ, ter Laak HJ, van Engelen BG, van Venrooij BG. Anti-Jo-1 positive inclusion body myositis with a marked and sustained clinical improvement after oral prednisone. J Neurol Neurosurg Psychiatry 2001;70(5):706.
16. Chinoy H, Fertig N, Oddis CV, Ollier WE, Cooper RG. The diagnostic utility of myositis autoantibody testing for predicting the risk of cancer-associated myositis. Ann Rheum Dis 2007;66(10):1345–9.
17. Targoff IN, Mamyrova G, Trieu EP, et al. A novel autoantibody to a 155-kd protein is associated with dermatomyositis. Arthritis Rheum 2006;54(11):3682–9.
18. Oddis CV, Fertig N, Goel A, et al. Clinical and serological characterization of the anti-MJ antibody in childhood myositis [Abstract]. Arthritis Rheum 1997;40:S139.
19. Betteridge Z, Gunawardena H, North J, Slinn J, McHugh N. Identification of a novel autoantibody directed against small ubiquitin-like modifier activating enzyme in dermatomyositis. Arthritis Rheum 2007;56(9):3132–7.
20. Sato S, Hirakata M, Kuwana M, et al. Autoantibodies to a 140-kd polypeptide, CADM-140, in Japanese patients with clinically amyopathic dermatomyositis. Arthritis Rheum 2005;52(5):1571–6.
21. Gunawardena H, Wedderburn LR, North J, et al. Clinical associations of autoantibodies to a p155/140 kDa doublet protein in juvenile dermatomyositis. Rheumatology 2008;47(3):324–8.
22. Gunawardena H, Wedderburn LR, Chinoy H, et al. Novel autoantibodies targeting a p140 protein are a major autoantigen system in juvenile dermatomyositis and a marker of calcinosis [Abstract]. Arthritis Rheum 2008;58:S923.
23. Kaji K, Fujimoto M, Hasegawa M, et al. Identification of a novel autoantibody reactive with 155 and 140 kDa nuclear proteins in patients with dermatomyositis: an association with malignancy. Rheumatology 2007;46(1):25–8.

24. Mierau R, Dick T, Bartz-Bazzanella P, Keller E, Albert ED, Genth E. Strong association of dermatomyositis-specific Mi-2 autoantibodies with a tryptophan at position 9 of the HLA-DR beta chain. Arthritis Rheum 1996;39:868–76.

25. Targoff IN, Trieu EP, Plotz PH, Miller FW. Antibodies to glycyl-transfer RNA synthetase in patients with myositis and interstitial lung disease. Arthritis Rheum 1992;35:821–30.

26. Schmidt WA, Wetzel W, Friedlander R, et al. Clinical and serological aspects of patients with anti-Jo-1 antibodies – an evolving spectrum of disease manifestations. Clin Rheumatol 2000;19(5):371–7.

27. Miller FW, Twitty SA, Biswas T, Plotz PH. Origin and regulation of a disease-specific autoantibody response: antigenic epitopes, spectrotype stability, and isotype restriction of anti-Jo-1 antibodies. J Clin Invest 1990;85:468–75.

28. Stone KB, Oddis CV, Fertig N, et al. Anti-Jo-1 antibody levels correlate with disease activity in idiopathic inflammatory myopathy. Arthritis Rheum 2007;56(9):3125–31.

29. Nishikai M, Reichlin M. Heterogeneity of precipitating antibodies in polymyositis and dermatomyositis: characterization of the Jo-1 antibody system. Arthritis Rheum 1980;23:881–8.

30. Targoff IN, Reichlin M. The association between Mi-2 antibodies and dermatomyositis. Arthritis Rheum 1985;28:796–803.

31. Reichlin M, Maddison PJ, Targoff IN, et al. Antibodies to a nuclear/nucleolar antigen in patients with polymyositis-overlap syndrome. J Clin Immunol 1984;4:40–4.

32. Targoff IN. Autoantibodies to aminoacyl-transfer RNA synthetases for isoleucine and glycine: two additional synthetases are antigenic in myositis. J Immunol 1990;144:1737–43.

33. Reeves WH, Nigam SK, Blobel G. Human autoantibodies reactive with the signal-recognition particle. Proc Natl Acad Sci U S A 1986;83:9507–11.

34. Tan EM, Smolen JS, McDougal JS, et al. A critical evaluation of enzyme immunoassays for detection of antinuclear autoantibodies of defined specificities. I. Precision, sensitivity, and specificity [see comments]. Arthritis Rheum 1999;42(3):455–64.

35. Hengstman GJ, van Brenk L, Vree Egberts WT, et al. High specificity of myositis specific autoantibodies for myositis compared with other neuromuscular disorders. J Neurol 2005;252(5):534–7.

36. Hengstman GJ, Vree Egberts WT, Seelig HP, et al. Clinical characteristics of patients with myositis and autoantibodies to different fragments of the Mi-2β antigen. Ann Rheum Dis 2006;65:242–5.

37. Mahler M, Raijmakers R, Dahnrich C, Bluthner M, Fritzler MJ. Clinical evaluation of autoantibodies to a novel PM/Scl peptide antigen. Arthritis Res Ther 2005;7(3):R704–13.

38. Kao AH, Lacomis D, Lucas M, Fertig N, Oddis CV. Anti-signal recognition particle autoantibody in patients with and patients without idiopathic inflammatory myopathy. Arthritis Rheum 2004;50(1):209–15.

39. Targoff IN, Johnson AE, Miller FW. Antibody to signal recognition particle in polymyositis. Arthritis Rheum 1990;33:1361–70.

40. Williams J, Lucas M, Fertig N, Medsger TA. Anti-Ku antibody in patients with systemic sclerosis: comparison of clinical features associated with anti-U1RNP, anti-U3RNP, and anti-PM-Scl antibodies [Abstract]. Arthritis Rheum 2005;52:S590–1.

41. Mathews MB, Bernstein RM. Myositis autoantibody inhibits histidyl-tRNA synthetase: a model for autoimmunity. Nature 1983;304:177–9.

42. Vazquez-Abad D, Rothfield NF. Sensitivity and specificity of anti-Jo-1 antibodies in autoimmune diseases with myositis. Arthritis Rheum 1996;39:292–6.

43. Shamim EA, Rider LG, Pandey JP, et al. Differences in idiopathic inflammatory myopathy phenotypes and genotypes between Mesoamerican mestizos and North American Caucasians: ethnogeographic influences in the genetics and clinical expression of myositis. Arthritis Rheum 2002;46(7):1885–93.

44. Mathews MB, Reichlin M, Hughes GRV, Bernstein RM. Anti-threonyl-tRNA synthetase, a second myositis-related autoantibody. J Exp Med 1984;160:420–34.

45. Bunn CC, Bernstein RM, Mathews MB. Autoantibodies against alanyl-tRNA synthetase and tRNAala coexist and are associated with myositis. J Exp Med 1986;163:1281–91.

46. Hirakata M, Suwa A, Nagai S, et al. Anti-KS: identification of autoantibodies to asparaginyl-transfer RNA synthetase associated with interstitial lung disease. J Immunol 1999;162(4):2315–20.

47. Betteridge Z, Gunawardena H, North J, Slinn J, McHugh N. Anti-synthetase syndrome: a new autoantibody to phenylalanyl transfer RNA synthetase (anti-Zo) associated with polymyositis and interstitial pneumonia. Rheumatology 2007;46(6):1005–8.

48. Targoff IN, Trieu EP, Miller FW. Reaction of anti-OJ autoantibodies with components of the multi-enzyme complex of aminoacyl-tRNA synthetases in addition to isoleucyl-tRNA synthetase. J Clin Invest 1993;91:2556–64.

49. Targoff IN, Arnett FC. Clinical manifestations in patients with antibody to PL-12 antigen (alanyl-tRNA synthetase). Am J Med 1990;88:241–51.

50. Brouwer R, Vree Egberts W, Jongen PH, van Engelen BG, van Venrooij WJ. Frequent occurrence of anti-tRNA(His) autoantibodies that recognize a conformational epitope in sera of patients with myositis. Arthritis Rheum 1998;41:1428–37.

51. Fathi M, Vikgren J, Boijsen M, et al. Interstitial lung disease in polymyositis and dermatomyositis: longitudinal evaluation by pulmonary function and radiology. Arthritis Care Res 2008;59(5):677–85.

52. Furuya T, Hakoda M, Tsuchiya N, et al. Immunogenetic features in 120 Japanese patients with idiopathic inflammatory myopathy. J Rheumatol 2004;31(9):1768–74.

53. Yamasaki Y, Yamada H, Nozaki T, et al. Unusually high frequency of autoantibodies to PL-7 associated with milder muscle disease in Japanese patients with polymyositis/dermatomyositis. Arthritis Rheum 2006;54(6):2004–9.

54. Rider LG, Miller FW, Targoff IN, et al. A broadened spectrum of juvenile myositis: myositis-specific autoantibodies in children. Arthritis Rheum 1994;37:1534–8.

55. Feldman BM, Reichlin M, Laxer RM, Targoff IN, Stein LD, Silverman ED. Clinical significance of specific autoantibodies in juvenile dermatomyositis. J Rheumatol 1996;23:1794–97.

56. Espada G, Confalone Gregorian M, Ortiz Z, et al. Serum autoantibodies in juvenile idiopathic inflammatory myopathies (IIM) in a cohort of Argentine patients [Abstract]. Arthritis Rheum 1997;40:S140.

57. Legault D, McDermott J, Crous-Tsanaclis AM, Boire G. Cancer-associated myositis in the presence of anti-Jo1 autoantibodies and the antisynthetase syndrome. J Rheumatol 2008;35(1):169–71.

58. Respicio G, Shwaiki W, Abeles M. A 58-year-old man with anti-Jo-1 syndrome and renal cell carcinoma: a case report and discussion. Conn Med 2007;71(3):151–3.

59. Mozaffar T, Pestronk A. Myopathy with anti-Jo-1 antibodies: pathology in perimysium and neighbouring muscle fibres. J Neurol Neurosurg Psychiatry 2000;68:472–8.

60. Friedman AW, Targoff IN, Arnett FC. Interstitial lung disease with autoantibodies against aminoacyl-tRNA synthetases in the absence of clinically apparent myositis. Semin Arthritis Rheum 1996;26:459–67.

61. Douglas WW, Tazelaar HD, Hartman TE, et al. Polymyositis-dermatomyositis-associated interstitial lung disease. Am J Respir Crit Care Med 2001;164(7):1182–5.

62. Clawson K, Oddis CV. Adult respiratory distress syndrome in polymyositis patients with the anti-Jo-1 antibody. Arthritis Rheum 1995;38(10):1519–23.

63. Hirakata M, Nagai S. Interstitial lung disease in polymyositis and dermatomyositis. Curr Opin Rheumatol 2000;12(6):501–8.

64. Oddis CV, Medsger TA Jr, Cooperstein LA. A subluxing arthropathy associated with the anti-Jo-1 antibody in polymyositis/dermatomyositis. Arthritis Rheum 1990;33:1640–5.

65. Romisch K, Miller FW, Dobberstein B, High S. Human autoantibodies against the 54 kDa protein of the signal recognition particle block function at multiple stages. Arthritis Res Ther 2006;8(2):R39.

66. Satoh T, Okano T, Matsui T, et al. Novel autoantibodies against 7SL RNA in patients with polymyositis/dermatomyositis. J Rheumatol 2005;32(9):1727–33.

67. Hengstman GJ, ter Laak HJ, Vree Egberts WT, et al. Anti-signal recognition particle autoantibodies: marker of a necrotising myopathy. Ann Rheum Dis 2006;65(12):1635–8.
68. Miller T, Al Lozi MT, Lopate G, Pestronk A. Myopathy with antibodies to the signal recognition particle: clinical and pathological features. J Neurol Neurosurg Psychiatry 2002;73(4):420–8.
69. Joffe MM, Love LA, Leff RL, et al. Drug therapy of the idiopathic inflammatory myopathies: predictors of response to prednisone, azathioprine, and methotrexate and a comparison of their efficacy. Am J Med 1993;94:379–87.
70. Dimitri D, Andre C, Roucoules J, Hosseini H, Humbel RL, Authier FJ. Myopathy associated with anti-signal recognition peptide antibodies: clinical heterogeneity contrasts with stereotyped histopathology. Muscle Nerve 2007;35(3):389–95.
71. Leff RL, Burgess SH, Miller FW, et al. Distinct seasonal patterns in the onset of adult idiopathic inflammatory myopathy in patients with anti-Jo-1 and anti-signal recognition particle autoantibodies. Arthritis Rheum 1991;34:1391–6.
72. Nilasena DS, Trieu EP, Targoff IN. Analysis of the Mi-2 autoantigen of dermatomyositis. Arthritis Rheum 1995;38:123–8.
73. Seelig HP, Renz M, Targoff IN, Ge Q, Frank MB. Two forms of the major antigenic protein of the dermatomyositis-specific Mi-2 autoantigen. Arthritis Rheum 1996;39:1769–71.
74. Ge Q, Nilasena DS, O'Brien CA, Frank MB, Targoff IN. Molecular analysis of a major antigenic region of the 240-kD protein of Mi-2 autoantigen. J Clin Invest 1995;96:1730–7.
75. Seelig HP, Moosbrugger I, Ehrfeld H, Fink T, Renz M, Genth E. The major dermatomyositis-specific Mi-2 autoantigen is a presumed helicase involved in transcriptional activation. Arthritis Rheum 1995;38:1389–99.
76. Zhang Y, Ng HH, Erdjument-Bromage H, Tempst P, Bird A, Reinberg D. Analysis of the NuRD subunits reveals a histone deacetylase core complex and a connection with DNA methylation. Genes Dev 1999;13:1924–35.
77. Zhang Y, LeRoy G, Seelig HP, Lane WS, Reinberg D. The dermatomyositis-specific autoantigen Mi2 is a component of a complex containing histone deacetylase and nucleosome remodeling activities. Cell 1998;95:279–89.
78. Wang HB, Zhang Y. Mi2, an auto-antigen for dermatomyositis, is an ATP-dependent nucleosome remodeling factor. Nucleic Acids Res 2001;29(12):2517–21.
79. Wade PA, Gegonne A, Jones PL, Ballestar E, Aubry F, Wolffe AP. Mi-2 complex couples DNA methylation to chromatin remodelling and histone deacetylation. Nat Genet 1999;23:62–6.
80. Hausmanowa-Petrusewicz I, Kowalska-Oledzka E, Miller FW, et al. Clinical, serologic, and immunogenetic features in Polish patients with idiopathic inflammatory myopathies. Arthritis Rheum 1997;40:1257–66.
81. Okada S, Weatherhead E, Targoff IN, Wesley R, Miller FW. International Myositis Collaborative Study Group. Global surface ultraviolet radiation intensity may modulate the clinical and immunologic expression of autoimmune muscle disease. Arthritis Rheum 2003;48(8):2285–93.
82. Brouwer R, Vree Egberts WT, Hengstman GJ, et al. Autoantibodies directed to novel components of the PM/Scl complex, the human exosome. Arthritis Res 2002;4(2):134–8.
83. Ge Q, Wu Y, Trieu EP, Targoff IN. Analysis of the specificity of anti-PM-Scl autoantibodies. Arthritis Rheum 1994;37(10):1445–52.
84. Alderuccio F, Chan EKL, Tan EM. Molecular characterization of an autoantigen of PM-Scl in the polymyositis/scleroderma overlap syndrome: a unique and complete human cDNA encoding an apparent 75-kD acidic protein of the nucleolar complex. J Exp Med 1991;173:941–52.
85. Raijmakers R, Renz M, Wiemann C, et al. PM-Scl-75 is the main autoantigen in patients with the polymyositis/scleroderma overlap syndrome. Arthritis Rheum 2004;50(2):565–9.
86. Schilders G, Egberts WV, Raijmakers R, Pruijn GJ. C1D is a major autoantibody target in patients with the polymyositis-scleroderma overlap syndrome. Arthritis Rheum 2007;56(7):2449–54.
87. Schnitz W, Taylor-Albert E, Targoff IN, Reichlin M, Scofield RH. Anti-PM/Scl autoantibodies in patients without clinical polymyositis or scleroderma. J Rheumatol 1996;23:1729–33.
88. Genth E, Mierau R, Genetzky P, et al. Immunogenetic associations of scleroderma-related antinuclear antibodies. Arthritis Rheum 1990;33:657–65.

89. Jablonska S, Blaszczyk M. Scleroderma overlap syndromes. Adv ExpMed Biol 1999;455:85–92.
90. Mimori T, Hinterberger M, Pettersson I, Steitz JA. Autoantibodies to the U2 small nuclear ribonucleoprotein in scleroderma-polymyositis overlap syndrome. J Biol Chem 1984;259:560–5.
91. Okano Y, Medsger TA Jr. Newly identified U4/6 snRNP-binding proteins by serum autoantibodies from a patient with systemic sclerosis. J Immunol 1991;146:535–42.
92. Okano Y, Targoff IN, Oddis CV, et al. Anti-U5 small nuclear ribonucleoprotein (snRNP) antibodies: a rare anti-U snRNP specificity. Clin Immunol Immunopathol 1996;81:41–7.
93. Tormey VJ, Bunn CC, Denton CP, Black CM. Anti-fibrillarin antibodies in systemic sclerosis. Rheumatology 2001;40(10):1157–62.
94. Frank MB, McCubbin VR, Trieu EP, Wu Y, Isenberg DA, Targoff IN. The association of anti-Ro52 autoantibodies with myositis and scleroderma autoantibodies. J Autoimmun 1999;12:137–42.
95. Watkins C, Fertig N, Lucas M, Burlingame RW, Oddis CV. The diagnostic utility of anti-52 kDa Ro/SSA autoantibody testing in patients with idiopathic inflammatory myopathy and other myopathic syndromes [Abstract]. Arthritis Rheum 2004.
96. Casciola-Rosen LA, Pluta AF, Plotz PH, et al. The DNA mismatch repair enzyme PMS1 is a myositis-specific autoantigen. Arthritis Rheum 2001;44(2):389–96.
97. Targoff IN, Trieu EP, Sontheimer RD. Autoantibodies to 155 kd and Se antigens in patients with clinically-amyopathic dermatomyositis [Abstract]. Arthritis Rheum 2000;43:S194.
98. Betteridge ZE, Gunawardena H, Chinoy H, Ollier WER, Cooper RG, McHugh NJ. Clinical and immunogenetic characteristics of patients with autoantibodies to small ubiquitin-like modifier activating enzyme in dermatomyositis [Abstract]. Arthritis Rheum 2008;58:S227–8.
99. Tillie-Leblond I, Wislez M, Valeyre D, et al. Interstitial lung disease and anti-Jo-1 antibodies: difference between acute and gradual onset. Thorax 2008;63(1):53–9.
100. Katsumata Y, Ridgway WM, Oriss T, et al. Species-specific immune responses generated by histidyl-tRNA synthetase immunization are associated with muscle and lung inflammation. J Autoimmunity 2007;29(2-3):174–86.
101. Casciola-Rosen L, Andrade F, Ulanet D, Wong WB, Rosen A. Cleavage by granzyme B is strongly predictive of autoantigen status: implications for initiation of autoimmunity. J Exp Med 1999;190:815–26.
102. Casciola-Rosen L, Nagaraju K, Plotz P, et al. Enhanced autoantigen expression in regenerating muscle cells in idiopathic inflammatory myopathy. J Exp Med 2005;201(4):591–601.
103. Targoff IN. Immune manifestations of inflammatory muscle disease. Rheum Dis Clin North Am 1994;20(4):863.
104. Targoff IN. Laboratory testing in the diagnosis and management of idiopathic inflammatory myopathies. Rheum Dis Clin North Am 2002;28:859–890.
105. Brouwer R, Pruijn GJ, van Venrooij WJ. The human exosome: an autoantigenic complex of exoribonucleases in myositis and scleroderma. Arthritis Research 2001;3(2):102–106.
106. Mahler M, Raijmakers R. Novel aspects of autoantibodies to the PM/Scl complex: clinical, genetic and diagnostic insights. Autoimmunity Reviews 2007;6(7):432–437.
107. Craft J, Mimori T, Olsen TL, Hardin JA. The U2 small nuclear ribonucleoprotein particle as an autoantigen. Analysis with sera from patients with overlap syndromes. J Clin Invest 1988; 81:1716–1724.
108. Arad-Dann H, Isenberg D, Ovadia E, Shoenfeld Y, Sperling J, Sperling R. Autoantibodies against a nuclear 56-kDa protein: a marker for inflammatory muscle disease. J Autoimmun 1989;2:877–888.
109. Targoff IN, Hanas J. The polymyositis-associated Fer antigen is elongation factor 1a. Arthritis & Rheumatism 32, S81. 1989. (Abstract)
110. Targoff IN, Arnett FC, Berman L, O'Brien CA, Reichlin M. Anti-KJ: a new antibody associated with the myositis/lung syndrome that reacts with a translation-related protein. J Clin Invest 1989;84:162–172.
111. Dagenais A, Bibor-Hardy V, Senecal JL. A novel autoantibody causing a peripheral fluorescent antinuclear antibody pattern is specific for nuclear pore complexes. Arthritis Rheum 1988;31(10):1322–1327.

# Chapter 11
# Antisynthetase Syndrome

**Galina S. Marder and Robert Greenwald**

**Abstract** Antisynthetase syndrome is a systemic, inflammatory, autoimmune disease characterized by myositis, polyarthritis, and interstitial lung disease and is associated with presence of autoantibodies to transfer RNA (tRNA) synthetases (antisynthetase antibodies). We review the current literature on the role of antisynthetase antibodies in the pathogenesis of this syndrome, mechanism of injury, clinical picture of the antisynthetase syndrome, and current approach to the management of the disease.

**Keywords** Antisynthetase syndrome • Myositis • Inflammatory arthritis • Interstitial lung disease • Antisynthetase antibodies

## Introduction

Antisynthetase syndrome is a systemic, inflammatory, autoimmune disease characterized by myositis, polyarthritis, and interstitial lung disease (ILD). It is usually associated with the presence of autoantibodies to transfer RNA (tRNA) synthetases (antisynthetase antibodies). ILD complicating polymyositis (PM) was initially described by Mills and Matthews in 1956 *(1)*. In 1974, Frazier and Miller *(2)* described the clinical, radiological, and pathological features of pulmonary fibrosis associated with polymyositis and dermatomyositis (DM). It was not until 1980, however, that the first antisynthetase antibody, anti-Jo-1 antibody, was discovered. Initially, it was thought to be a marker of inflammatory myopathy alone, but in 1983 Yoshida and others *(3)* reported the association of these antibodies with the presence of pulmonary fibrosis in patients with myositis. These antibodies were

G.S. Marder (✉) and R. Greenwald
The Myositis and Vasculitis Center, North Shore Long Island Jewish Health System,
Albert Einstein College of Medicine, Lake Success, NY, USA

L.J. Kagen (ed.), The Inflammatory Myopathies,
DOI: 10/1007/978-1-60327-827-0_11,
© Humana Press. a part of Springer Science + Business Media, LLC 2009

subsequently acknowledged to be a principal component of a distinct syndrome called *antisynthetase syndrome*. Moreover, these antibodies appear to be important in the pathogenesis of this syndrome, and they may serve as surrogate biomarkers because their serum levels correlate with disease activity and may even appear prior to disease onset *(4–7)*. This chapter reviews the suggested pathogenesis and clinical and current approach to management of antisynthetase syndromes.

## Antisynthetase Autoantibodies and Their Targets

Aminoacyl-transfer RNA synthetases (ARSs) are a family of cytoplasmic enzymes that catalyze amino acid attachment to corresponding aminoacyl-tRNAs during the translation phase of protein synthesis *(8)*. They are divided into two classes (I and II) based on sequence motifs, molecular structure, and the site of aminoacylation *(9)*. While class II tRNA synthetases are present in cytoplasm in a free form, class I tRNA synthetases are associated in a multienzyme complex of nine synthetases that function together. All of the known antisynthetase antibodies, except anti-isoleucyl-tRNA, are against single class II tRNA enzymes found freely in the cytoplasm *(9–12)*.

Most studies have shown that autoantibodies to one synthetase do not cross-react with other synthetases *(13)*, and that they interact with the tRNA synthetase itself, not the tRNA *(12)*. Exceptions are Jo-1 antibodies, which have both activities *(12,14)*, and anti-alanyl-tRNA synthetase (PL-12), which also targets tRNA directly *(11)*. Isoleucyl-tRNA synthetase, which is a class I tRNA synthetase, exists and functions together with seven to nine other synthetases (those for glutamine, leucine, methionine, glutamic acid, arginine, lysine, and sometimes aspartic acid or proline) and is recognized by OJ autoantibodies. These OJ antibodies can recognize any individual component of the enzyme complex *(12,14)*. An antisynthetase autoantibody inhibits the enzymatic activity of the target synthetase antigen in vitro *(13)*, but it is unknown if this action plays any role in vivo.

Although eight antisynthetase antibodies have been reported to date, only six have been fully described *(4,12,13,15–18)*, and commercial assays are available for just five of them. Antibodies against tyrosyl-tRNA synthetase have been identified only in preliminary reports *(17)*. Two other antibodies, anti-KS (anti-asparaginyl-tRNA synthetase) *(8,9)* and anti-Zo (antiphenylalanyl-tRNA synthetase) *(17)*, have been described in a small number of cases, and although they have been accepted in the research community, assays for their detection are not available for routine practice.

In 1989, Targoff et al. *(19)* isolated antibodies to KJ antigen in two patients with a syndrome clinically similar to the antisynthetase syndrome, but the antigen appeared to be a translation factor, functionally similar to a tRNA synthetase but not actually a true synthetase. The clinical features of the syndrome and the functional similarity of the KJ antigen to a true tRNA synthetase strongly suggest a relationship between this unique autoantibody and the clinical syndrome.

Antibodies against synthetases are the most common among all myositis-specific antibodies, with reported frequencies up to 23–38% in some series *(7,20)*. Histidyl-tRNA synthetase (anti-Jo-1, HisRS) has the highest frequency among antisynthetases itself in myositis populations and is found in almost 15–25% of patients with myositis across various population selections *(7,12,20,21)*. OJ antibodies and EJ antibodies are observed infrequently, with occurrence in less than 2% of cases *(9,12,15)*. A list of the antisynthetase antibodies, their frequency, and clinical associations can be found in Table 11.1*(12)*.

## The Role of Jo-1 Autoantibodies in Pathogenesis

The close relationship between antisynthetase antibodies and the clinical syndrome has been a major focus of attention in the last three decades. Initially, the presence of these autoantibodies was attributed to the discovery of picornavirus RNA interaction with HisRS, causing a breach of tolerance with possible formation of antibodies to the self-antigen, that is, anti-Jo-1 *(3)*. However, further work has elucidated the pleotropic functions of these enzymes, synthetases, including their

**Table 11.1**  Types of antisynthetase antibodies

|            | Antigens                                        | Frequency                              | PM or DM | Myositis/ILD                                          | References      |
|------------|-------------------------------------------------|----------------------------------------|----------|-------------------------------------------------------|-----------------|
| Anti-Jo-1  | 1. Histidyl-tRNA 2. Histidyl-tRNA synthetase    | 25%                                    | PM > DM  | Subacute myositis in 95% and ILD in 80%               | *(4,12)*        |
| Anti-PL-7  | Threonyl-tRNA synthetase                        | 3–4% 17% in Japanese patients          | PM < DM  | Similar to Jo-1 profile                               | *(7,12,16,35)*  |
| Anti-PL-12 | 1. Alanyl-tRNA 2. Alanyl-tRNA synthetase        | 3–4%                                   | PM < DM  | ILD without myositis is more common, sclerodactyly    | *(12,36)*       |
| Anti-OJ    | Isoleucyl-tRNA, multienzyme complex             | <2%                                    | PM < DM  | Similar to Jo-1                                       | *(12,15)*       |
| Anti-EJ    | Glycyl-tRNA synthetase                          | <2%, but more common in Asians         | PM < DM  | ILD without myositis common                           | *(12,18)*       |
| Anti-KS    | Asparaginyl-tRNA synthetase                     |                                        | PM < DM  | Most with ILD without myositis                        | *(9,8,12)*      |
| Anti-Zo    | Phenylalanyl-tRNA synthetase                    | n/a                                    |          |                                                       | *(12,17)*       |
| KJ         | Translation factor Tyrosyl-tRNA synthetase      | n/a n/a; only one case reported        |          |                                                       | *(12,19)* *(17)* |

Modified from **Ref. *12***
*PM/DM* polymyositis/dermatomysitis

potential role in perpetuating humoral and cellular immune responses *(6,7,11,22–24)*. Three comprehensive reviews by Ascherman, Targoff, and Hengstman et al. *(6,7,24)* offered an in-depth analysis of many years of research on the possible role of Jo-1 antigen and its autoantibodies in the pathogenesis of myositis and associated lung disease.

Early studies by Miller et al. *(25)* showed that anti-Jo-1 immunoglobulin (Ig) G$_1$ levels correlate with disease activity independent of total IgG or IgG subclass and demonstrate immunoglobulin class switching of the antibodies over time, suggesting an antigen-driven mechanism. The striking association of anti-Jo-1 levels with disease activity was further confirmed in a large cross-sectional study and smaller longitudinal observations by Stone et al. *(5)*. The lack of cross-reactivity between antisynthetase antibodies also indicates a specific antigen-driven process rather than an epiphenomenon response to tissue injury when antibodies to multiple specificities would be expected *(6)*.

Further evidence implicating antisynthetases in the pathogenesis of the syndrome comes from induction of muscle and lung inflammation in mice in response to murine Jo-1 immunization, as demonstrated by the work of Katsumata *(26)*. In a mouse model developed by Nagaraju et al. *(27)*, major histocompatibility complex (MHC) class I upregulation in the skeletal muscles led to inflammatory myopathy with characteristics similar to human myositis, with high frequency of Jo-1 positivity. Moreover, Levine and others *(28)* demonstrated myositis-specific autoantigens present at higher levels in muscle tissue of patients with myositis compared with control subjects. Because MHC class I molecules present peptides from cytosolic proteins to cytotoxic T lymphocytes, it is conceivable that expression of the Jo-1 antigen could be intimately related to the MHC I upregulation in the muscle tissue, triggering cytotoxicity. Furthermore, studies demonstrated the existence of antigen-specific T cells directed against Jo-1 in peripheral blood of patients with antisynthetase syndrome *(22)*. These cells can promote cell-mediated cytolysis of muscle cells as well as anti-Jo-1 antibody formation in selected patients with polymyositis *(6,22)*.

The ability of aminoacyl-tRNA synthetases to function as regulators and signaling molecules in addition to taking part in protein translation was a fascinating discovery *(23)*. Several synthetases were capable of eliciting different chemotactic responses, as was demonstrated by the work of Howards and colleagues *(29)*. Tyrosyl tRNA was shown to have two distinct cytokine activities when released from apoptotic cells *(30)*. Additional functions (e.g., blocking apoptosis, signaling functions, and serving as a component of an interferon gamma [INFγ]-activated inhibitor of translation complex) have been attributed to various synthetases *(23)*. This evidence is complemented by clinical work that demonstrated significantly higher expression of IFN-inducible chemokines, such as CXCL9 and CXCL10, which are involved in the process of activated T-cell recruitment in Jo-1-positive patients *(31)*.

A higher level of expression of cleavable and noncleavable forms of HisRSs was detected in the alveolar epithelial layer of normal lungs compared with other tissues, further linking target tissues in the antisynthetase syndrome *(28)*.

These findings, coupled with the ability of HisRS and asparaginyl-tRNA synthetase to induce migration of T cells and monocytes to target tissue through interaction with chemokine receptors CCR3 and CCR5 *(29)*, provide an auxiliary explanation for the combination of clinical features of myositis and ILD in this syndrome. Furthermore, in patients with inflammatory myopathies, restricted accumulation of T lymphocytes expressing T-cell receptor (TCR) BV gene segments in lung and the muscle but not in peripheral blood was observed by Englund et al. *(32)*, also offering a possible explanation for a shared mechanism of injury targeting two key organs in antisynthetase syndrome.

In summary, although the initiating stimulus is not known, an extrinsic (i.e., picornavirus) or intrinsic factor causing apoptosis may lead to alteration of ARSs or their fragments and their expression in association with MHC class I molecule upregulation on the surface of the myocyte, alveolar cell, or monocyte. Later, the released antigen could be processed via antigen-presenting cells and presented to B cells, triggering antisynthetase antibody formation. In addition, released synthetases and their fragments functioning as chemokines generate T-cell and monocyte migration to the site and further perpetuate the inflammatory process (Fig. 11.1)*(6,11,23,24)*.

Shamim, Rider, and Miller *(33)* published a comprehensive review of currently available data on genetic associations in idiopathic inflammatory myopathies. In the isolated Jo-1-positive group, a strong association of HLA-DQA1*0501 or *0401 was demonstrated across three ethnic groups: whites, Hispanics, and blacks. HLA-DRB1*0301, DOB1*0201, and HLA DR3 were present in Jo-1-positive white patients *(12)*.

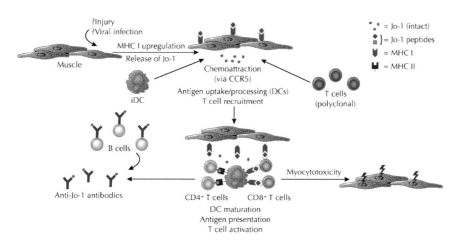

**Fig. 11.1** Proposed pathogenesis of antisynthetase syndrome. (From **Ref. 6**. Reprinted from *Current Rheumatology Reports*. Used with permission from Current Medicine Group, LLC, Philadelphia)

## Clinical Manifestations and Prognosis

The clinical picture of patients with antisynthetase syndromes has been evaluated in a number of small prospective studies as well as some large retrospective studies, most of which focused on Jo-1 antibody-associated cases. Other synthetases are much less common; therefore, the clinical information is based on small case series. Although the frequency of different clinical features of the syndrome varies considerably, the overall specificity of all described antisynthetases is high, and they have similar clinical associations *(11)*. Among the features most common for antisynthetase syndromes are myositis, arthritis, and ILD (Table 11.2).

## *Myositis*

Myositis associated with this syndrome has clinical characteristics similar to idiopathic inflammatory myositis not associated with antisynthetases. Overall reported frequency of myositis varies from 78 to 91% in Jo-1 antibody-associated cases *(34)*. Variability in reported results depends on the patient population, that is, if the subjects are exclusively from a myositis cohort or selected by antibody screening in a wider population. Myositis frequently is not the first symptom of the antisynthetase syndrome and in some cases may follow initial symptoms years later. Anti-Jo-1 antibodies have been found even before the onset of clinically detectable myositis *(25)*.

**Table 11.2** Principal clinical features of antisynthetase syndrome (*34,39–41*)

| Clinical manifestations | Reported incidence (%) | Clinical descriptors | Comments |
|---|---|---|---|
| ILD | 90 | NSIP, cellular and fibrotic<br>BOOP<br>DAD<br>UIP | May precede myositis |
| Myositis | 78–91 | Acute, subacute, sub-clinical or late onset, or absent | Incidence for Jo-1-associated cases, less common in PL-12- and KS-positive patients |
| Raynaud's | 62 | More common than in IIM | Usually severe sclerodactyly not reported |
| Arthritis | 94 | 1. Nonerosive polyarthritis<br>2. Erosive arthropathy | Subluxations reported |
|  | 64–83 | 3. Unspecified arthritis |  |
| Fever | 20 | At onset or during flares up to 87% |  |
| Mechanic's hands | 17–71 | Fissured hyperkeratotic skin over palmar surface and fingers | 1. Not a specific feature<br>2. One case of mechanic's feet is reported |

Analysis of the clinical picture of nine available cases of OJ-associated antisynthetase syndrome has demonstrated striking similarity to Jo-1-associated patients *(15)*. Anti-PL-7 and anti-PL-12 are found in fewer than 3% of all patients with idiopathic inflammatory myositis *(12,16)*. PL-7 antibody has been observed at higher prevalence in Japanese patients, and most of these patients had significantly milder muscle disease *(10,35)*. The EJ antibody-associated syndrome clinically resembles that of anti-Jo-1-associated cases, although dermatomyositis was reported more frequently than polymyositis *(7,15)*. According to Hirakata et al. *(8,9)*, KS antibodies have a much stronger association with ILD than with myositis and were more common with dermatomyositis in the small number of patients reported. Similarly, in PL-12-positive patients, myositis is significantly less frequent than ILD, with high occurrence of amyopathic antisynthetase syndrome *(12,36)*.

Myositis in antisynthetase syndrome has distinct histopathologic characteristics in anti-Jo-1-positive patients. Mozaffar and Pestronk *(37)* described distinct features of fragmentation of perimysial connective tissue with the inflammation, predominantly by macrophages, and significant perifascicular atrophy. This pattern is characteristic of dermatomyositis pathology but without the significant drop in capillary density that is usually associated with the vasculopathy of dermatomyositis (Table 11.3). Five of eleven patients in Späth's *(38)* cohort of anti-Jo-1-positive patients with myositis also had perifascicular atrophy with mononuclear perimysial infiltrate. The sparse pathological data require further corroboration.

## *Cutaneous*

The frequency of anti-Jo-1 antibodies is significantly higher in patients with polymyositis than in dermatomyositis *(34)*, but the reverse is true for all other antisynthetase antibodies. Characteristic scaly, fissured, hyperkeratotic skin changes

**Table 11.3** Characteristic histopathological features of myositis in antisynthetase syndrome based on Mozaffar and Pestronk's data (37)

| | Antisynthetase syndrome | Polymyositis | Dermatomyositis |
|---|---|---|---|
| Fragmentation of perimysial connective tissue | +++++[a] | + | + |
| Inflammation | | | |
|   Perimysial | +++++[a] Macrophage predominant | + | ++ |
|   Endomysial | + | +++ | + |
|   Perivascular | ½+ | +++ | +++ |
| Capillary distribution | Normal | Normal | Decreased density[a] |
| Perifascicular atrophy | +++++ | Absent | +++++ |

[a]Statistically significant difference

on the lateral and palmar surface of hands and fingers ("mechanic's hands") have been reported with a higher association in this syndrome but are not specific for this condition. These changes can also be found in some patients with dermatomyositis with other myositis-specific antibodies, such as Mi-2 and PM-Scl. The highest association of mechanic's hands with antisynthetase syndrome was reported in earlier studies with a frequency of 71%, but in all following studies the incidence was significantly lower, such as 17% in the study by Schmidt et al. *(34)* and 7% as reported by Mielnik and colleagues *(39)* (similar to the incidence in an anti-Jo-1-negative group).

## *Arthritis*

Other clinical manifestations, such as arthritis and Raynaud's phenomenon, are associated with antisynthetase syndrome at a higher frequency compared to patients with inflammatory myopathy without Jo-1 antibodies *(39)*. Sclerodactyly was also seen in at a higher frequency according to analysis by Schmidt and coworkers *(34)*, but the frequency was not statistically significant. It was however significantly higher in the study by Marguerie and colleagues *(40)*. Arthritis has been reported with a frequency of 64–83%, compared to only 18% in the serologically negative group *(34,39)*. Oddis et al. *(41)* evaluated patterns of arthritis in a Pittsburgh anti-Jo-1-positive cohort. They distinguished two distinct patterns: deforming nonerosive subluxing arthropathy (especially involving thumbs) and nondeforming arthropathy, primarily affecting small joints of the hands, wrists, shoulders and knees. An additional report of deforming arthritis and calcinosis in the absence of myositis associated with antisynthetase syndrome has been published *(42)*. Schmidt et al. *(34)* compiled data from their own cohort and cumulative results from various series and single cases available in print. They reported the combined frequency of erosive arthropathy was 16%, deforming arthritis was 18%, and unspecified arthritis was represented in 74% of collective patients.

## *Interstitial Lung Disease*

Interstitial lung disease is the most devastating symptom of antisynthetase syndrome. In the same Pittsburgh cohort of 98 patients with antisynthetase syndrome, ILD was reported in 64% of cases *(43)*. ILD can follow or precede the diagnosis of myositis and in some cases can present as the sole manifestation. Marguerie et al. *(40)* evaluated the clinical and laboratory features of 29 patients with Jo-1, anti-PL-12, and anti-PL-7 antibodies. Pulmonary fibrosis was seen in 23 of 29 patients, including 15 of 19 patients with Jo-1-positive antibodies, and only 16 of these patients had myositis. Friedman, Targoff, and Arnett *(44)* demonstrated that, in patients with antisynthetase antibodies with ILD and no myositis ($n = 10$), anti-PL-12 were the most common antibodies at 60%, followed by anti-Jo-1 and anti-OJ, with equal distribution. They also observed a more favorable response to corticosteroids as compared with idiopathic ILD, thus suggesting that patients with idiopathic ILD should be screened for antisynthetase antibodies because their prompt recognition could improve outcome.

When Yoshifuji et al. *(45)* stratified 41 cases of polymyositis or dermatomyositis associated with ILD/myositis into ILD-preceding, simultaneous, and myositis-preceding groups, antisynthetase antibodies were found more commonly in the ILD-preceding group ($p < 0.0$). They demonstrated that the presence of antisynthetases was predictive of a recurrent course and late-onset myopathy, although these patients had better responses to corticosteroids. These authors introduced the term SALID, seropositive amyopathic ILD. Because it is likely that new antisynthetase antibodies are to be discovered, the incidence of SALID could be much higher than was originally suspected *(45)*.

The ILD in patients with antisynthetase syndrome can dominate the disease course; it can be rapidly progressive, refractory to therapy, and occasionally fatal. Some cases may present as an acute respiratory syndrome (ARDS) *(46,47)*. The Tillie-Leblond group *(48)* conducted a multicenter retrospective analysis of patients with anti-Jo-1 antibody-associated ILD to study characteristics and long-term outcome of these patients. There were 32 patients enrolled; 47% of them presented with acute respiratory failure, and 53% had gradual onset of ILD. Patients who had received therapy for myositis before they presented with ILD were excluded from analysis. Median duration between symptoms, diagnosis, and acute respiratory failure in the acute group was 5 weeks and was 26 weeks in the group with gradual onset. Both fever on admission and acute respiratory insufficiency were seen in 47% of patients in this cohort and were observed more commonly in the acute group. The presence of myositis at the time of respiratory symptoms had no impact on prognosis. More patients presenting acutely with ILD improved at 3 months, 87 versus 53% in the gradual-onset group. They confirmed the original observation that relapses are common, and additional chronic immunosuppression is required *(48)*.

Chest radiography and pulmonary function tests are routinely used for evaluation of patients with suspected pulmonary involvement. Chest X-ray is not always sufficiently sensitive. High-resolution chest computed tomography (CT) provides much more information and is widely used in clinical practice. It is believed that the ground glass pattern in high-resolution CT (HRCT) indicates inflammatory reversible disease, and a reticular pattern correlates with pulmonary fibrosis. However, most of the early antisynthetase syndrome reports lack radiological findings in detail. Progress in imaging techniques has allowed the further characterization of pulmonary involvement, and more recent reports have closed the gap in the earlier literature on antisynthetase syndrome. Hara, Inoue, and Sato *(49)* described air space consolidation with traction bronchiectasis and ground glass opacities predominantly in lower lobes as the most frequent radiological findings in nine cases of ILD patients with positive EJ, PL-7, and anti-Jo-1 antibodies. According to Tillie-Leblond and colleagues *(48)*, three types of findings on chest HRCT can be seen: diffuse patchy ground glass attenuation, basal predominance of irregular linear opacities, and basal consolidation. These patterns were observed in 80% of patients with acute onset and 35% of patients with gradual onset. Schnabel et al. *(50)* observed that ground glass opacities on HRCT were associated with a progressive disease course.

Lung biopsy in ILD associated with dermatomyositis and polymyositis may show cellular or fibrotic forms of nonspecific interstitial pneumonia (NSIP), bronchiolitis obliterans organizing pneumonia (BOOP), pulmonary capillaritis associated with diffuse alveolar damage (DAD), and usual interstitial pneumonia (UIP) (Table 11.4) *(48,51,52)*. Multiple investigators have demonstrated a predominance of CD8 lymphocytes in broncholaveolar lavage and lung tissue immunostaining in patients with ILD associated with antisnthetase antibodies. *(46,53)*. Sauty et al. *(53)* reported NSIP in lung biopsy with CD8-positive lymphocytic alveolar inflammation in three of four patients with anti-Jo-1 antibodies who had no myositis during follow-up. NSIP was seen in 5 of 11 cases reported by Tillie-Leblond et al. *(48)*. In addition, diffuse alveolar damage and cryptogenic organizing pneumonia were observed only in the group of patients

**Table 11.4** Types of ILD observed in antisynthetase syndrome

| | | Clinical course | | | |
|---|---|---|---|---|---|
| Type | Histological finding | Acute | Chronic progressive | Asymptomatic | Prognosis |
| NSIP | Cellular-interstitial lympho-plasmocytic infiltrate and intraalveolar macrophages | + | + | + | More favorable |
| | Fibrotic-interstitial fibroblastic proliferation, collagen deposition, broadening of interstitial space, minimal lymphocytic infiltrate | | + | + | Poor |
| BOOP | Inflammatory lesion in terminal bronchioles and surrounding connective tissue with extension into distal airways | + | | + | More favorable |
| DAD | Pulmonary capillaritis associated or bland alveolar hemorrhage | + | | | Poor |
| UIP | Septal thickening and distortion with honeycombing, only mild or moderate degree of mononuclear inflammation | | + | + | Poor |

who presented with acute pulmonary distress, whereas usual interstitial pneumonitis was seen in the group presenting with gradual onset. It can be specu-
lated that a more inflammatory type of lung involvement (as seen in cellular
NSIP, BOOP, and DAD) leads to a more acute process with a better chance of
response to corticosteroids. Interstitial fibrotic changes with only mild or moderate degrees of mononuclear inflammation and honeycombing (such as in UIP
or fibrotic NSIP) are likely to have a more gradual, progressive course and be
resistant to corticosteroids alone *(51,54,55)*. Therefore, histopathological
evaluation is essential in patients with ILD and could be of prognostic value.

Pulmonary hypertension has been reported in association with ILD. Handa et al.
*(56)* reported a case of pulmonary hypertension with diffuse fibrosing interstitial
pneumonia in a patient with PL-12 antibody. Histological studies showed moderate
intimal proliferation in the muscular pulmonary arteries, suggestive of direct
inflammatory vascular lesions independent of vasoconstriction secondary to ILD-
induced hypoxia.

In addition to the extramuscular manifestations mentioned, serositis, carditis,
and cardiomyopathy have been reported *(52)*. Pericarditis was in 18% of Jo-1-
positive patients found in the series by Schmidt et al. *(34)*, but only a few additional
cases of pericardial and pleural effusion have been reported since *(57)*.

## Prognosis and Treatment

The clinical course of Jo-1 and other synthetase antibody-positive patients was
monocyclic with full recovery within 2 years in 21–31%, but the majority of
patients had polycyclic relapsing (27–28%) or a chronic course (31–35%) as
reported in analysis of a Mediterranean cohort *(21)*. Mortality in this syndrome is
reported to be 12%–40% *(21,38,48,58)*. According to the analysis by Tillie-Leblond
and others *(48)*, patients presenting acutely had 6% mortality during the first 3
months compared to 18% overall mortality during 62 months of follow-up. Overall
prognosis of patients with the antisynthetase syndrome was significantly worse
compared with patients with myositis without antibodies, mostly because of ILD.
Interestingly, outcome was good in both the antisynthetase-positive and -negative
groups in a retrospective review by Mielnik et al. *(39)*, probably because of significant underrepresentation of patients with ILD. Survival of patients with ILD positive for Jo-1 antibodies was 85% at 1 year, 74% at 3-year follow-up, and 60% at
6-year follow-up according to observations by Douglas et al. *(54)*. There was no
statistically significant difference between serologically positive and negative
groups that allowed the conclusion that the presence of positive Jo-1 antibody has
no prognostic value on survival.

Likewise, in a retrospective review of long-term outcome in polymyositis
and dermatomyositis by Bronner et al. *(58)*, patients with Jo-1 antibodies did

not do worse than serologically negative patients in either disability or quality of life, but they did require longer courses of immunosuppressive therapy. Yoshifuji and colleagues *(45)* investigated the response of ILD to corticosteroids in 41 cases of polymyositis or dermatomyositis with ILD and compared the responses between the serologically positive and negative groups. Although the response rate of ILD to corticosteroids was significantly better in the seropositive group ($p < 0.01$), the recurrence rate was also significantly higher ($p < 0.01$). Nevertheless, a 2-year prognosis of pulmonary function was similar in both groups.

Corticosteroids remain the mainstay first-line therapy for myositis and ILD. They are usually used at an initial dose of 1 mg/kg and slowly tapered over a period of months. In rare cases presenting with acute respiratory failure, pulse steroids should be considered. An individualized approach in each case is extremely important. The manifestations at disease onset may determine the dose and length of the initial therapy with corticosteroids and the need for the addition of an immunosuppressive agent. Although myositis and arthritis respond to corticosteroids favorably, ILD, despite a good initial response to corticosteroids alone, frequently recurs as corticosteroids are tapered and requires long-term immunosuppression. Tillie-Leblond et al. *(48)* demonstrated higher mortality and a higher rate of progression in the group treated with corticosteroid alone.

There is no consensus regarding a steroid-sparing agent, regimen of induction, and length of maintenance. Although some data have been compiled on the use of immunosuppressive agents, most of the data come from case reports and series and retrospective reviews *(39,43,46,48,53–55,59–61)*. Cyclophosphamide, azathioprine, mycophenolate mofetil, cyclosporine, and tacrolimus are most frequently used.

Wilkes et al. *(43)* conducted a retrospective review of 13 charts of patients with antisynthetase-associated ILD and idiopathic inflammatory myopathy (IIM) to evaluate the efficacy of tacrolimus. All but one (positive for PL-12) had Jo-1 antibodies. The majority previously failed immunosuppressive therapy with methotrexate, azathioprine, or cyclophosphamide. Twenty percent (3 of 13) were treated with tacrolimus as the first choice of immunosuppressive therapy. A significant improvement in pulmonary function tests paralleled statistically significant reduction in steroid dosage. A few cases of antisynthetase syndrome treated successfully with rituximab were reported Table 11.5 *(61,62)*.

# Conclusion

Prospective therapeutic trials focusing on pulmonary morbidity and long-term outcome are needed. Further understanding of the pathophysiology of the syndrome will allow development of a targeted therapeutic approach.

**Table 11.5** Treatment of antisynthetase-associated ILD cases reported in the literature

| Year | Design | N | Clinical features | Therapy | Outcome | References |
|---|---|---|---|---|---|---|
| 1996 | Retrospective analysis | 10 | PL-12-6 OJ-2 Jo-1-2 | Steroids ± 3-cytoxan, 2-Azathioprine (2-AZA) | 6/10 resolved or improved | (44) |
| 1997 | Case series | 4 | Jo-1 + ILD | Steroids (high dose) + cyclosporine | 4/4 improved | (53) |
| 1999 | Case report | 1 | Jo-1-positive BOOP with DM | Cytoxan + steroids | Improved | (55) |
| 2001 | Retrospect multi-center | 32 | Percentage of Jo-1 positivity not reported | Cyclosporine + steroids | Survival was better with combination treatment than corticos-teroids alone | (48) |
| 2001 | Case report | 1 | ILD as initial manifestation Jo-1 positive | Cytoxan (CTX) + prednisolone | ILD and myosi-tis improved | (60) |
| 2005 | Case report | 1 | Jo-1 + refractory myositis, ILD Failed MTX | Steroids and Rituxan | Improved | (62) |
| 2005 | Retrospective analysis | 13 | Jo-1–12 PL-12-1 | Steroids and tacrolimus | Improved | (43) |
| 2006 | Case report | 1 | Jo-1 + synovitis and myositis, ILD failed Methotrexate (MTX) | Steroids and Rituxan | Improved but relapsed, responded with re-treat-ment | (61) |
| 2006 | Case report | 1 | Jo-1 positive | Steroids and Leflunomide | Improved | (63) |
| 2006 | Case report | 1 | Jo-1 + multiple pulmonary nodules, mechanic's foot | Steroids and cytoxan for induction and cyclosporine for mainte-nance | Improved with partial resolution of Nodules | (57) |
| 2007 | Case report | 2 | Jo-1 + acute respiratory failure | Steroids + cyclosporine | Improved | (64) |
| 2007 | Case report | 1 | Jo-1 + ILD and deforming arthritis, cal-cinosis | Steroids and tac-rolimus | Improved | (42) |
| 2008 | Case report | 1 | Jo-1 + ARDS, NSIP on biopsy | Steroids + tac-rolimus | Rapidly improved | (46) |

# References

1. Mills ES, Matthews WH. Interstitial pneumonitis in dermatomyositis. JAMA 1956; 160:1467–70.
2. Frazier AR, Miller RD. Interstitial pneumonitis in association with polymyositis and dermatomyositis. Chest 1974;65:403–7.
3. Yoshida S, Akizuki M, Imori T, et al. The precipitating antibody to an acidic nuclear protein antigen, the Jo-1, in connective tissue diseases. A marker for a subset of polymyositis with interstitial pulmonary fibrosis. Arthritis Rheum 1983;26:604–11.
4. Mathews MB, Bernstein RM.Myosmitis autoantibody inhibit histidyl-tRNA synthetase: a model for autoimmunity. Nature 1983;304:177–9.
5. Stone KB, Oddis CV, Fertig N, et al. Anti-Jo-1 antibody levels correlate with disease activity in idiopathic inflammatory myopathy. Arthritis Rheum 2007;56(9):3125–31.
6. Ascherman D. The role of Jo-1 in the immunopathogenesis of polymyositis: current hypotheses. Curr Rheumatol Rep 2003;1523(3774):426–30.
7. Targoff IN. Autoantibodies and their significance in myositis. Curr Rheumatol Rep 2008;10(4):333–40.
8. Hirakata M, Suwa A, Takada T, et al. Clinical and immunogenetic features of patients with autoantibodies to asparaginyl-transfer RNA synthetase. Arthritis Rheum 2007;56:1295–303.
9. Hirakata M, Suwa A, Nagai S, et al. Anti KS: identification of autoantibodies to asparaginyl-transfer RNA synthetase associated with interstitial lung disease. J Immunol 1999;162:2315–20.
10. Matsushita T, Hasegawa M, Fujimoto M, et al. Clinical evaluation of anti-aminoacyl tRNA synthetase antibodies in Japanese patients with dermatomyositis. J Rheumatol 2007;34:1012–18.
11. Targoff IN. Update on myositis-specific and myositis-associated autoantibodies. Curr Opin Rheumatol 2000;12(6):475–81.
12. Targoff IN. Laboratory testing in the diagnosis and management of idiopathic inflammatory myopathies. Rheum Dis Clin North Am 2002;28:859–90.
13. Plotz PN, Rider LG, Targoff IN, Raben N, O'Hanlon TP, Miller FW. NIH conference. Myositis: immunologic contributions to understanding cause, pathogenesis, and therapy. Ann Intern Med 1995;122(9):715–24.
14. Brouwer R, Egberts WV, Jongen PH, Van Engelen BGM, Vendrooij WJ. Frequent occurrence of anti RNA-his autoantibodies that recognize a conformational epitope in sera of patients with myositis. Arthritis Rheum 1998;41(8):1428–37.
15. Targoff IN, Trieu EP, Miller FW. Reaction of anti-OJ autoantibodies with components of the multi-enzyme complex of aminoacyl-tRNA synthetases in addition to isoleucyl-tRNA synthetase. J Clin Invest 1993;9:2556–64.
16. Mathew M, Reichlin M, Hughes GRV, Bernstein RM. PL-7 anti-threonyl-tRNA synthetase, a second myositis related autoantibody. J Exp Med 1984;160:420–34.
17. Betteridge Z, Gunawardena H, North J, Slinn J, McHugh N. Anti-synthetase syndrome: a new autoantibody to phenylalanyl transfer RNA synthetase (anti Zo) associated with polymyositis and interstitial pneumonia. Rheumatology (Oxford) 2007;46:1005–8.
18. Hirakata M, Suwa A, Tkeda Y, et al. Autoantibodies to glycyl-transfer RNA synthetase in myositis. Arthritis Rheum 1996;39(1):146–51.
19. Targoff IN, Arnett FC, Berman L, O'Brien C, Reichlin M. Anti KJ—a new antibody associated with the syndrome of polymyositis and interstitial lung disease. J Clin Invest 1989;84:162–72.
20. Brouwer R, Hengstman GJD, Egberts WV, et al. Autoantibody profiles in the sera of European patients with myositis. Ann Rheum Dis 2001;60:116–23.
21. Selva-O'Callaghan A, Labrador-Horrilllo M, Solans-Laque R, Pilar Simeon-Aznar C, Martinez-Gomez X, Viardell-Tarres M. Myositis-specific and myositis-associated antibodies in a series of eighty-eight Mediterranean patients with idiopathic inflammatory myopathy. Arthritis Rheum 2006;55(5):791–8.

22. Ascherman DP, Oriss TB, Oddis CV, Wright TM. Critical requirements for professional APC in eliciting T cell response to novel fragments of histidyl tRNA synthetase (Jo-1) in Jo-1 positive polymyositis. J Immunol 2002;169:7127–34.
23. Park SG, Kim HJ, Min YH, et al. Human lysyl-tRNA synthetase is secreted to trigger proinflammatory response. Proc Natl Acad Sci U S A 2005;102(18):6356–61.
24. Hengstman GJD, van Engelen BGM, van Venrooij WJ. Myositis specific autoantibodies: changing insights in pathophysiology and clinical associations. Curr Opin Rheumatol 2004;16:692–9.
25. Milller FW, Twitty SA, Biswas T, Plotz PH. Origin and regulation of a disease-specific autoantibody response. Antigenic epitopes, spectrotype restriction of anti-Jo-1 autoantibodies. J Clin Invest 1990;85:468–75.
26. Katsumata Y. Species-specific immune response generated by histidyl-tRNA synthetase immunization are associated with muscle and lung inflammation. J Autoimmun 2007;29(2–3):174–86.
27. Nagaraju K, Raben N, Loeffler L, et al. Conditional up-regulation of MHC class I in skeletal muscle leads to self sustaining autoimmune myositis- myositis specific autoantibodies. Proc Natl Acad Sci U S A 2000;97(16):9209–14.
28. Levine SM, Raben N, Xie D, et al. Novel conformation of histidyl-transfer RNA synthetase in the lung. The target tissue in Jo1 autoantibody-associated myositis. Arthritis Rheum 2007;56(8):2729–39.
29. Howard OMZ, Dong HF, Yang D, et al. Histidyl-tRNA synthetase and asparaginyl-tRNA synthetase, autoantigens in myositis, activate chemokine receptors on T lymphocytes and immature dendritic cells. J Exp Med 2002;196(6):781–91.
30. Casciola-Rosen L. Autoimmune myositis: new concepts for disease initiation and propagation. Curr Opin Rheumatol 2005;17:699–700.
31. Eggebeen A, Rosas I, Kaminski N, Richards T, Oddis C, Ascherman D. Serum biomarkers of interstitial lung disease in Jo-1 antibody-positive myositis patients. Arthritis Rheum Abstract Supplement, 2007 Annual Scientific Meeting.
32. Englund PWJ, Fathi M, Rasmussen E, Grunewald J, Tornling G, Lundberg IE. Restricted TCR BV gene usage in lungs and muscle tissue of patients with idiopathic inflammatory myopathies. Arthritis Rheum 2007;56:372–83.
33. Shamim EA, Rider LG, Miller FW. Update on the genetics of the idiopathic inflammatory myopathies. Curr Opin Rheumatol 2000;12:482–91.
34. Schmidt WA, Wetzel W, Friedlander R, et al. Clinical and serological aspects of patients with anti-Jo-1 antibodies-an evolving spectrum of disease manifestations. Clin Rheumatol 2000;19:371–7.
35. Yamasaki Y, Yamada H, Nozaki T, et al. Unusually high frequency of autoantibodies to PL-7 associated with milder muscle disease in Japanese patients with polymyositis/dermatomyositis. Arthritis Rheum 2006;54(6):2004–9.
36. Targoff IN, Arnett FC. Clinical manifestations in patients with antibody to PL12 antigen. Am J Med 1990;88(3):241–51.
37. Mozaffar T, Pestronk A. Myopathy with anti Jo-1 antibodies: pathology in perimysium and neighbouring muscle fibers. J Neurol Neurosurg Psychiatry 2000;68:472–8.
38. Späth M, Schroder M, Schlotter-Weigel B, et al. The long term outcome of anti Jo-1 positive inflammatory myopathies. J Neurol 2004;251:859–64.
39. Mielnik P, Wiesik-Szewczyk E, Olesinka M, Chwalinska-Sadowska H, Zabek J. Clinical features and prognosis of patients with idiopathic inflammatory myopathies and anti Jo-1 antibodies. Autoimmunity 2006;39(3):243–7.
40. Marguerie C, Bunn CC, Beynon HLC, et al. Polymyositis, pulmonary fibrosis and autoantibodies to aminoacyl-tRNA synthetase enzymes. Q J Med 1990;77(282):1019–38.
41. Oddis CV, Medsger TA Jr, Cooperstein LA. A subluxing arthropathy associated with the anti-Jo-1 antibody in polymyositis/dermatomyositis. Arthritis Rheum 1990;33(11):1640S.
42. Ozrturk MA, Unverdi S, Goker B, Haznedaroglu S, Tunc L. A patient with antisynthetase syndrome associated with deforming arthritis and periarticular calcinosis sine myositis. Scand J Rheumatol 2007;36(3):239–41.
43. Wilkes MR, Sereika SM, Fertig N, Lucas MR, Oddis CV. Treatment of antisynthetase-associated interstitial lung disease with tacrolimus. Arthritis Rheum 2005;52(8):2439–46.

44. Friedman AW, Targoff IN, Arnett FC. Interstitial lung disease with autoantibodies against aminoacyl-tRNA synthetases in the absence of clinically apparent myositis. Semin Arthritis Rheum 1996;26(1):459–67.

45. Yoshifuji H, Fujii T, Kobayashi S, et al. Anti-aminoacyl-tRNA synthetase antibodies in clinical course prediction of interstitial lung disease complicated with idiopathic inflammatory myopathies. Autoimmunity 2006;39(3):233–41.

46. Gugliemi S, Merz TM, Gugger M, Suter C, Nicod LP. Acute respiratory distress syndrome secondary to antisynthetase syndrome is reversible with tacrolimus. Eur Respir J 2008;31:213–7.

47. Clawson K, Oddis CV. Adult respiratory distress syndrome in polymyositis patients with the anti-Jo-1 antibody. Arthritis Rheum 1995;38(10):1519–23.

48. Tillie-Leblond I, Wislez M, Valeyre D, et al. Interstitial lung disease and anti-Jo-1 antibodies: difference between acute and gradual onset. Thorax 2008;63(1):53–9.

49. Hara H, Inoue Y, Sato T. [Clinical and pathological findings of patients with interstitial lung disease associated with antisynthetase] [Abstract]. Nihon Kokyuki Gakkai Zasshi 2005;43(11):652–63.

50. Schnabel A, Reuter M, Biederer J, Richter C, Gross WL. Interstitial lung disease in polymyositis and dermatomyositis: clinical course and response to treatment. Semin Arthritis Rheum 2003;32(5):273–84.

51. Schwarz MI. The lung in polymyositis. Clin Chest Med 1998;19:701–71.

52. Fathi M. Interstitial lung disease in polymyositis and dermatomyositis. Stockholm: Karolinska Institutet, 2006.

53. Sauty A, Rochat T, Schoch D, et al. Pulmonary fibrosis with predominant CD8 lymphocytic alveolitis and anti-Jo-1 antibodies. Eur Respir J 1997;10:2907–12.

54. Douglas WW, Tazelaar HD, Hartman TE, et al. Polymyositis-dermatomyositis-associated interstitial lung disease. Am J Respir Crit Care Med 2001;164(7):1182–5.

55. Knoell KA, Hook M, Griece DP, Hendrix JD. Dermatomyositis associated with bronchiolitis obliterans organizing pneumonia (BOOP). J Am Acad Dermatol 1999;40(2):328–30.

56. Handa T, Nagai S, Kawabata D, et al. Long-term clinical course of a patient with anti PL-12 antibody accompanied by interstitial pneumonia and severe pulmonary hypertension. Intern Med 2005;44(4):319–25.

57. Mogulkoc N, Kabasakal Y, Ekren P, Bishop P. An unusual presentation of anti-Jo-1 syndrome, mimicking lung metastases, with massive pleural and pericardial effusions. J Clin Rheumatol 2006;12(2):90–2.

58. Bronner IM, van der Meulen MFG, de Visser M, et al. Long-term outcome in polymyositis and dermatomyositis. Ann Rheum Dis 2006;65:1456–61.

59. Kenji N, Masayoshi H, Masako H, Yasuyuki Y, Takao K, Nobuyuki M. Efficacy of cyclosporine treatment to interstitial pneumonitis associated with polymyositis and dermatomyositis. Arthritis Rheum 2001;44(9):S353 (Abstract 1804).

60. Lumpa J, Nennesma I, Einarsdottir H, Lundberg I. MRI-guided muscle biopsy confirmed polymyositis diagnosis in a patient with interstitial lung disease. Ann Rheum Dis 2001;60(4):423–6.

61. Brulhart L, Waldburger JM, Gabay C. Rituximab in the treatment of antisynthetase syndrome. Ann Rheum Dis 2006;65:974–5.

62. Labotte O, Kotb R, Maigne G, Blanc FX, Goujard C, Delfraissy JF. Efficacy of rituximab in refractory myositis. J Rheumatol 2005;32(7):1369–70.

63. Lange U, Piegsa M, Muller-Ladner U, Strunk J. Anti Jo-1 antibody positive polymyositis-successful therapy with leflunomide. Autoimmunity 2006;39(3):261–4.

64. Jordan Greco AS, Metrailler JC, Dayer E. The antisynthetase syndrome: a cause of rapidly progressive interstitial lung disease [Abstract]. Rev Med Suisse 2007;3(134):2675–6, 2679–81.

# Chapter 12
# Pulmonary Manifestations of Inflammatory Myopathy

**Eun Ha Kang and Yeong Wook Song**

**Abstract** Pulmonary manifestations are common findings in polymyositis and dermatomyositis and substantially contribute to morbidity and mortality. Interstitial lung disease (ILD) is the most frequent type of pulmonary manifestation, followed by aspiration pneumonia and hypoventilation. The clinical course of ILD in myositis varies from asymptomatic to rapidly progressive, and treatment response is variable depending on underlying histopathologic patterns. These observations suggest that different mechanisms are involved in the pathogenesis of myositis-associated ILD. Histopathologic patterns of ILD are broad in myositis, and nonspecific interstitial pneumonia is the pattern most frequently encountered. An initial lung evaluation should be performed in all myositis patients because a significant number of patients are asymptomatic. High-resolution computed tomography and pulmonary function tests are useful for assessing disease extent and activity. Bronchoalveolar lavage and lung biopsies can help exclude infectious causes and determine prognoses. No optimal treatment has been established for ILD in myositis. Despite a lack of controlled studies, corticosteroid therapy has been widely used as initial treatment; immunosuppressive agents are added later if response is unsatisfactory. However, the early administration of immunosuppressive agents can improve treatment response, particularly in patients who present with rapidly progressive ILD. Because of its heterogeneous clinical course, not all ILD patients need immunosuppression, and a substantial proportion of patients shows stable ILD, requiring only monitoring or mild-to-moderate treatment. Opportunistic lung infections should be considered in the differential diagnosis when response to aggressive treatment is inadequate.

**Keywords** Polymyositis • Dermatomyositis • Myositis • Interstitial lung disease

E.H. Kang and Y.W. Song (✉)
Department of Internal Medicine, Division of Rheumatology,
Seoul National University Hospital, Seoul, Korea

L.J. Kagen (ed.), *The Inflammatory Myopathies*,
DOI 10.1007/978-1-60327-827-0_12,
© Humana Press, a part of Springer Science+Business Media, LLC 2009

# Introduction

Polymyositis (PM) and dermatomyositis (DM) are systemic autoimmune diseases in which muscle is the primary target of immune-mediated inflammation. Although histological evidence suggests that PM and DM result from different immunopathogenesis, they share most clinical manifestations except skin rashes (e.g., Gottron's papules or heliotrope rash), which are observed only in DM *(1)*. In addition to muscle inflammation and dysfunction, systemic complications shared by PM and DM involve vessels, joints, gastrointestinal tracts, cardiac tissues, and lungs. In particular, damage to lung parenchyma, which manifests as interstitial lung disease (ILD), is a major prognostic factor that substantially contributes to morbidity and mortality *(2,3)*.

Interstitial lung disease develops in 23.1-65% of myositis patients *(3,4)*. Prevalence estimates vary depending on whether clinical, functional, radiographic, or histologic criteria are used to define ILD. With the introduction of modern technologies, such as, high-resolution computed tomography (HRCT) and pulmonary function testing, the prevalence is as high as 65% *(4)*. The strongest predictive factor for ILD in myositis is the presence of positivity for anti-aminoacyl-tRNA (transfer RNA) synthetase antibodies (anti-synthetase antibodies), of which the anti-histidyl-tRNA synthetase (anti-Jo-1) antibody is the most commonly encountered and is found in approximately 20% of myositis patients *(5)*. The reported frequency of ILD in patients with anti-Jo-1 antibodies exceeds 70% *(3,4,6)*.

Although ILD is the most common form of lung involvement in PM and DM, there are a number of other disease components of myositis that also result in secondary pulmonary complications (i.e., ventilatory failure due to respiratory muscle weakness, aspiration pneumonia due to esophageal dysfunction, pulmonary edema caused by cardiac involvement, and vascular disease in the form of pulmonary hypertension) (Table 12.1) *(3,7–9)*. Furthermore, it should also be emphasized that in addition to

**Table 12.1** Pulmonary manifestations in PM and DM

Primary lung involvements
  Interstitial lung disease
    Nonspecific interstitial pneumonia
    Unusual interstitial pneumonia
    Diffuse alveolar damage
    Bronchiolitis obliterans organizing pneumonia
    Others
Secondary lung involvements
  Aspiration pneumonia
  Infection (opportunistic and conventional)
  Respiratory muscle failure
  Pulmonary edema due to congestive heart failure
  Pulmonary arterial hypertension
  Vasculitis

the pulmonary manifestations associated with myositis itself, treatment-related infections are another important source of pulmonary manifestations in PM and DM patients *(10)*.

# Interstitial Lung Disease

## *Clinical Manifestations*

Interstitial lung disease can appear with, before, or after the onset of skin or muscle manifestations but tends to be a component of early myositis *(3,6,11–13)*. Cough and dyspnea are the most commonly reported symptoms *(3,4,11,13)*. ILD occurring in the context of myositis has been described to adopt one of three clinical patterns based on symptoms at presentation: rapidly progressive form with acute onset symptoms, subacute form with slowly progressive symptoms, and asymptomatic or subclinical form with an abnormal chest radiograph or an abnormal pulmonary function test but without any pulmonary complaints *(3,7)*. However, ILD that initially presents as a slowly progressive or asymptomatic pattern can transform into the rapidly progressive pattern during the later course of the disease *(14)*.

A slowly progressive pattern presenting with insidious onset dyspnea and a nonproductive cough is the most common variant. Constitutional symptoms are unremarkable in this subset of patients. The acute forms occur in less than 20% of PM and DM patients with ILD *(3)* and are often accompanied by constitutional symptoms, such as fever and malaise. Treatment response is highly variable depending on underlying histopathologic processes. Because the acute clinical course often rapidly progresses to respiratory failure, ruling out infection before initiating immunosuppressive treatment is the major challenge in this form of ILD. Rapidly progressive ILD was noted in patients with so-called amyopathic dermatomyositis (ADM), who have the typical rash of DM (Gottron's papules or heliotrope rash) but without muscle symptoms *(15–18)*. ILD in these patients characteristically responds poorly to even aggressive treatment and progresses rapidly to respiratory failure *(16–18)*.

Up to 30% of PM and DM patients seem to have subclinical or asymptomatic ILD *(3,18)*. Complaints associated with another organ disease may overwhelm subtle pulmonary discomforts in these patients. Alternatively, these patients may not have exertional dyspnea because of limited physical activity due to musculoskeletal involvements. This lack of overt symptoms emphasizes the need for pulmonary screening in all myositis patients, especially those with anti-Jo-1 antibody.

Overall 5-year survival rates of patients with myositis-associated ILD are around 70% *(3,19)*, but ILD in the context of ADM often adopts a clinical course of acute presentation, a histologic pattern of diffuse alveolar damage (DAD), and a poor treatment response and is associated with high mortality rates *(16–18)*.

## *Histopathology and Radiologic Findings*

A broad range of histologic patterns have been reported in patients with myositis-associated ILD, such as bronchiolitis obliterans organizing pneumonia (BOOP; or cryptogenic organizing pneumonia), DAD, nonspecific interstitial pneumonia (NSIP), and usual interstitial pneumonia (UIP) *(20)*. Furthermore, ILD in myositis tends to exhibit a mixture of more than one histological pattern *(21)*. Since the classification of idiopathic ILD was newly standardized to categorize NSIP as a distinct histologic pattern *(22)*, studies have shown that NSIP is the most frequent pattern in PM and DM *(13,19,21)*. NSIP is distinguished from UIP by a distinct inflammatory component, whereas UIP is characterized by numerous fibroblast foci disseminated in a temporally heterogeneous fibrotic background (Fig. 12.1) *(22)*. The main features of NSIP are a temporally uniform, diffuse, or patchy mixture of interstitial inflammation and fibrosis with a varying ratio (Fig. 12.2a) *(22)*. Treatment response of ILD varies depending on the underlying histological pattern. BOOP responds favorably to corticosteroids, whereas DAD and UIP respond poorly to immunosuppressive therapies, including corticosteroids, and exhibit poor prognoses *(3,20)*. The response of NSIP to corticosteroids depends on degrees of inflammation and fibrosis *(19,21)*. A broad range of histopathologic patterns and the varying degrees of responsiveness to treatment that are dependent on underlying histopathology suggest that the mechanisms to develop ILD could be heterogeneous in myositis.

HRCT has become the preferred imaging technique to detect the early stages of ILD due to its much higher sensitivity than simple chest radiography. Furthermore, HRCT distinctly visualizes various histopathologies of ILD and provides useful information on disease activity *(22–24)*. For example, a reticular

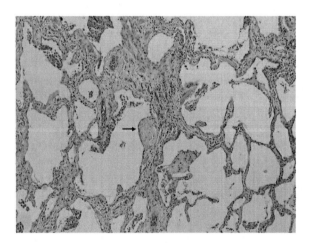

**Fig. 12.1** The fibroblastic foci (*arrow*) are present adjacent to areas of established dense fibrosis, which represent the characteristic "temporal heterogeneity," the cardinal feature of UIP. Mild-to-moderate interstitial inflammation and microscopic honeycomb change are also observed.

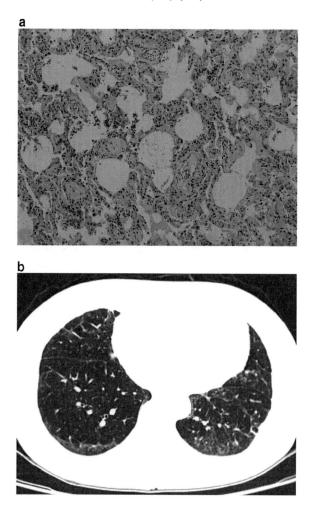

**Fig. 12.2** Nonspecific interstitial pneumonia (NSIP). (**a**) There are chronic inflammatory infiltrates and fibrosis in the interstitium, which are diffuse and temporally uniform in contrast to the temporal heterogeneity of the UIP pattern. (**b**) Ground glass opacities are the predominant finding of NSIP. It is mostly bilateral, symmetrical, and subpleural predominant as shown in this case. Irregular linear and reticular opacities are also present.

HRCT pattern indicates a histologic finding of fibrosis, whereas a ground glass pattern suggests reversible inflammatory disease and a better prognosis *(23,25)*. The most common HRCT pattern in myositis-associated ILD of subacute onset is a combination of ground glass opacities and septal/reticular opacities in the absence of prominent honeycombing *(3,6,13,19,26,27)*, which corresponds to the findings of NSIP (Fig. 12.2b) *(22,28)*. Small areas of consolidation may be observed, but extensive consolidation argues against NSIP *(22,28)*. In contrast to NSIP, UIP

**Fig. 12.3** HRCT image of a PM patient shows basal predominant reticular opacities and honey combing, indicating UIP as an underlying pathology. Traction bronchiectasis (not shown) is also common.

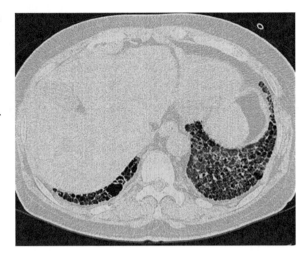

features prominent honeycombing together with septal/reticular opacities, but ground glass opacities are inconspicuous (Fig. 12.3) *(22)*. HRCT findings associated with acute-onset ILD are focal consolidations that tend to be located subpleurally or at bronchovascular bundles together with focal ground glass opacities. These findings are commonly seen in BOOP (Fig. 12.4a, b) *(22)*. DAD is another histopathologic pattern observed in acute-onset ILD *(20)*, particularly in association with ADM *(16–18)*. The characteristic HRCT findings of DAD are extensive consolidation together with prominent ground glass opacities without showing any regional predilection (Fig. 12.5a, b) *(22)*. Acute-onset ILD with the initial HRCT findings of BOOP could prove to be early DAD in histopathology *(18,29)*. Therefore, despite favorable initial HRCT findings, sustained attention is required in patients who present with rapidly progressive symptoms to allow a timely lung biopsy and immediate aggressive immunosuppression.

## Pulmonary Function Testing

Clinical respiratory symptoms are unreliable for detecting ILD in patients with myositis because a substantial proportion of patients are asymptomatic *(3,4,18)*. The most useful diagnostic tests for ILD are noninvasive pulmonary function tests as these provide an objective assessment of respiratory symptoms and allow estimation of disease severity and response to therapy. Typically, ILD patients demonstrate a restrictive ventilatory defect with decreased total lung capacity (TLC), functional residual capacity, residual volume (RV), forced expiratory volume in 1 s (FEV1), and forced vital capacity (FVC) but have a normal or elevated FEV1/

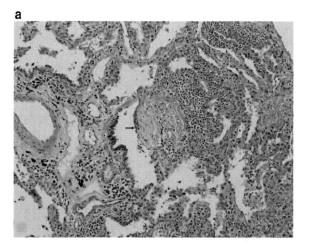

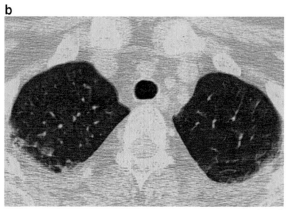

**Fig. 12.4** (**a**) The lung architecture is typically preserved in BOOP. Variable degrees of lymphoplasma cell and histiocyte infiltrates are present in the interstitium. Note the patchy fibroblast plug in the airway (*arrow*). (**b**) The HRCT of a DM patient demonstrates air space consolidation and ground glass opacities around bronchovascular bundles, particularly in the subpleural area, which is a typical finding of BOOP.

FVC ratio and a decreased diffusing capacity of the lung for carbon monoxide (DLCO). However, not all of these abnormalities are found in every patient. The most sensitive finding appears to be a decreased DLCO, although this is not a specific finding of myositis-associated ILD. Furthermore, reduced lung volumes (TLC, FVC) can be partially or entirely caused by respiratory muscle weakness. The following findings can help determine that reduced lung volumes are due to respiratory muscle weakness: reduced maximal inspiratory or expiratory pressures, reduced maximal voluntary ventilation, and increased RV with a normal FEV1/FVC ratio.

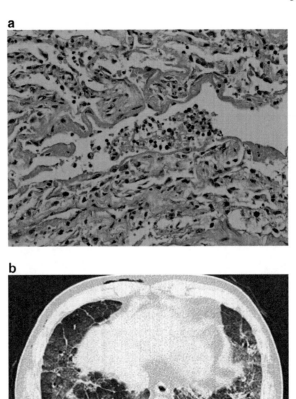

**Fig. 12.5** (**a**) Eosinophilic proteinaceous exudate, referred to as hyaline membrane, outlines the alveolar spaces along with accumulated cellular debris within air spaces, which is the most characteristic finding of the exudative phase of DAD. (**b**) The HRCT image of DAD shows extensive ground glass opacities with areas of focal sparing of lung lobules, giving a geographic appearance. Patchy consolidations, bronchial dilations, and reticular opacities due to organizing fibrosis are also observed.

## Bronchoalveolar Lavage

Myositis-associated ILD does not have a specific bronchoalveolar lavage (BAL) cell profile. Although it has been reported that BAL can be useful for detecting asymptomatic ILD in connective tissue diseases, its significance is unclear *(30)*.

The most important roles of BAL in ILD are (1) to identify other causes that mimic ILD, such as infections, drug-induced reactions, and malignancies; and (2) to predict clinical course based on cellular profiles of BAL fluid. The BAL fluid of ILD in PM and DM commonly shows elevated lymphocyte counts *(3,6,13)*. The presence of neutrophilia (defined as a differential count >5%) irrespective of lymphocyte count is associated with ILD progression and a poor prognosis *(3,6)*. Patients with nonprogressive ILD commonly show septal/reticular opacities in HRCT scans and a low neutrophil count with a variable lymphocyte count in BAL fluid. On the other hand, patients with progressive ILD show dominant ground glass opacities and BAL fluid neutrophilia *(6)*. However, because ground glass opacities indicate active inflammatory components that are likely to respond to treatment, it remains to be determined whether BAL fluid neutrophilia predict a poor treatment outcome in addition to ILD progression.

## *Serological Markers*

Autoantibody profiles are useful for predicting the presence of ILD in myositis. Of the various myositis-specific autoantibodies, antisynthetase antibodies are strongly associated with ILD. Furthermore, anti-Jo-1 antibody, the most common antibody in this group, is found in 20-30% of all PM and DM patients *(5)*. The reported frequency of ILD in patients with anti-Jo-1 antibodies is more than 70% *(3,4,6)*.

Sato et al. *(31)* used a radioimmunoprecipitation method to screen the sera of 298 patients with various connective diseases for autoantibodies and found that 8 of 42 DM patients immunoprecipitated an unknown polypeptide of approximately 140 kDa. All eight had been diagnosed as having ADM, and four of the eight had rapidly progressive ILD, which suggests that this novel autoantibody might be a useful marker for a subset of patients with ADM and rapidly progressive ILD.

It has also been suggested that Krebs von den Lungen-6 (KL-6), a glycoprotein expressed on type II alveolar pneumocytes and bronchiolar epithelial cells, and serum surfactant protein D are useful markers of ILD activity in myositis *(32–34)*. Both were found to be overexpressed in myositis-associated ILD and to be inversely correlated with VC and DLCO. However, their diagnostic or prognostic value should be studied further in larger patient cohorts before they are used in clinical practice.

## Prognosis

Clinical patterns at presentation, HRCT changes, pulmonary function test results, BAL profiles, and lung biopsy findings can be of value in terms of predicting progression or prognosis in myositis-associated ILD. Of these variables, histopathologic type appears to best predict therapeutic responses and survival *(3,19–21)*.

**Table 12.2**  Poor prognostic factors of myositis-associated ILD

| Prognostic factors | Features | References |
|---|---|---|
| Acute onset with rapidly progressive presentation<br>Associated with ADM<br>Diffuse alveolar damage<br>Unusual interstitial pneumonia | Acute presentation and histology of diffuse alveolar damage are often seen in interstitial lung disease associated with amyopathic dermatomyositis | *(3,16–18)* |
| Extensive fibrosis in HRCT | This finding indicates irreversible parenchymal lung damage and portends unresponsiveness to treatment | *(6)* |
| Initial low FVC (<60%), initial low DLCO (<45%) | Low initial FVC and DLCO indicate extensive parenchymal involvement | *(3,18)* |
| Neutrophilic BAL | BAL neutrophilia is associated with ILD deterioration | *(3,6)* |

Table 12.2 summarizes factors that have been associated with poor prognosis (i.e., acute onset with a rapidly progressive presentation, ADM, extensive fibrotic change by HRCT, initial low FVC or DLCO, neutrophilic BAL, and histologic UIP or DAD) *(3,6,16–18,20)*. On the other hand, dominant ground glass opacities in HRCT images have been shown to predict ILD progression *(6)* but with a better treatment response *(3,26)*.

## Treatment

No optimal treatment has been established for myositis-associated ILD. Controlled studies are lacking because of the heterogeneous clinical courses and treatment responses in these patients. High-dose corticosteroid therapy ($\geq 1$ mg/kg) is the first-line treatment for myositis with or without ILD. However, responses can differ for myositis and ILD; ILD response may be inadequate despite marked improvements in muscle inflammation. Because the clinical courses of myositis-associated ILD are highly variable, not all patients need immunosuppressive agents in addition to corticosteroid. Patients with progressive ILD, particularly those with acute-onset ILD, require combined immunosuppressive agents, whereas a significant number of patients show stable ILD and require only monitoring in addition to moderate treatment aimed at controlling extrapulmonary manifestations *(6)*. Therefore, patients with asymptomatic or slowly progressive onset ILD should be carefully monitored for progression to avoid treatment delays and unnecessary treatment.

It has been estimated that about 50% of myositis patients affected by ILD respond favorably to initial corticosteroid treatment *(7,11)*. Adding an immunosuppressive agent when corticosteroid therapy fails to improve ILD has been a widely accepted strategy. However, initial aggressive treatment with corticosteroid and immunosuppressive agents should be considered for those who have rapid progression and poor prognostic factors because early treatment initiation can improve response rate. The immunosuppressive drugs that have been found to be effective in myositis-associated ILD typically include cyclophosphamide, azathioprine, and methotrexate *(3,6,19)*. Good responses have been reported for T-cell targeted therapies based on cyclosporine A *(35–38)* or tacrolimus *(39,40)* in patients refractory to other immunosuppressive agents, especially during early disease stage. Of note, tacrolimus was found to improve ILD in anti-Jo-1-positive patients who failed to respond to other combination treatments, including cyclosporine A *(39,40)*. Mycophenolate mofetil has been introduced as a treatment for refractory myositis, but assessments of its efficacy have focused on myositis rather than on ILD *(41,42)*. Rituximab was also found to improve myositis and associated ILD in an open-label study *(43)*. An international, multicenter trial has been initiated to evaluate the efficacy of rituximab in DM and PM patients, including those with ILD.

Therapeutic regimens against myositis-associated ILD have been effective in only a limited number of patients, which suggests that different mechanisms are involved in the pathogenesis of ILD. Experiences with more recent agents that have been reported to be effective in refractory cases are limited; thus, prospective randomized controlled trials are needed to confirm their efficacies. Moreover, the duration of immunosuppressive treatment has not been determined, and its beneficial effects must be balanced versus the risks of serious side effects associated with long-term immunosuppression.

Autologous stem cell transplantation (ASCT) has been tried in several refractory autoimmune diseases and showed promising results *(44,45)*. The proposed mechanisms of action of ASCT include induction of intense immune suppression, eradication of autoreactive T-cell clones, and thymic reeducation *(46)*. The attractive feature of ASCT is that it can potentially cure disease by inducing tolerance. Successful treatment of myositis-associated ILD has been reported with ASCT *(47–49)*. However, because of its high treatment-related mortality *(45)*, ASCT is likely to be saved for refractory patients who have failed to respond to other medical treatments.

Lung transplantation has been tried only anecdotally in myositis-associated ILD *(50,51)*. Due to scarcity of cases, knowledge of the outcome after transplantation is lacking, especially with respect to ILD relapse. However, lung transplantation remains as a viable option for patients who show progressive deterioration on medical treatment, particularly those with rapidly progressive ILD that leads to severe respiratory failure despite combined immunosuppression *(51)*.

## Secondary Pulmonary Complications

The prevalence of secondary pulmonary manifestations (Table 12.1) is difficult to estimate due to a lack of reports. However, these alternative sources of lung dysfunction should always be suspected because treatment options are greatly different from those for ILD. Of the various mechanisms involved, infection (with or without aspiration), and hypoventilation are the major types of secondary pulmonary complications *(7,10)*. In a study of 156 myositis patients, infection was reported in 33.3% (52/156), and 73.1% (38/52) of these were lung infections (aspiration pneumonia in 27, opportunistic lung infection in 8, and conventional pneumonia in 3) *(10)*. Fungal infections, especially by *Pneumocystis carinii*, are the most common cause of opportunistic lung infections *(10)*. Immunosuppressive treatment is implicated in high susceptibility to infection. In patients with aspiration pneumonia, esophageal dysfunction and impaired airway protection appear to be common *(7)*. Frank respiratory insufficiency, due to respiratory muscle weakness, appears to occur in approximately 5% of PM and DM patients, while physiologic evidence of impaired ventilatory mechanics has been found in a substantial number of myositis patients *(7)*.

Clinically evident myocardial involvement is rare in PM and DM patients, but subclinical cardiac dysfunction may be more common *(8)*. Dyspnea, hypoxia, and parenchymal opacities in chest roentgenograms may be due to congestive heart failure and need to be distinguished from ILD or respiratory muscle disease by echocardiography and pulmonary function testing. Pulmonary arterial hypertension, which is commonly seen in systemic sclerosis, is also observed in a few myositis patients *(9)* and may occur secondary to congestive heart failure, alveolar hypoventilation, or ILD. Doppler echocardiography, arterial blood gas analysis, and pulmonary function tests (including DLCO) provide valuable means of differentiating primary and secondary pulmonary arterial hypertension. However, definitive diagnoses require catheterization and direct pulmonary artery pressure measurements.

## Conclusion

Pulmonary manifestations are common findings in PM and DM and substantially contribute to morbidity and mortality. All myositis patients should be screened for ILD at initial evaluation because a substantial proportion of patients are asymptomatic, or pulmonary symptoms can be overwhelmed by limited physical activity due to severe muscle weakness. HRCT and pulmonary function tests are useful for assessing disease extent and activity, while BAL and lung biopsies can help exclude infectious causes and determine prognosis. No optimal treatment has been established for ILD in myositis patients, and controlled studies are needed to confirm the efficacies of immunosuppressive drugs that have been used to treat ILD in myositis.

## References

1. Nagaraju K, Plotz PH, Miller FW. Etiology and pathogenesis of inflammatory muscle disease. In: Hochberg MC, Silman AJ, Smolen JSet al, eds. Rheumatology. 3rd ed. Philadelphia: Mosby, 2003:1523–36.
2. Arsura EL, Greenberg AS. Adverse impact of interstitial pulmonary fibrosis on prognosis in polymyositis and dermatomyositis. Semin Arthritis Rheum 1988;18:29–37.

3. Marie I, Hachulla E, Cherin P, et al. Interstitial lung disease in polymyositis and dermatomyositis. Arthritis Rheum 2002;47:614–22.

4. Fathi M, Dastmalchi M, Rasmussen E, et al. Interstitial lung disease, a common manifestation of newly diagnosed polymyositis and dermatomyositis. Ann Rheum Dis 2004; 63:297–301.

5. Targoff IN. Humoral immunity in polymyositis/dermatomyositis. J Invest Dermatol 1993;100:116–23S.

6. Schnabel A, Reuter M, Biederer J, et al. Interstitial lung disease in polymyositis and dermatomyositis: clinical course and response to treatment. Semin Arthritis Rheum 2003; 32:273–84.

7. Dickey BF, Myers AR. Pulmonary disease in polymyositis/dermatomyositis. Semin Arthritis Rheum 1984;14:60–76.

8. Denbow CE, Lie JT, Tancredi RG, Bunch TW. Cardiac involvement in polymyositis. Arthritis Rheum 1979;22:1088–92.

9. Bunch TW, Tancredi RG, Lie JT. Pulmonary hypertension in polymyositis. Chest 1981;79:105–7.

10. Marie I, Hachulla E, Cherin P, et al. Opportunistic infections in polymyositis and dermatomyositis. Arthritis Rheum 2005;53:155–65.

11. Schwarz MI, Matthay RA, Sahn SA, et al. Interstitial lung disease in polymyositis and dermatomyositis: analysis of six cases and review of the literature. Medicine (Baltimore) 1976;55:89–104.

12. Friedman AW, Targoff IN, Amett FC. Interstitial lung disease with autoantibodies against aminoacyl-tRNA synthetases in the absence of clinically apparent myositis. Semin Arthritis Rheum 1996;26:459–67.

13. Cottin V, Thivolet-Bejui F, Reynaud-Gaubert M, et al. Interstitial lung disease in amyopathic dermatomyositis, dermatomyositis and polymyositis. Eur Respir J 2003;22:245–50.

14. Park GM, Choi CM, Um SW, et al. Clinical features of dermatomyositis/polymyositis with lung involvement. Tuberc Respir Dis 2001;51:354–63 (Korean).

15. Euwer RL, Sontheimer RD. Amyopathic dermatomyositis (dermatomyositis sine myositis). Presentation of six new cases and review of the literature. J Am Acad Dermatol 1991;24: 959–66.

16. Ito M, Kaise S, Suzuki S, et al. Clinico-laboratory characteristics of patients with dermatomyositis accompanied by rapidly progressive interstitial lung disease. Clin Rheumatol 1999; 18:462–7.

17. Lee CS, Chen TL, Tzen CY, et al. Idiopathic inflammatory myositis with diffuse alveolar damage. Clin Rheumatol 2002;21:391–6.

18. Kang EH, Lee EB, Shin KC, et al. Interstitial lung disease in patients with polymyositis, dermatomyositis and amyopathic dermatomyositis. Rheumatology (Oxford) 2005;44: 1282–6.

19. Douglas WW, Tazelaar HD, Hartman TE, et al. Polymyositis-dermatomyositis-associated interstitial lung disease. Am J Respir Crit Care Med 2001;164:1182–5.

20. Tazelaar HD, Viggiano RW, Pickersgill TV, Colby TV. Interstitial lung disease in polymyositis and dermatomyositis. Am Rev Respir Dis 1990;141:727–33.

21. Tansey D, Wells AU, Colby TV, et al. Variations in histological patterns of interstitial pneumonia between connective tissue disorders and their relationship to prognosis. Histopathology 2004;44:585–96.

22. American Thoracic Society/European Respiratory Society International Multidisciplinary Consensus Classification of the Idiopathic Interstitial Pneumonias. Am J Respir Crit Care Med. 2002;165:277–304.

23. Muller NL, Miller RR, Webb WR, et al. Fibrosing alveolitis: CT-pathologic correlation. Radiology 1986;160:585–8.

24. Muller NL, Staples CA, Miller RR, et al. Disease activity in idiopathic pulmonary fibrosis: CT and pathologic correlation. Radiology 1987;165:731–4.

25. Lee JS, Im JG, Ahn JM, et al. Fibrosing alveolitis: prognostic implication of ground-glass attenuation at high-resolution CT. Radiology 1992;184:451–4.
26. Ikezoe J, Johkoh T, Kohno N, et al. High-resolution CT findings of lung disease in patients with polymyositis and dermatomyositis. J Thorac Imaging 1996;11:250–9.
27. Mino M, Noma S, Taguchi Y, et al. Pulmonary involvement in polymyositis and dermatomyositis: sequential evaluation with CT. Am J Roentgenol 1997;169:83–7.
28. Arakawa H, Yamada H, Kurihara Y, et al. Nonspecific interstitial pneumonia associated with polymyositis and dermatomyositis: serial high-resolution CT findings and functional correlation. Chest 2003;123:1096–103.
29. Ichikado K, Johkoh T, Ikezoe J, et al. Acute interstitial pneumonia: high-resolution CT findings correlated with pathology. Am J Roentgenol 1997;168:333–8.
30. Wallaert B, Hatron PY, Grosbois JM, et al. Subclinical pulmonary involvement in collagen-vascular diseases assessed by bronchoalveolar lavage. Relationship between alveolitis and subsequent changes in lung function. Am Rev Respir Dis 1986;133:574–80.
31. Sato S, Hirakata M, Kuwana M, et al. Autoantibodies to a 140-kd polypeptide, CADM-140, in Japanese patients with clinically amyopathic dermatomyositis. Arthritis Rheum 2005; 52:1571–6.
32. Kubo M, Ihn H, Yamane K, et al. Serum KL-6 in adult patients with polymyositis and dermatomyositis. Rheumatology (Oxford) 2000;39:632–6.
33. Fukaya S, Oshima H, Kato K, et al. KL-6 as a novel marker for activities of interstitial pneumonia in connective tissue diseases. Rheumatol Int 2000;19:223–5.
34. Ihn H, Asano Y, Kubo M, et al. Clinical significance of serum surfactant protein D (SP-D) in patients with polymyositis/dermatomyositis: correlation with interstitial lung disease. Rheumatology (Oxford) 2002;41:1268–72.
35. Maeda K, Kimura R, Komuta K, Igarashi T. Cyclosporine treatment for polymyositis/ dermatomyositis: is it possible to rescue the deteriorating cases with interstitial pneumonitis.? Scand J Rheumatol 1997;26:24–9.
36. Gruhn WB, Diaz-Buxo JA. Cyclosporine treatment of steroid resistant interstitial pneumonitis associated with dermatomyositis/polymyositis. J Rheumatol 1987;14:1045–7.
37. Nawata Y, Kurasawa K, Takabayashi K, et al. Corticosteroid resistant interstitial pneumonitis in dermatomyositis/polymyositis: prediction and treatment with cyclosporine. J Rheumatol 1999;26:1527–33.
38. Levi S, Hodgson HJ. Cyclosporin for dermatomyositis. Ann Rheum Dis 1989;48:85–6.
39. Oddis CV, Sciurba FC, Elmagd KA, Starzl TE. Tacrolimus in refractory polymyositis with interstitial lung disease. Lancet 1999;353:1762–3.
40. Wilkes MR, Sereika SM, Fertig N, et al. Treatment of anti-synthetase-associated interstitial lung disease with tacrolimus. Arthritis Rheum 2005;52:2439–46.
41. Majithia V, Harisdangkul V. Mycophenolate mofetil (CellCept): an alternative therapy for autoimmune inflammatory myopathy. Rheumatology (Oxford) 2005;44:386–9.
42. Pisoni CN, Cuadrado MJ, Khamashta MA, et al. Mycophenolate mofetil treatment in resistant myositis. Rheumatology (Oxford) 2007;46:516–8.
43. Levine TD. Rituximab in the treatment of dermatomyositis: an open-label pilot study. Arthritis Rheum 2005;52:601–7.
44. Burt RK, Traynor AE, Pope R, et al. Treatment of autoimmune disease by intense immuno-suppressive conditioning and autologous hematopoietic stem cell transplantation. Blood 1998;92:3505–14.
45. Gratwohl A, Passweg J, Bocelli-Tyndall C, et al. Autologous hematopoietic stem cell transplantation for autoimmune diseases. Bone Marrow Transplant 2005;35:869–79.
46. Bingham SJ, Snowden J, Morgan G, Emery P. High dose immunosuppressive therapy and stem cell transplantation in autoimmune and inflammatory diseases. Int Immunopharmacol 2002;2:399–414.
47. Baron F, Ribbens C, Kaye O, et al. Effective treatment of Jo-1-associated polymyositis with T-cell-depleted autologous peripheral blood stem cell transplantation. Br J Haematol 2000;110:339–42.

48. Oryoji K, Himeji D, Nagafuji K, et al. Successful treatment of rapidly progressive interstitial pneumonia with autologous peripheral blood stem cell transplantation in a patient with dermatomyositis. Clin Rheumatol 2005;24:637–40.
49. Tsukamoto H, Nagafuji K, Horiuchi T, et al. A phase I-II trial of autologous peripheral blood stem cell transplantation in the treatment of refractory autoimmune disease. Ann Rheum Dis 2006;65:508–14.
50. Selva-O'Callaghan A, Labrador-Horrillo M, Muñoz-Gall X, et al. Polymyositis/dermatomyositis-associated lung disease: analysis of a series of 81 patients. Lupus 2005;14:534–42.
51. Kim J, Kim YW, Lee SM, et al. Successful lung transplantation in a patient with dermatomyositis and acute form of interstitial pneumonitis. Clin Exp Rheumatol 2009;27:168–9.

# Chapter 13
# Dermatological Manifestations of Dermatomyositis

Mark Kagen

**Abstract** The rash of dermatomyositis can be extremely characteristic. It is generally manifest over the face and hands but may be widespread. In approximately one-third of patients, rash precedes the occurrence of overt myopathy. In most patients, however, the two manifestations become evident at about the same time. Histological examination of affected skin reveals degeneration of the basal keratinocyte layer, characteristic of interface dermatitis. There is also dermal edema and a perivascular mononuclear cell infiltrate, containing T lymphocytes and dendritic cells. Calcifications in the skin, which may be seen at areas of trauma, occur particularly in juvenile dermatomyositis. Therapeutic approaches employ measures used to treat systemic disease. In addition, protection from sun exposure is recommended, and topical agents containing corticosteroids may provide benefit.

**Keywords** Rash • Amyopathic dermatomyositis • Hypomyopathic dermatomyositis • Interface dermatitis

## Rash

The rash of dermatomyositis is often most noticeable on the face and hands but can be quite widespread, appearing on the scalp, neck, trunk, and both upper and lower extremities. It may be photosensitive and pruritic. Its appearance is characteristic and, in the right clinical setting, strongly suggestive of the diagnosis (1).

Its manifestations on the face are marked by periorbital edema with a deep violet-red coloration. On occasion, it has been confused with an allergic reaction to topical cosmetics. It is most marked over the upper eyelids, where scaling may occur. Its violaceous appearance has been termed the *heliotrope sign* or *lilac suffusion*. This heliotrope rash may also extend over the cheeks, including the area of the

M. Kagen
Riverchase Dermatology, Naples, FL, USA

L.J. Kagen (ed.), *The Inflammatory Myopathies*,
DOI 10.1007/978-1-60327-827-0_13,
© Humana Press. a part of Springer Science+Business Media, LLC 2009

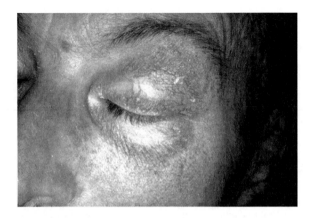

**Fig. 13.1** Violaceous periorbital rash: the heliotrope sign

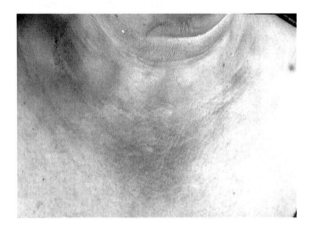

**Fig. 13.2** Erythematous rash over the anterior neck and chest: the V sign in a sun-exposed area

nasolabial folds. This is in contrast to the rash of cutaneous lupus erythematosus, which generally spares the area of the nasolabial folds. Although the heliotrope sign is virtually pathognomonic, it is not always absolutely diagnostic. Similar changes have been noted in allergic reactions, during the course of trichinosis, as well as in a patient with sarcoidosis *(2)*. Over the scalp, the erythematous rash is often scaly and distressingly pruritic (Figs. 13.1 and 13.2) *(3)*.

At the extremities, a deeply red, slightly raised rash can be present over extensor surfaces, particularly at the dorsum of the hands and fingers. *Gottron sign* is the term used to describe the violaceous discoloration of the knuckles, elbows, knees, and medial malleoli of the ankles (Fig. 13.3). In these areas, the rash may be heaped up and plaque-like and is then called *Gottron papules*. The rash at the dorsum of the fingers is present over the knuckles (Fig. 13.4). This is in contrast to the rash of

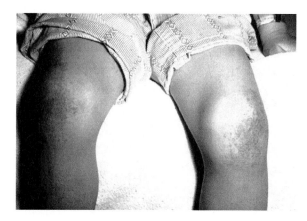

**Fig. 13.3** Gottron sign, violaceous discoloration of the knees

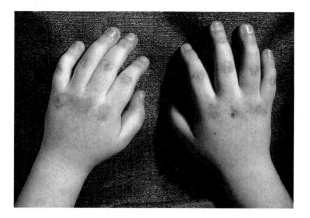

**Fig. 13.4** Gottron papules over bony prominences of the dorsum of the hands. (From **Ref.** *12*. Reprinted with permission from Lippincott Williams and Wilkins [Walters Kluwer, Philadelphia].)

cutaneous lupus erythematosus, which appears at interphalangeal areas. The nail beds and periungual areas display hyperemia, telangiectasia, and ischemic areas. In severe instances, destruction of the periungual architecture may occur and lead to what is termed *ragged cuticles* (Fig. 13.5). There may also be chronic eczematous changes of the hands, with roughening and fissuring, most noticeable at the radial surfaces of the fingers, "mechanic's hands."

A deeply erythematous to brownish rash can be seen at the anterior surface of the neck and over the sun-exposed surface of the chest, the *V sign*. Similar skin changes over the upper posterior thorax are known as the *shawl sign*. Plaque-like areas of erythema may also be seen at the upper outer thighs. In addition to its diffuse redness, the rash of dermatomyositis is poikilodermic; that is, it may be mottled and variegated in its appearance, with areas of hypo- and hyperpigmentation.

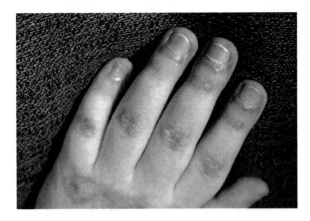

**Fig. 13.5** Gottron papules overlying the metacarpophalangeal (MCP), proximal interphalangeal (PIP), and distal interphalangeal (DIP) joints of the hands, and periungual changes of erythema and ragged cuticles. (From **Ref.** *12*. Reprinted with permission from Lippincott Williams and Wilkins [Walters Kluwer, Philadelphia].)

*Poikiloderma atrophicans vasculare* is the term applied to the manifestation of these signs of poikiloderma with telangiectasia and atrophy, often noted especially over the neck and torso.

At the feet, Gottron papules may be seen at the medial malleoli of the ankles, and similar changes to those of the fingers may be seen at the toes. In approximately 30% of patients, the rash may precede the occurrence of overt myopathy by months or even years in some cases *(4)*. The terms *amyopathic dermatomyositis* or *dermatomyositis sine myositis* have been used to describe this situation. However, myopathy will usually become evident over time. Moreover, in most cases of amyopathic dermatomyositis, if an extensive evaluation is performed, subtle evidence of an underlying myopathy, such as the presence of slightly elevated serum enzymes or myoglobin or a slight abnormality of the electromyogram, will be detected. In these cases, the term *hypomyopathic dermatomyositis* has been applied *(5,6)*. In approximately 60% of patients, rash and myopathy become evident at the same time. Rarely, perhaps in as many as 10% of cases, the rash may appear after the onset of myopathy *(7)*.

The severity of rash, particularly over the trunk and abdomen, where skin ulceration and breakdown may occur, has been associated with the presence of an underlying malignancy.

## Histology

Histological examination of affected skin demonstrates epidermal atrophy and liquefactive vacuolar degeneration of the basal keratinocyte layer characteristic of paucicellular interface dermatitis (Fig. 13.6). In addition, perivascular infiltrates of lymphocytes with macrophages and dendritic cells may be seen. A few polymorphonuclear leukocytes and occasional areas of lymphocytic infiltration can also be

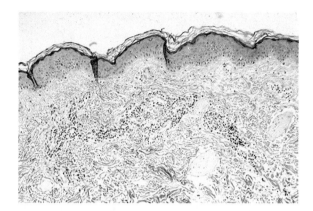

**Fig. 13.6** Skin biopsy; notable is a perivascular mononuclear cell infiltrate. There is also a subtle vacuolization of basal keratinocytes

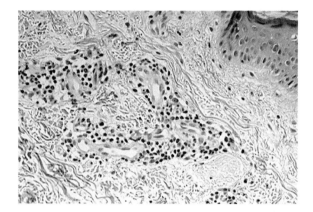

**Fig. 13.7** Skin biopsy, at higher power, demonstrating mononuclear cell perivascular infiltrate

seen around the pilosebaceous apparatus. Dermal edema with increased deposits of mucin can also be apparent. Cytotoxic CD8 T lymphocytes are present in the dermis and are thought to be important mediators of tissue injury. Dendritic cells and CD4 lymphocytes are also found in this skin layer (Fig. 13.7).

## Calcinosis

Calcification can occur in and under the skin, often at areas of pressure or trauma. It may appear as hard, gritty, painful nodules at the fingers or elbows, which may then erupt on to the surface (Figs. 13.8 and 13.9). Less commonly, soft masses of

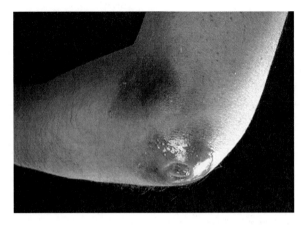

**Fig. 13.8** Infected area of calcinosis erupting onto the skin at the elbow. (From **Ref.** *12*. Reprinted with permission from Lippincott Williams and Wilkins [Walters Kluwer, Philadelphia].)

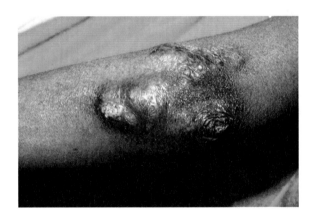

**Fig. 13.9** Multiple calcific eruptions onto the skin at the elbow. These areas were not infected

cheesy, or even milky, substance may be present, particularly at the posterior thigh. Calcinosis is found most commonly in juvenile dermatomyositis, with possibly up to 40% of children with this disorder so affected. It can also occur in adults, but less frequently *(8)*. Rarely, areas of calcification of the skin may become infected and present a situation that is difficult to treat. In addition to the skin, calcification may occur in deeper layers of the connective tissue, particularly investing the fascia of muscles and muscle fibers. In these locations, it may present a severe impediment to mobility and normal muscle function (Figs. 13.10 and 13.11).

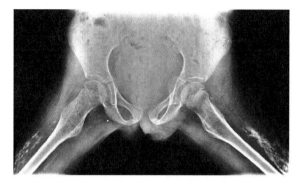

**Fig. 13.10**   Calcium deposits in the skin and deeper layers of the thigh.

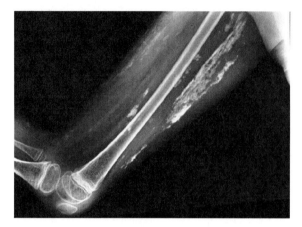

**Fig. 13.11**   Calcium deposits in the skin and deeper layers of the thigh and leg (From **Ref.** *12*. Reprinted with permission from Lippincott Williams and Wilkins [Walters Kluwer, Philadelphia].)

# Therapy

The measures used in the treatment of the systemic manifestations of dermatomyositis will also be useful for its skin manifestations. In addition, protection from sun exposure is important. This involves modification of outdoor activities and the use of sunscreens and sun-protective clothing. Topical measures such as corticosteroid preparations, topical tacrolimus *(9)*, and emollients may provide some benefit.

Hydroxychloroquine, chloroquine, and quinacrine have been helpful, but caution must be used since the use of these antimalarial compounds may entail risk of drug eruption *(10,11)*.

Treatment methods for calcinosis are generally unsatisfactory. A number of agents, including corticosteroids, calcium channel blockers (such as diltiazem), diphosphonates,

EDTA (ethylenediaminetetraacetic acid), aluminum hydroxide, and low-dose warfarin have been tried. Localized masses may be removed surgically, but generalized involvement remains a distressing problem. Sometimes, calcium deposits reabsorb spontaneously.

# References

1. Callen JP, Wortmann RL. Dermatomyositis. Clin Dermatol 2006;24:363–73.
2. Itoh J, Akiguchi I, Midorikawa R, Kameyama M. Sarcoid myopathy with typical rash of dermatomyositis. Neurology 1980;30:1118–21.
3. Kasteler JS, Callen JP. Scalp involvement in dermatomyositis. JAMA 1994;272:1939–41.
4. Krain L. Dermatomyositis in 6 patients without initial muscle involvement. Arch Dermatol 1975;111:241–5.
5. el-Azhary RA, Pakzad SY. Amyopathic dermatomyositis: retrospective review of 37 cases. J Am Acad Dermatol 2002;46:560–5.
6. Euwer RL, Sontheimer RD. Amyopathic dermatomyositis (dermatomyositis sine myositis). J Am Acad Dermatol 1991;24:959–66.
7. Sontheimer RD. Skin manifestations of systemic autoimmune connective tissue disease: diagnostics and therapeutics. Best Pract Res Clin Rheumatol 2004;18:429–62.
8. Weinel S, Callen JP. Calcinosis cutis complicating adult-onset dermatomyositis. Arch Dermatol 2004;140:365–6.
9. Ueda M, Makinodan R, Matsumura M, Ichihashi M. Successful treatment of amyopathic dermatomyositis with topical tacrolimus. Br J Dermatol 2003;148:595–6.
10. Woo TY, Callen JP, Voorhees JJ, Bickers DR, Hanno R, Hawkins C. Cutaneous lesions of dermatomyositis are improved by hydroxychloroquine. J Am Acad Dermatol 1984;10:592–600.
11. Pelle MT, Callen JP. Adverse cutaneous reactions to hydroxychloroquine are more common in patients with dermatomyositis than in patients with cutaneous lupus erythematosus. Arch Dermatol 2002;138:1231–3.
12. Kagen LJ. Polymyositis/Dermatomyositis in Arthritis and Allied conditions. In: McCarty DJ and Koopman WJ, eds. Lea and Febiger Philadelphia 1993: 1225–1252 Twelfth Edition.

# Chapter 14
# The Differential Diagnosis of Inflammatory Myopathy

**Michael Rubin and Asaf Klein**

**Abstract** The differential diagnosis of idiopathic inflammatory myopathy is broad, encompassing a variety of disorders affecting the motor unit. Primary muscle disorders that must be considered include congenital myopathy, hereditary metabolic disorders, and muscular dystrophy. Secondary muscle disorders include those associated with collagen vascular disease or malignancy or due to infection, drugs, or toxins. Disorders of the neuromuscular junction, such as myasthenia gravis, and anterior horn cell disease may also present as proximal muscle weakness.

**Keywords** Myositis • Muscular • Myopathy • Dystrophy • Weakness

## Introduction

If the correct diagnosis is not idiopathic inflammatory myopathy, what else might it be? Polymyositis, dermatomyositis, and inclusion body myositis encompass the idiopathic inflammatory myopathies, presenting with proximal weakness of the legs more so than the arms. The pathognomonic skin lesion for dermatomyositis is Grotton's papule or sign, whereas myopathic histologic abnormalities are sought for inclusion body myositis. Diagnosis of polymyositis is assisted by the demonstration of serum anti-aminoacyl-tRNA (transfer RNA) synthetase antibodies *(1)*. When evaluation fails to yield one of these diagnoses, what else must be considered (Table 14.1)?

M. Rubin (✉) and A. Klein
Department of Neurology, Division of Neuromuscular Disease,
Weill Cornell Medical College, New York, NY, USA

L.J. Kagen (ed.), *The Inflammatory Myopathies*,
DOI 10.1007/978-1-60327-827-0_14,

**Table 14.1** Differential diagnosis of inflammatory myopathy

Muscular dystrophy
Congenital myopathy
Metabolic myopathy
   Glycogenoses
   Disorders of lipid metabolism
Mitochondrial myopathy
Endocrine myopathies
Muscle disorders associated with electrolyte disturbance
Infiltrative myopathy
   Amyloid
   Sarcoid
   Behçet's disease
Myositis associated with malignancy
Infections
Myositis associated with collagen vascular disease
Drug induced
Toxin induced
Nutritional deficiency
Neuromuscular junctionopathy
Anterior horn cell disease

# Congenital Myopathies and Muscular Dystrophies

Although both congenital myopathies and muscular dystrophies are inherited, the former result from genetic abnormalities in the contractile apparatus of muscle, with fixed, unique histochemical or ultrastructural changes on muscle biopsy, whereas the latter affect the stability of the sarcolemmal membrane and demonstrate ongoing muscle degeneration and regeneration on muscle biopsy.

## *Congenital Myopathies*

Most congenital myopathies present as congenital hypotonia with delayed motor milestones and are not discussed here. Those that may resemble idiopathic inflammatory myopathy are mentioned briefly (Table 14.2).

Six genes, all related to thin-filament proteins, have thus far been shown to result in nemaline myopathy *(2, 3)*, the most common congenital myopathy. Although its clinical presentation is typically hypotonia during the first year of life, adult onset in the fifth or sixth decade is reported, resembling limb-girdle muscular dystrophy, affecting lower extremities much more than upper, with associated neck extensor weakness and lumbar lordosis. Inheritance is either autosomal dominant or recessive, but sporadic cases are frequent. Disease course is static or slowly progressive.

**Table 14.2** The congenital myopathies with known gene defects

|  | Gene | Gene locus | Inheritance | Protein |
|---|---|---|---|---|
| Nemaline rods and nemaline | ACTA1 | 1q42 | AD or AR | Skeletal α-actin |
| myopathy | NEB | 2q2 | AR | Nebulin |
|  | TPM3 | 1q2 | AD | α-Tropomyosin |
|  | TPM2 | 9p13 | AD | β-Tropomyosin |
|  | TNNT1 | 19q13 | AR | Troponin T |
|  | CFL2 | 14q12 | AD | Cofilin-2 |
| *Other myopathies with abundant rods* |  |  |  |  |
| Rods and cores | RYR1 | 19q13 | AD | Ryanodine receptor |
| Rods and caps | TPM2 | 9q13 | AD | β-Tropomyosin |
| *Congenital myopathies with cores* |  |  |  |  |
| Central core disease | RYR1 | 19q13 | AD or AR | Ryanodine receptor |
| Multiminicore disease | SEPN1 | 1p36 | AR | Selenoprotein N1 |
| Congenital myopathy and | TTN | 2q31 | AR | Titin |
| fatal cardiomyopathy |  |  |  |  |
| *Central nuclei and centronuclear myopathies* |  |  |  |  |
| Myotubular myopathy | MTM1 | Xq28 | XLR | Myotubularin |
| Centronuclear myopathy | DNM2 | 19p13 | AD | Dynamin 2 |
|  | BIN1 | 2q14 | AR | Amphiphysin |
|  | RYR1 | 19q13 | AD | Ryanodine receptor |
| Congential myopathy and | TTN | 2q31 | AR | Titin |
| fatal cardiomyopathy |  |  |  |  |
| *Surplus protein congenital myopathies* |  |  |  |  |
| Actin aggregation myopathy | ACTA1 | 1q42 | AD | Skeletal α-actin |
| Hyaline body myopathy | MYH7 | 14q11 | AD | Slow/β-cardiac myosin heavy- |
| Cap disease | TPM2 | 9q13 | AD | chain β-tropomyosin |
| Reducing body myopathy | FHL1 | Xq26 | XLD/R | Four-and-a-half lim |
|  |  |  |  | domain-1 protein |
| Spheroid body myopathy | MYOT | 5q23 | AD | Myotilin |
| Congenital fiber-type disproportion |  |  |  |  |
|  | ACTA1 | 1q42 | AD | Skeletal α-actin |
|  | SEPN1 | 1p36 | AR | Selenoprotein N1 |
|  | TPM3 | 1q2 | AD | α-Tropomyosin |
| *Congenital myopathies characterized by distal involvement, distal arthrogryposis, or both* |  |  |  |  |
|  | NEB | 2q2 | AR | Nebulin |
|  | TPM2 | 9q13 | AD | β-Tropomyosin |
|  | **MYH3** | **17p13** | **AD** | **Myosin heavy chain 3** |
|  | MYH8 | 17p13 | AD | Perinatal myosin |
|  | TNNI2 | 11p15 | AD | Troponin I |
|  | TNNT3 | 11p15 | AD | Troponin T3 |

*ACTA* alpha-skeletal actin; *BIN1* bridging integrator 1; *CFL2* cofilin; *DNM* dynamin; *FHL* four-and-a-half lim domain protein; *MYH* myosin heavy chain; *NEB* nebulin; *RYR1* ryanodine receptor type 1; *SEPN1* selenoprotein; *TNNT* troponin T; *TPM* tropomyosin; *TTN* titin
Reprinted from **Ref. 2**. Used with permission from Lippincott Wilkins & Williams

Core myopathies are characterized by regions (cores), peripheral or central, focal, multiple, or extensive, where oxidative enzyme staining is absent *(2)*. Central core myopathy, the first congenital myopathy to be identified *(4)*, demonstrates large cores and is caused by mutations in the RYR1 (ryanodine receptor type 1) gene encoding the skeletal muscle ryanodine receptor. It is often diagnosed in hypotonic children but may first express itself in the adult, usually with nonprogressive proximal limb weakness. Pain is frequent, and creatine kinase may be increased tenfold. Inheritance is usually autosomal dominant, but recessive and sporadic forms exist, and the disease is allelic to the malignant hyperthermia syndrome. Some patients are severely affected and wheelchair bound.

Centronuclear myopathy, so named because the myonuclei are at the geometric center of many muscle fibers, may rarely become symptomatic after age 30 years, usually as a slowly progressive limb-girdle syndrome primarily affecting the legs. Ambulation is usually maintained to the fifth decade. Inheritance is autosomal dominant or recessive, the former having adult onset with mild weakness and slow progression, and related to DNM2 gene mutations that encode dynamin-2, involved in endocytosis, actin assembly, and centrosome cohesion *(5)*.

Myotubular myopathy is rare (1 in 50,000 live births), X-linked, and like centronuclear myopathy, demonstrates centrally located nuclei. However, weakness is more severe, often requiring ventilatory assistance, with substantial early mortality. Milder forms survive to adulthood. Previously lumped together due to similar myopathology, genetic studies have revealed different mutations in myotubular and centronuclear myopathy.

Hyaline body myopathy may be autosomal dominant or recessive and is clinically heterogeneous, with onset from childhood to the fifth decade, presenting as a generally nonprogressive scapuloperoneal or limb-girdle distribution weakness.

## *Muscular Dystrophies*

Duchenne muscular dystrophy, the result of a dystrophin gene mutation on the X chromosome that causes production of less than 5% of the normal quantity of dystrophin, is the most common form of muscular dystrophy *(6)*. In almost all patients, disease is evident by 5 years of age, with wheelchair dependence by age 13 years.

Becker muscular dystrophy, demonstrating at least 20% of the normal quantity of dystrophin, presents after age 5 years, and patients remain ambulatory by age 16 years, clinically differentiating this milder dystrophinopathy from Duchenne muscular dystrophy. Isolated quadriceps myopathy represents a *forme fruste* of Becker muscular dystrophy *(7)*. Female carriers may demonstrate mild weakness with elevated creatine kinase, and 50% will have no family history of neuromuscular disease *(8)* (Table 14.3).

Myotonic dystrophy type 1 (Steinert's disease, DM1), the most common adult form of muscular dystrophy, is autosomal dominant and best considered a multisystem disease. Frontal balding; cataracts; retinal degeneration; cardiomyopathy with conduction defects; endocrinopathy; gonadal atrophy; mental changes; smooth muscle involvement affecting the esophagus, colon, and uterus; in addition to the characteristic myotonia and predominantly distal muscle wasting and weakness allow this condition to be recognized and differentiated from other muscular dystrophies, inflammatory

**Table 14.3**  Muscular dystrophies

Congenital muscular dystrophy
Duchenne muscular dystrophy
Becker's muscular dystrophy
Myotonic muscular dystrophy
Facioscapulohumeral muscular dystrophy
Emery-Dreifuss muscular dystrophy
Limb-girdle muscular dystrophy
Oculopharyngeal muscular dystrophy

myositides, or myopathies. Diagnosis is confirmed by documenting expansion of the triplicate (CTG) repeat sequence (normal <50 copies) in the myotonin-protein kinase gene on chromosome 19q and is 100% accurate (9).

Myotonic dystrophy type 2 (DM2, proximal myotonic myopathy (PROMM)) maps to chromosome 3q21 with expansion of a CCTG repeat and demonstrates muscle weakness and myotonia with less commonly occurring cardiac conduction defects, cataracts, diabetes mellitus, and testicular failure.

Emery-Dreifuss muscular dystrophy, caused by mutation of the emerin (Xq28) or lamin A/C gene (1q21), demonstrates weakness and wasting in a humeroperoneal distribution, affecting the biceps and triceps and sparing the deltoid, and is associated with elbow and Achilles heel contracture, cardiomyopathy, and arrhythmias. Onset is in later childhood or adulthood, and diagnosis of the X-linked or autosomal form is by DNA analysis.

Facioscapulohumeral muscular dystrophy typically has a childhood or young adult onset, with facial weakness and inability to smile, whistle, or fully close the eyes. However, it is shoulder-girdle weakness with arm elevation difficulty that usually brings the patient to medical attention. Biceps and triceps may be severely weak, with strong deltoids, and wrist extension is weaker than flexion. Foot drop is an early manifestation, and pelvic girdle weakness develops in 20%. Other organ systems are spared. DNA testing for deletion of a 3.3-kb repeat sequence on chromosome 4 (D4Z4) is 95–98% positive.

First described in 1954 by Walton and Natrass (10), 21 (or more) forms of limb-girdle muscular dystrophy, 6 dominant and 15 recessive (Table 14.4), are currently recognized (11). Distinguishing between them can be difficult. Recessive cases are usually of earlier onset with more rapid progression, and they have higher serum creatine kinase levels than the dominant forms. Diagnosis requires muscle histology, immunocytochemistry, Western blot analysis, and genetic testing for specific proteins.

Oculopharyngeal muscular dystrophy, autosomal dominant and most often seen in French Canadians, is caused by expansion of a GCG repeat on chromosome 14q11 (poly-A binding protein 2 [PABP2]) and presents in the fourth to sixth decade, usually with asymmetric ptosis, dysphagia, and progressive external ophthalmoplegia. Some cases demonstrate limb weakness. Diagnosis is confirmed by demonstration of the repeat expansion.

**Table 14.4** Molecular classification and clinical features of autosomal recessive limb-girdle muscular dystrophy

| Disease | Protein | Gene | Relative prevalence/ founder mutations | Creatine kinase levels[a] | Age of onset | Respiratory involvement | Cardiac involvement | Clinical clues |
|---|---|---|---|---|---|---|---|---|
| LGMD2A | Calpain3 | CAPN3 | One of the most common forms of AR-LGMD worldwide; founder mutations in Basques (2362_2363delinsT-CATCT) and in eastern Europeans (550delA) | Normal to 50× | First to second decade (2–40 years) | – | – | Preferential involvement of posterior thigh muscles; ankle contractures; scapular winging |
| LGMD2B | Dysferlin | DYSF | More common in southern than northern Europe; founder mutations in several populations | 10–100× | Second to third decade (10–73 years) | ± | – | Distal weakness and wasting; muscle pain or swelling; good athletic performance in childhood; inflammatory cells in muscle biopsy |
| LGMD2C | γ-Sarcoglycan | SGCG | Present worldwide; founder mutations in North Africans (521delT) and gypsies (848G > A) | 10–100× | First decade (3–20 years) | + | + | Calf hypertrophy; scapular winging |
| LGMD2D | α-Sarcoglycan | SGCA | Present worldwide; most frequent sarcoglycan form in all populations; common mutation (229C > T), especially in northern Europe | 10–100× | First decade (3–40 years) | + | Rare | Calf hypertrophy; scapular winging |
| LGMD2E | β-Sarcoglycan | SGCB | Common in northern and southern Indiana Amish | 10–100× | First decade (3–20 years) | + | + | Calf hypertrophy or hypotrophy; distal leg weakness |
| LGDM2F | δ-Sarcoglycan | SGCD | Rare all over the world; common mutation (del656C) in African-Brazilian | 10–100× | First decade (3–20 years) | + | + | Calf hypertrophy |

| LGMD | Protein | Gene | Distribution | CK level[a] | Age of onset | | | Clinical features |
|---|---|---|---|---|---|---|---|---|
| LGMD2G | Telethonin | TCAP | Rarely reported outside Brazil | Normal to 30× | Second decade (9–15 years) | – | ± | Calf hypertrophy or hypotrophy; distal leg weakness |
| LGMD2H | TRIM32 | TRIM32 | Only recently reported outside Hutterite population of Canada | Normal to 20× | Second decade (1–44 years) | – | ± | Possible mild facial weakness; small vacuoles in muscle fibers |
| LGMD2I | Fukutin-related protein | FKRP | Relatively frequent in northern Europe; founder mutation in northern Europeans (826C > A) | 10–100× | First to second decade (1–40 years) | + | + | Calf hypertrophy; myoglobinuria; muscle pain |
| LGMD2J | Titin | TTN | Reported only in Finland | Normal to 25× | First decade (5–20 years) | – | – | Distal weakness described; proximal–distal myopathy with associated cardiomyopathy recently described |
| LGMD2K | O-Mannosyl transferase-1 | POMT1 | Few reported LGMD cases (Turkish and English families) | 10–50× | Birth to 6 years | + | – | Microcephaly and cognitive impairment; muscle hypertrophy (thigh and calf) |
| LGMD2L[b] | Fukutin | FKTN | Few reported LGMD cases | 5–100× | <1 years | ? | – | Motor function deterioration during infections |
| LGMD2M[b] | O-Mannose β-1, 2-N-acetyl-glucosaminyl transferase | POMGn1 | Only one reported LGMD case | 20–60× | 12 years | ? | ? | Rapidly progressive |
| LGMD2N[b] | O-Mannosyl transferase-2 | PMOT2 | Few reported LGMD cases | 15× | <2 years | ? | –/? | Calf hypertrophy; possible cognitive impairment |
| LGMD?[b] | ? | 11p13 | Reported in French Canadian families | Normal to 30× | Third decade (11–50 years) | ? | - | Quadriceps atrophy |

Reprinted from **Ref. 103**. Used with permission from Lippincott Williams & Wilkins

*LGMD* limb-girdle muscular dystrophy

[a]In UI/L

[b]No international agreement has been reached for the nomenclature of this LGMD

# Metabolic Myopathies

## Glycogenoses

Patients with glycogenoses, generally children or teenagers but not uncommonly adults, usually complain of random muscle aching and cramps associated with intermittent attacks of rhabdomyolysis and myoglobinuria. However, progressive muscle weakness is a well-recognized presentation, and it is these patients whose diagnosis may be confused with inflammatory myopathy. Diagnosis can be further confounded because, in both groups, serum creatine kinase levels can be elevated, needle electromyography and muscle histology may be myopathic without characteristic inflammatory changes, and even Bohan and Peter criteria for polymyositis *(12)* may be satisfied *(13)*.

McArdle's disease (glycogenosis type V, myophosphorylase deficiency), the most common of the glycogenoses, can begin at any age, including adults, and may present with progressive proximal muscle weakness *(14)*. Over 90% of patients demonstrate elevated serum creatine kinase levels, indicating ongoing muscle destruction, which is felt to be responsible for the fixed weakness these patients can develop in later years. Phosphofructokinase deficiency (glycogenosis type VII, Tarui's disease) is less common than McArdle's disease but is clinically indistinguishable without biochemical analysis.

Debrancher deficiency (glycogenosis type III, Cori-Forbes disease) can present as weakness in the third or fourth decade but affects distal leg and intrinsic hand muscles. It is thus more likely to be confused with motor neuron disease or peripheral neuropathy than with inflammatory myopathy. Brancher deficiency (glycogenosis type IV) typically presents in infancy with hepatic failure, but adult-onset proximal myopathy is reported *(15)*.

Phosphoglycerate kinase deficiency (glycogenosis type X), presenting as a primary myopathy, has been reported in only a handful of individuals. Hemolytic anemia and mental retardation are the usual presentation. Aldolase A deficiency (glycogenosis type XII) has been reported in a child with myopathy and fever-associated exercise intolerance and weakness *(16)*.

Acid maltase deficiency, invariably fatal by age 2 years when presenting as infantile-onset Pompe disease, may present in adults as polymyositis or limb-girdle muscular dystrophy or, in approximately a third, as progressive respiratory failure *(17)*. Acid maltase is a lysosomal enzyme whose deficiency would not be expected to interfere with energy metabolism; thus, the biochemical basis for this myopathy remains a puzzle.

## Disorders of Lipid Metabolism

Disorders of beta-oxidation, the process by which fatty acids, in the form of acyl-coenzyme A (CoA) molecules, are broken down in mitochondria or in peroxisomes

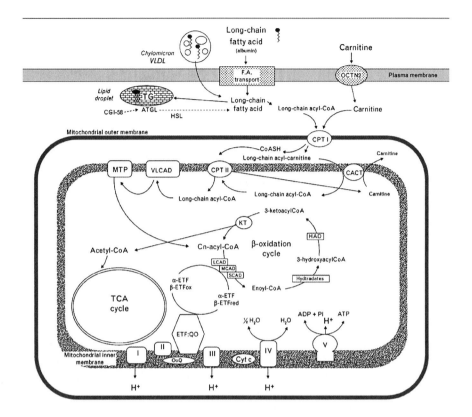

**Fig. 14.1** Scheme of selected metabolic pathways of fatty acid transport and oxidation. *ATGL* adipose triglyceride lipase; *ATP* adenosine-50-triphosphate; *CACT* carnitine/acylcarnitine translocase; *CGI-58* comparative gene identification-58; *CoA* coenzyme A; *CoASH* coenzyme A; *CoQ* coenzyme Q; *CPT I* carnitine palmitoyltransferase I; *CPT II* carnitine palmitoyltransferase II; *ETF* electron-transfer flavoprotein; *ETF-QO* ETF:coenzyme Q oxidoreductase; *HAD* 1-3-hydroxyacyl-CoA dehydrogenase; *HSL* hormone-sensitive lipase; *LCAD* long-chain acyl-CoA dehydrogenase; *MCAD* medium-chain acyl-CoA dehydrogenase; *MTP* mitochondrial trifunctional protein; *OCTN2* sodium-dependent carnitine transporter; *SCAD* short-chain acyl-CoA dehydrogenase; *TCA* tricarboxylic acid; *VLCAD* very long-chain acyl-CoA dehydrogenase; *VLDL* very-low-density lipoprotein; *I, II, III, IV, V*, respiratory chain complex I, II, III, IV, and V, respectively. (From **Ref. 104**. Reprinted from *Current Opinion in Neurology*. Used with permission from Lippincott Williams & Wilkins)

to generate acetyl-CoA (see Fig. 14.1), present with fairly similar clinical features. Most patients die in childhood, but in adults metabolic crises cease, and proximal myopathy develops. Muscle histochemistry demonstrates lipid excess.

Carnitine, crucial to long-chain fatty acid oxidation, controls their influx into mitochondria. Carnitine deficiency may result in primary carnitine myopathy, presenting as a slowly progressive symmetric myopathy. Exercise-induced rhabdomyolysis does not occur, but stress, such as pregnancy, may exacerbate the weakness.

Muscle carnitine levels are low, serum levels are variable, and liver and heart concentrations are normal. Systemic carnitine deficiency results in muscle weakness with hypertrophic cardiomyopathy and attacks of hypoketotic hypoglycemia (Reye's syndrome) and is differentiated from the myopathic form by low carnitine in tissues other than muscle *(18)*. Secondary carnitine deficiency has a clinical presentation similar to systemic carnitine deficiency and is seen in patients with decreased carnitine intake (e.g., malnutrition, malabsorption, strict vegetarian diet), decreased carnitine synthesis (e.g., cirrhosis), decreased body stores (e.g., prematurity), or increased carnitine loss (organic aciduria, renal Fanconi's syndrome, hemodialysis).

Other disorders of beta-oxidation are extremely rare and even less frequently present as myopathy. Included in this group are short-chain, medium-chain, long-chain, and very long-chain acyl-CoA synthetase dehydrogenase deficiency. Lipid storage myopathy was reported in a single adult case of short-chain dehydrogenase deficiency *(19)*, and 16% of medium-chain dehydrogenase deficiency patients demonstrated weakness in a large retrospective study *(20)*.

## Mitochondrial Myopathies

Mitochondrial myopathies represent a group of disorders resulting from impairment of the mitochondrial respiratory chain, the process by which adenosine triphosphate (ATP) is generated in the mitochondrial inner membrane through five complexes (I–V) (see Fig. 14.1). In a northeast England population study, a prevalence of 9.2/100,000 was documented, making this group one of the most common inherited neuromuscular disorders *(21)*.

Defects in either mitochondrial or nuclear DNA can result in mitochondrial myopathies, the former including mutations in tRNAs, ribosomal RNAs (rRNAs), or protein-coding genes, the last encompassing mutations in respiratory chain subunits or ancillary proteins, including coenzyme Q10 deficiency and mutations affecting the structure or abundance of mitochondrial DNA *(22)*. Several well-defined syndromes are associated with multisystem involvement and thus are not likely to be confused with inflammatory myopathy. These are mentioned in passing and include Kearns-Sayre syndrome (KSS); chronic progressive external ophthalmoplegia (CPEO); mitochondrial encephalomyopathy with lactic acidosis and stroke-like episodes (MELAS); Leber hereditary optic neuropathy (LHON); neuropathy, ataxia, retinitis pigmentosa (NARP); myoclonic epilepsy with ragged red fibers (MERRF); mitochondrial neurogastrointestinal encephalomyopathy (MNGIE); and autosomal recessive cardiomyopathy ophthalmoplegia (ARCO). Isolated myopathy may occur due to mitochondrial or nuclear DNA mutation, and diagnosis is facilitated when histopathology reveals the characteristic ragged red fibers on Gomori trichrome stain. Some mitochondrial myopathies are secondary, such as following exposure to toxins, including zidovudine (AZT) and clofibrate *(23,24)*.

CoQ10 (ubiquinone) acts as an electron shuttle between complexes I and III and between II and III. CoQ10 deficiency has been associated not only with different syndromes, some multisystem, but also with isolated myopathy *(25–27)*. Ragged red fibers, consistent with mitochondrial myopathy, and lipid storage are seen on muscle biopsy, and muscle CoQ10 concentration is markedly decreased. Improvement follows oral CoQ10 supplementation.

Controversy exists regarding the pathogenesis of myopathy following statin usage, an iatrogenic disorder ranging from benign elevation of serum creatine kinase to myalgia, muscle cramps, fixed weakness, and even acute rhabdomyolysis and myoglobinuria *(28)*. Muscle CoQ10 deficiency has been raised as a possible cause because statins inhibit the synthesis of mevalonate, a precursor of CoQ10. However, among 18 patients with statin-related myopathy, no significant difference in CoQ10 concentration was found between patients and control subjects (see "Drug- and Toxin-Induced Myopathy") *(29)*.

Mitochondrial DNA mutation involving tRNA resulted in pure myopathy in several patients *(30–32)*, probably as a result of "skewed heteroplasmy," that is, a preferential accumulation of the mutation in skeletal muscle. Mutations in mitochondrial DNA involving protein-coding genes may also cause pure myopathy *(33)*.

## Drug- and Toxin-Induced Myopathy

Due to its high metabolic activity, muscle is sensitive to the effects of drugs and toxins. The exact incidence of toxic myopathies is unknown, but early diagnosis is important because treatment entails removing the offending agent *(34)*. Necrotizing myopathy, characterized by acute or subacute muscle pain or weakness or both, is the most common myotoxic syndrome. Lipid-lowering agents are often implicated, including HMG-CoA reductase inhibitors, fibric acid derivatives such as clofibrate and gemfibrozil, and nicotinic acid *(35–37)*. With standard doses of statins, the incidence of myopathy is typically about 1/10,000 patients/year, but it increases with higher doses *(38, 39)*. Serum creatine kinase levels may be normal or elevated; in some instances, muscle biopsy has shown necrosis and mononuclear cell infiltration. A genomewide association study has presently identified at least one common variant in the SLCO1B1 gene on chromosome 12 strongly associated with an increased risk of statin-induced myopathy *(40)*. SLCO1B1 encodes the organic anion-transporting polypeptide OATP1B1, which mediates the hepatic uptake of various drugs, including most statins and statin acids *(41)*. Genotyping these variants may help achieve the benefits of statin therapy more safely and effectively. Other agents associated with necrotizing myopathy include cyclosporine, labetalol, and propofol.

Alcohol abuse also causes acute necrotizing myopathy with muscle pain, swelling, weakness, and serum creatine kinase elevation, but more often, chronic alcoholic myopathy is the result, with insidious onset, predominantly proximal, lower extremity, limb-girdle weakness. Unexplained elevation of serum creatine kinase may be an incidental finding in asymptomatic alcoholics, perhaps the result of subclinical necrotizing myopathy, hypokalemia, or muscle trauma *(42)*.

Chloroquine, used to treat malaria, lupus, and rheumatoid arthritis, may cause slowly progressive proximal muscle weakness and atrophy, more so in the legs than arms, and serum creatine kinase is usually elevated. Hydroxychloroquine (structurally related to chloroquine) and amiodarone may cause a similar although less-severe picture, the latter associated with tremor and ataxia.

Colchicine inhibits polymerization of tubulin into microtubular structures and, over several months, may cause myopathy, more often in patients with chronic renal failure. Vincristine has a similar mechanism of action, usually resulting in severe axonal neuropathy, but myopathy with myalgias and proximal muscle weakness may occur as well *(43)*.

Inflammatory myopathy may be toxin induced. L-Tryptophan products manufactured by a Japanese company were, in the late 1980s, associated with outbreak of the eosinophilia-myalgia syndrome, comprising muscle pain, tenderness, weakness, skin changes, and striking blood eosinophilia, with normal serum creatine kinase and sedimentation rate. Suspicion fell on some contaminant suspected to cause an allergic reaction *(44)*. Muscle biopsies revealed perimysial inflammation. Removal of the product and administration of high-dose steroid was usually curative. Toxic oil syndrome, restricted to ingestion of a particular rapeseed oil, illegally marketed in Spain in 1981, caused a similar syndrome *(45)*. D-Penicillamine, phenytoin, procainamide, interferon-alpha, imatinib mesylate (Gleevec), and lamotrigine may also cause myositis.

Steroid administration, the most common cause of iatrogenic myopathy, occurs more commonly in women than men (2:1 ratio), more so with doses above 30 mg/day than below and more so with fluorinated (dexamethasone and triamcinolone) than nonfluorinated glucocorticoids *(46)*. Weakness usually requires chronic administration but may begin within weeks. Following high-dose intravenous steroids, with or without concomitant use of neuromuscular blocking agents, acute quadriplegic myopathy (critical illness myopathy) causing severe generalized weakness may occur *(47)*. Critically ill patients with sepsis or multisystem failure are also prone to this syndrome, even in the absence of intravenous steroid administration *(48, 49)*.

## Endocrine Myopathies

Adrenal insufficiency causes generalized weakness and muscle cramping with normal serum creatine kinase levels and electromyographic examination. Cortisol, renin, and ACTH (corticotropin) assays and ACTH stimulation testing provide the diagnosis.

Proximal muscle weakness, often out of proportion to the degree of muscle wasting, associated with myalgia, fatigue, and exercise intolerance characterize hyperthyroid myopathy. The serum creatine kinase level is usually normal. Inflammatory myositis may rarely coexist with hyperthyroidism, requiring corticosteroid therapy *(50)*. Hypothyroidism causes muscle stiffness, mild proximal weakness, myalgia, and myoedema in most and severe weakness and muscle hypertrophy in some. It is tenfold more common in women than men.

Hyperparathyroidism variably causes proximal muscle weakness and wasting, and severely affected patients have gait difficulties. Hypoparathyroidism is occasionally associated with chronic myopathy, but tetany is the muscle symptom most frequently encountered.

Slowly progressive proximal muscle weakness with impaired exercise tolerance occurs in 50% of patients with acromegaly. Muscle wasting is not prominent, and serum creatine kinase levels are mildly elevated.

Panhypopituitarism results in severe weakness with preserved muscle bulk and is the consequence of thyroid and adrenal hormone insufficiency.

## Muscle Disorders Associated with Electrolyte Disturbance

Rapid-onset weakness (over hours to days) generally occurs with electrolyte abnormalities and would not be confused with idiopathic inflammatory myopathy. Hypokalemic myopathy can be manifest in one of three forms, but only one, a syndrome of proximal, flaccid, transient, or persistent weakness with preserved reflexes and sensation, usually with markedly elevated serum creatine kinase, mimics inflammatory myopathy. Other presentations, which would not enter the differential diagnosis, include attacks resembling familial periodic paralysis with areflexia and, rarely, severe muscle necrosis with myoglobinuria. Hyperkalemic weakness similarly results in rapid-onset generalized weakness and must be differentiated from hyperkalemic periodic paralysis. Ascending paralysis mimicking Guillain-Barre syndrome has been reported *(51)*.

Hypernatremia and hypermagnesemia cause rapidly developing generalized weakness. Hypomagnesemia has been reported with mitochondrial myopathy in two cases *(52)*, and hypophosphatemia may present as chronic proximal myopathy, although acute and subacute generalized weakness mimicking Guillain-Barre syndrome is recorded.

## Infections Associated with Myopathy

Among infectious agents that may cause myositis, viruses are the most likely to produce a generalized muscle disorder resembling inflammatory myopathy, most commonly influenza A and B in the United States, more so B, and more so in school-aged children *(53–55)*. HIV infection may cause myopathy, polymyositis, and rhabdomyolysis *(56, 57)*. Case reports have also associated polymyositis with hepatitis B and C viral infection (Table 14.5) *(58)*.

*Staphylococcus aureus* may occasionally cause diffuse myositis with rhabdomyolysis *(59)*. Group A streptococci may cause a variety of muscle infections, of which group A streptococci necrotizing myositis is the most severe, beginning with flu-like symptoms, including rash and myalgias, and evolving to intense muscle pain with

**Table 14.5** Infections associated with inflammatory myopathy

| |
|---|
| Viral |
|   HIV |
|   Human T-lymphotropic virus (HTLV) |
|   Hepatitis B and C |
| Bacterial |
|   *Staphylococcus aureus* |
|   Streptococci |
|   *Escherichia coli* |
|   *Legionella* |
| Fungal |
|   Candida |
|   Cryptococcus |
|   Histoplasmosis |
| Parasitic |
|   Protozoa |
| Cestodes (tapeworms) |
|   Nematodes |

multiple sites of involvement due to bacteremia and seeding of the muscles. This disease has a rapidly progressive course over 1–4 days and may be fatal *(60)*.

Fungal involvement of muscle is unusual, with most cases involving immuno-compromised patients. Candida is the most commonly reported cause of fungal myositis, with fever, rash, and muscle tenderness in candidemic patients suggesting myositis, most often due to diffuse, multiple microabscesses *(61)*. Cryptococcus infection may rarely present with infectious myositis *(62)*, but most such infections are asymptomatic. Histoplasmosis, endemic to the Ohio and Mississippi River valleys, occurs via fungal microconidia inhalation into the lungs and is also usually asymptomatic, but dissemination may occur and reports of myositis exist *(63)*.

*Trichinella* (trichinosis), *Taenia solium* (cysticercosis), and *Toxoplasma gondii* (toxoplasmosis) are the most commonly reported parasitic causes of myositis *(64)*. Trichinosis follows ingestion of undercooked meat of domestic or wild animals containing *Trichinella*-encysted larvae, usually undercooked pork, but increasingly undercooked wild game, including polar bear, wild boar, walrus, cougar, and fox *(65)*. Most cases are subclinical, but muscle invasion may cause myalgia, swelling, and weakness. Extraocular muscles are affected initially, followed by the masseters, diaphragm, neck, and larynx, as well as limb muscles *(66)*. Rarely, cases have included severe proximal muscle weakness simulating polymyositis *(67)*.

Involvement of muscle with the pork tapeworm *Taenia solium*, cysticercosis is usually asymptomatic, an incidental finding of calcified cysts on radiographs. Occasional cases of myopathy have been reported *(68)*. Rare cases of polymyositis have been reported with *Toxoplasma gondii*, mainly among immunocompromised hosts *(69, 70)*.

## Myopathy Associated with Collagen Vascular Disease

Polyarteritis nodosa is a systemic vasculitis affecting multiple organ systems, including muscle, resulting in myalgia and weakness, but peripheral nerve involvement is much more common, seen in about 50% of patients overall (Table 14.6) *(71)*. In fact, when weakness is present, it is usually due to neuropathy. Other systemic vasculitides that preferentially affect nerve over muscle include Churg-Strauss, microscopic polyangiitis and Wegener's granulomatosis. Mixed cryoglobulinemia, defined by the presence of a serum protein that precipitates in the cold, produces peripheral neuropathy in up to 60% *(72)* Nonsystemic vasculitis of peripheral nerve produces neuropathy with evidence of vasculitis on nerve or muscle biopsy but not elsewhere *(73)*. Polymyalgia rheumatica produces axial stiffness and myalgia, but weakness (unrelated to pain) is rare, and muscle biopsy shows type II muscle cell atrophy but not myositis. Giant cell arteritis is a related condition, seen with poly-myalgia rheumatica in over a third of cases *(74)*, causing granulomatous inflammation of large arteries with headache, visual symptoms, and jaw or limb claudication *(75)*.

Rheumatoid arthritis and Sjogren's syndrome each affect 1% of the population and predominantly affect nerve rather than muscle *(76)*. Chronic rheumatoid arthritis may be associated with proximal muscle weakness and atrophy due to coexistent polymyositis or dermatomyositis, but other conditions, including spinal cord compression due to the concomitant arthritis or toxic myopathy due to steroid or other medication use, must be excluded *(77)*. Sjogren's syndrome, an autoimmune disease of exocrine glands, may be associated with mild muscle pain or weakness, but if significant proximal weakness develops, serious consideration must be given to possible concomitant idiopathic inflammatory polymyositis. The same may be said for patients with systemic lupus erythematosus *(78)* and progressive systemic sclerosis *(79)*.

**Table 14.6**  Collagen vascular diseases associated with myositis

Polyarteritis nodosum
Wegener's granulomatosis
Systemic lupus erythematosus
Rheumatoid arthritis
Scleroderma
Sjogren's syndrome
Leukocytoclastic vasculitis
Hypersensitivity vasculitis
Polymyalgia rheumatica
Mixed connective tissue disease
Adult Still's disease

# Cancer and Myopathy

Although not considered paraneoplastic diseases, dermatomyositis and polymyositis are nevertheless associated with an increased risk of malignancy, up to 45% in the former, less so in the latter *(80, 81)*. Men and women are equally affected (those over 40 years of age having the higher risk), and lung, colon, and ovarian cancer are the most common associated malignancies.

Necrotizing myopathy may occur, presumably as a paraneoplastic syndrome, with the acute or insidious onset of proximal muscle weakness, myalgia, and elevated serum creatine kinase *(82)*. Gastrointestinal adenocarcinoma and small-cell and non-small-cell lung cancers are the most frequent underlying malignancy but, unlike paraneoplastic syndromes, are usually diagnosed simultaneously with the myopathy.

Cachexia, muscle atrophy, and proximal leg weakness are often seen with cancer, but serum creatine kinase and electromyographic study are usually normal. Potential causes of this myopathy include poor nutrition, disuse atrophy, increased catabolism due to cancer, and side effects of chemotherapy *(83)*.

Whether pure motor neuronopathy occurs as a paraneoplastic syndrome remains controversial as the association may be coincidental rather than causative. Case-control or population-based studies have yet to answer the question. In most instances, the symptoms, signs, and course of the motor nerve disease are identical to that of amyotrophic lateral sclerosis (ALS) *(84)*.

Weakness, areflexia or hyporeflexia, and autonomic dysfunction characterize Lambert-Eaton myasthenic syndrome (LEMS), a neuromuscular junctionopathy due to antibodies directed against the presynaptic P/Q-type voltage-gated calcium channels *(85)*. About half are associated with small-cell lung cancer, and proximal leg weakness is a common presenting symptom. Repetitive nerve stimulation studies demonstrate the characteristic incremental response, and serum antibody titers confirm the diagnosis *(86)*. Myasthenia gravis is a post-synaptic junctionopathy due to antibodies directed against the nicotinic acetylcholine receptor. Not considered a paraneoplastic syndrome as most have no underlying malignancy, 10% have thymoma *(87)*, and 5% have inflammatory myopathy, usually with thymoma *(88, 89)*.

# Infiltrative Myopathy

Primary amyloidosis results from deposition of amyloid fibrils, composed of insoluble immunoglobulin light chains (AL), in multiple organs, including kidney, heart, liver, and skin. Neurologic consequences are usually neuropathic, including carpal tunnel syndrome, sensorimotor neuropathy, and autonomic neuropathy *(90)*. Myopathy is uncommon, but amyloid may present with proximal weakness and fatigue.

Sarcoidosis results from the deposition of noncaseating granulomas in multiple organs, including the lungs, thoracic lymph nodes, eyes, and skin and in 5%, it affects the nervous system *(91)* (most commonly the facial nerve but also the meninges, hypothalamus, pituitary gland, spinal cord, and peripheral nerves) *(92)*.

Muscle involvement is uncommon but may occur as a proximal myopathy, chiefly affecting women over age 50 years (93). Less-common muscle presentations include subacute myositis with proximal weakness, myalgias, fever, and nodular sarcoid myopathy with palpable nodes but usually without pain or impaired function (94, 95).

Behçet disease, a chronic multisystem inflammatory disorder of unknown etiology affecting men more than women in the third and fourth decades of life, usually presents with oral and genital ulcers. Ocular involvement, usually recurrent anterior uveitis, is its most serious complication, but involvement of the joints, lungs, and vascular system also occurs (96). Muscle involvement is unusual (97), but myopathy, both clinical and subclinical, is reported (98).

## Nutritional Deficiency and Myopathy

With the increasing number of gastric restriction operations performed for morbid obesity, particularly Roux-en-Y gastric bypass or gastroplasty, the effects of impaired nutrition are increasingly encountered. Among 500 patients who over a 5-year period underwent such surgery (predominantly Roux-en-Y gastric bypass), 4.6% ($n = 23$) developed neurologic complications (99), most often peripheral neuropathy, with posterolateral myelopathy and Wernicke-Korsakoff encephalopathy seen less often. None developed myopathy, but it is described following partial gastrectomy for peptic ulcer disease (100) as well as in a case report following Roux-en-Y gastric bypass (101). Starvation, today best exemplified by anorexia nervosa, causes a purely starvation-induced myopathy resulting from severe dietary restriction that improves with adequate nutrition (102).

## Motor Neuron Disease

Chronic spinal muscular atrophy, a hereditary disease affecting the lower motor neuron, may begin in childhood (Kugelberg-Welander) or adult life, presenting with slowly progressive limb-girdle weakness. Chronic lower motor neuron disease in children may also have a scapuloperoneal, facioscapuloperoneal, or predominantly distal distribution. ALS may demonstrate predominantly proximal weakness, but the presence of upper motor neuron signs, including spasticity, brisk deep tendon reflexes, and Babinski signs, differentiates it from myopathy.

## Conclusion

Various conditions can mimic idiopathic inflammatory myopathy. A thorough history, more so than the physical examination, will be most useful in determining the correct diagnosis, but ancillary studies including serology, electromyography, muscle biopsy, and genetic studies may also be needed.

**Acknowledgment** We would like to thank Salvatore DiMauro for reviewing portions of the transcript and for helpful comments and suggestions.

# References

1. Zampieri S, Ghirardello A, Iaccarino L, et al. Anti-Jo-1 antibodies. Autoimmunity 2005;38:73–8.
2. Sewry CA, Jimenez-Mallebrera C, Muntoni F. Congenital myopathies. Curr Opin Neurol 2008;21:569–75.
3. D'Amico A, Bertini E. Congenital myopathies. Curr Neurol Neurosci Rep 2008;8:73–9.
4. Magee KR, Shy GM. A new congenital non-progressive myopathy. Brain 1956;79:610–21.
5. Bitoun M, Maugenre S, Jeannet PY, et al. Mutations in dynamin 2 cause dominant centronuclear myopathy. Nat Genet 2005;37:1207–9.
6. Cardamone M, Darras BT, Ryan MM. Inherited myopathies and muscular dystrophies. Semin Neurol 2008;28:250–9.
7. Sunohara N, Arahata K, Hoffman EP, et al. Quadriceps myopathy: forme fruste of Becker muscular dystrophy. Ann Neurol 1990;28:634–9.
8. Hoffman EP, Arahata K, Minetti C, et al. Dystrophinopathy in isolated cases of myopathy in females. Neurology 1992;42:967–72.
9. Brook JD, McCurrach ME, Harley HG, et al. Molecular basis of myotonic dystrophy: expansion of the trinucleotide (CTG) repeat at the 3′ end of a transcript encoding a protein kinase family member. Cell 1992;68:799–808.
10. Walton J, Natrass F. On the classification, natural history and treatment of the myopathies. Brain 1954;77:169–231.
11. Norwood F, de Visser M, Eymard B, et al. EFNS guideline on diagnosis and management of limb girdle muscular dystrophies. Eur J Neurol 2007;14:1305–12.
12. Bohan A, Peter JB. Polymyositis and dermatomyositis. N Engl J Med 1975;292:344–7.
13. Wortmann RL, DiMauro S. Differentiating idiopathic inflammatory myopathies from metabolic myopathies. Rheum Dis Clin North Am 2002;28:759–78.
14. DiMauro S, Lamperti C. Muscle glycogenosis. Muscle Nerve 2001;24:984–99.
15. DiMauro S, Servidei S, Tsujino S. Disorders of carbohydrate metabolism: glycogen storage diseases. In: Rosenberg RN, Prusiner SB, DiMauro S, Barchi RL, eds. The molecular and genetic basis of neurological disease. Boston: Butterworth-Heinemann, 1997:1067–97.
16. Kreuder J, Borkhardt A, Repp R, et al. Inherited metabolic myopathy and hemolysis due to a mutation in aldolase A. N Engl J Med 1996;334:1100–4.
17. Engel AG, Gomez MR, Seybold ME, et al. The spectrum and diagnosis of acid maltase deficiency. Neurology 1973;23:95–101.
18. Karpati G, Carpenter S, Engel AG. The syndrome of systemic carnitine deficiency: clinical, morphological, biochemical, and pathophysiological features. Neurology 1975;25:16–23.
19. Turnbull DM, Bartlett K, Stevens DL, et al. Short-chain acyl-CoA dehydrogenase deficiency associated with a lipid storage myopathy and secondary carnitine deficiency. N Engl J Med 1984;311:1232–6.
20. LaFolla AK, Thompson RJ, Roe CR. Medium-chain acyl-coenzyme A dehydrogenase deficiency: clinical course in 120 affected children. J Pediatr 1994;124:409–15.
21. Schaefer AM, McFarland R, Blakely EL, et al. Prevalence of mitochondrial DNA disease in adults. Ann Neurol 2008;63:35–9.
22. DiMauro S. Mitochondrial myopathies. Curr Opin Rheumatol 2006;18:636–41.
23. Bardosi A, Scheidt P, Goebel H. Mitochondrial myopathy: a result of clofibrate/etiofibrate treatment. Acta Neuropathol (Berl) 1985;68:164–8.
24. Chariot P, Monnet J, Mouchet M, et al. Determination of the blood lactate: pyruvate ratio as a noninvasive test for the diagnosis of zidovudine myopathy. Arthritis Rheum 1994;37:583–6.

25. Lalani S, Vladutiu GD, Plunkett K, et al. Isolated mitochondrial myopathy associated with muscle coenzyme Q10 deficiency. Arch Neurol 2005;62:317–20.
26. Horvath R, Schneiderat P, Schoser BGH, et al. Coenzyme Q10 deficiency and isolated myopathy. Neurology 2006;66:253–5.
27. Gempel K, Topaloglu H, Beril T, et al. The myopathic form of coenzyme Q10 deficiency is caused by mutations in the electron-transferring-flavoprotein dehydrogenase (EFTDH) gene. Brain 2007;130:2037–44.
28. Owczarek J, Jasinska M, Orszulak-Michalak D. Drug-induced myopathies: an overview of the possible mechanisms. Pharmacol Rep 2005;57:23–34.
29. Lamperti C, Naini AB, Lucchini V, et al. Muscle coenzyme Q10 in statin-related myopathy. Arch Neurol 2005;62:1709–12.
30. Moraes CT, Ciacci F, Bonilla E, et al. Two novel pathogenic mitochondrial DNA mutations affecting organelle number and protein synthesis. J Clin Invest 1993;92:2906–15.
31. Hadjigeorgiou GM, Kim SH, Fischbeck KH, et al. A new mitochondrial DNA mutation (A3288G) in the tRNALeu(UUR) gene associated with familial myopathy. J Neurol Sci 1999;164:153–7.
32. Pulkes T, Liolitsa D, Eunson LH, et al. New phenotypic diversity associated with the mito-chondrial tRNASer(UCN) gene mutation. Neuromuscul Disord 2005;15:364–71.
33. Hays AP, Oskoui M, Tanji K, et al. Mitochondrial neurology II: myopathies and peripheral neuropathies. In: DiMauro S, Hirano M, Schon EA, eds. Mitochondrial medicine. London: Informa Healthcare, 2006:45–74.
34. Walsh RJ, Amato AA. Toxic myopathies. Neurol Clin 2005;23:397–428.
35. DeGirolami U, Chucrallah A, Freeman R, et al. Lovastatin myopathy [Abstract]. J Neuropathol Exp Neurol 1991;50:352.
36. Katsilambros N, Braaten J, Ferguson BD, et al. Muscular syndrome after clofibrate. N Engl J Med 1972;282:1110–6.
37. Litin SC, Anderson CF. Nicotinic acid associated myopathy: a report of three cases. Am J Med 1989;86:481–3.
38. Law M, Rudnicka AR. Statin safety: a systematic review. Am J Cardiol 2006;97(Suppl): 52C–60C.
39. Armitage J. The safety of statins in clinical practice. Lancet 2007;370:1781–90.
40. The SEARCH Collaborative Group. SLCO1B1 variants and statin-induced myopathy – a genomewide Study. N Engl J Med 2008;359:789–99.
41. König J, Seithel A, Gradhand U, et al. Pharmacogenomics of human OATP transporters. Naunyn Schmiedebergs Arch Pharmacol 2006;372:432–43.
42. Amato AA, Dumitru D. Acquired myopathies. In: Dumitru D, Amato AA, Zwarts MJ, eds. Electrodiagnostic medicine. 2nd ed. Philadelphia, PA: Hanley and Belfus, 2002:1414–5.
43. Bradley WG, Lassman LP, Pearce GW, et al. The neuromyopathy of vincristine in man: clinical, electrophysiological, and pathological studies. J Neurol Sci 1970;10:107–31.
44. Belongia EA, Hedberg CW, Gleich GJ, et al. An investigation of the cause of the eosinophilia-myalgia syndrome associated with tryptophan use. N Engl J Med 1990;323:357–65.
45. Kilbourne EM, Rigau-Perez JG, Heath CW, et al. Clinical epidemiology of toxic oil syndrome; manifestations of a new illness. N Engl J Med 1983;309:1408–14.
46. Faludi G, Gotlieb J, Meyers J. Factors influencing the development of steroid-induced myopathies. Ann N Y Acad Sci 1966;138:62–72.
47. Lacomis D, Petrella JT, Giuliani MJ. Causes of neuromuscular weakness in the intensive care unit: a study of ninety-two patients. Muscle Nerve 1998;21:610–7.
48. Deconinck N, Van Parijs V, Beckers-Bleukx G, et al. Critical illness myopathy unrelated to corticosteroids or neuromuscular blocking agents. Neuromuscul Disord 1998;8:186–92.
49. Bolton CF. Neuromuscular manifestations of critical illness. Muscle Nerve 2005;32:140–63.
50. Hardman O, Molloy F, Brett F, et al. Inflammatory myopathy in thyrotoxicosis. Neurology 1997;48:339–41.
51. Evers S, Engelien A, Karsch V, et al. Secondary hyperkalemic paralysis. J Neurol Neurosurg Psychiatry 1998;64:249–52.

52. Klingberg W, Bender A, Riggs J. Mitochondrial myopathy and hypomagnesemia: two cases. Neurology 1983;33(Suppl):167.
53. Yoshino M, Suzuki S, Adachi K, et al. High incidence of acute myositis with type A influenza virus infection in the elderly. Intern Med 2000;39:431–2.
54. Hu JJ, Kao CL, Lee PI, et al. Clinical features of influenza A and B in children and association with myositis. J. Microbiol Immunol Infect 2004;37:95–8.
55. Agyeman P, Duppenthaler A, Heininger U, et al. Influenza-associated myositis in children. Infection 2004;32:199–203.
56. Dalakas MC, Pezeshkpour GH, Gravell M, et al. Polymyositis associated with AIDS retrovirus. JAMA 1986;256:2381–3.
57. Johnson RW, Williams FM, Kazi S, et al. Human immunodeficiency virus-associated polymyositis: a longitudinal study of outcome. Arthritis Rheum 2003;49:172–8.
58. Nojima T, Hirakata M, Sato S, et al. A case of polymyositis associated with hepatitis B infection. Clin Exp Rheumatol 2000;18:86–8.
59. Adamski GB, Garin EH, Ballinger WE, et al. Generalized nonsuppurative myositis with staphylococcal septicemia. J Pediatr 1980;96:964–7.
60. Subramanian KN, Lam KS. Malignant necrotising streptococcal myositis: a rare and fatal condition. J Bone Joint Surg Br 2003;85:277–8.
61. Jarowski CI, Fialk MA, Murray HW, et al. Fever, rash, and muscle tenderness A. distinctive clinical presentation of disseminated candidiasis. Arch Intern Med 1978;138:544–6.
62. Flagg SD, Chang YJ, Masuell CP, et al. Myositis resulting from disseminated cryptococcosis in a patient with hepatitis C cirrhosis. Clin Infect Dis 2001;32:1104–7.
63. Goel D, Prayaga AK, Rao N, et al. Histoplasmosis as a cause of nodular myositis in an AIDS patient diagnosed on fine needle aspiration cytology. A case report. Acta Cytol 2007;51:89–91.
64. Crum-Cianflone NF. Bacterial, fungal, parasitic, and viral myositis. Clin Microbiol Rev 2008; 21:473–94.
65. Roy SL, Lopez AS, Schantz PM. Trichinellosis surveillance: United States, 1997–2001. MMWR Surveill Summ 2003;52:1–8.
66. Capo V, Despommier DD. Clinical aspects of infection with *Trichinella* spp. Clin Microbiol Rev 1996;9:47–54.
67. Durán-Ortiz JS, García-de la Torre I, Orozco-Barocio G, et al. Trichinosis with severe myopathic involvement mimicking polymyositis. Report of a family outbreak. J Rheumatol 1992;19:310–2.
68. McGrill RJ. Cysticercosis resembling myopathy. Lancet 1948;6:728–30.
69. Rowland LP, Greer M. Toxoplasmic polymyositis. Neurology 1961;11:367–70.
70. Pollock JL. Toxoplasmosis appearing to be dermatomyositis. Arch Dermatol 1979;115:736–7.
71. Lovshin LL, Kernohan JW. Peripheral neuritis in periarteritis nodosa. Arch Int Med 1948;82: 321–38.
72. Gemignani F, Pavesi G, Fiocchi A, et al. Peripheral neuropathy in essential mixed cryoglobulinemia. J Neurol Neurosurg Psychiatry 1992;55:116–20.
73. Davies L, Spies JM, Pollard JD, McLeod JG. Vasculitis confined to peripheral nerves. Brain 1996;119:1441–8.
74. Salvarani C, Hunder GG. Musculoskeletal manifestations in a population-based cohort of patients with giant cell arteritis. Arthritis Rheum 1999;42:1259–66.
75. Rosenbaum R. Neuromuscular complications of connective tissue diseases. Muscle Nerve 2001;24:154–69.
76. Andonopoulos AP, Lagos G, Drosos AA, et al. The spectrum of neurological involvement in Sjogren's syndrome. Br J Rheumatol 1990;29:21–3.
77. Miro O, Pedrol E, Casademont J, et al. Muscle involvement in rheumatoid arthritis: clinicopathological study of 21 symptomatic patients. Semin Arthritis Rheum 1996;25:421–8.
78. Estes D, Christian CL. The natural history of systemic lupus erythematosus by prospective analysis. Medicine 1971;50:85–95.
79. Clements PJ, Furst DE, Campion DS, et al. Muscle disease in progressive systemic sclerosis. Arthritis Rheum 1978;21:62–71.

80. Sigurgeirsson B, Lindelöf B, Edhag O, et al. Risk of cancer in patients with dermatomyositis or polymyositis: a population based study. N Engl J Med 1992;326:363–7.
81. Callen JP. Relationship of cancer to inflammatory muscle diseases: dermatomyositis, polymyositis, and inclusion body myositis. Rheum Dis Clin North Am 1994;20:943–53.
82. Levin MI, Mozaffar T, Al-Lozi MT, et al. Paraneoplastic necrotizing myopathy: clinical and pathologic features. Neurology 1998;50:764–7.
83. Briemberg HR, Amato AA. Neuromuscular complications of cancer. Neurol Clin 2003;21:141–65.
84. Gordon PH, Rowland LP, Younger DS, et al. Lymphoproliferative disorders and motor neuron disease: an update. Neurology 1997;48:1671–8.
85. O'Neill JH, Murray NM, Newsom-Davis J. The Lambert-Eaton myasthenic syndrome: a review of 50 cases. Brain 1988;111:577–96.
86. Tim RW, Massey JM, Sanders DB. Lambert-Eaton myasthenic syndrome: electrodiagnostic findings and response to treatment. Neurology 2000;54:2176–8.
87. Lovelace RE, Younger DS. Myasthenia gravis with thymoma. Neurology 1997;48(Suppl 5): S76–81.
88. Pascuzzi RM, Roos KL, Phillips LH. Granulomatous inflammatory myopathy associated with myasthenia gravis: a case report and review of the literature. Arch Neurol 1986;43:621–3.
89. Mygland A, Vincent A, Newsom-Davis J, et al. Autoantibodies in thymoma-associated myasthenia gravis with myositis or neuromyotonia. Arch Neurol 2000;57:527–31.
90. Friedman Y, Paul JT, Turley J, Hazrati LN, Munoz D. Axial myopathy due to primary amyloidosis. Muscle Nerve 2007;36:542–6.
91. Scott TF. Neurosarcoidosis: progress and clinical aspects. Neurology 1993;43:8–12.
92. Delaney P. Neurologic manifestations in sarcoidosis: review of the literature, with a report of 23 cases. Ann Intern Med 1977;87:336–45.
93. Sepulveda-Sanchez JM, Villarejo-Galende A, Cabello A, et al. Miopatia sarcoidea. Presentacion de dos casos y revision de la bibliografia. Rev Neurol 2005;41:159–62.
94. Stjernberg N, Cajander S, Truedsson H, et al. Muscle involvement in sarcoidosis. Acta Med Scand 1981;209:213–6.
95. Berger C, Sommer C, Meinck HM. Isolated sarcoid myopathy. Muscle Nerve 2002; 26:553–6.
96. Haghighi AB, Pourmand R, Nikseresht AR. Neuro-Behçet disease: a review. Neurologist 2005;11:80–9.
97. Worthmann F, Bruns J, Turker T, et al. Muscular involvement in Behçet's disease: case report and review of the literature. Neuromuscul Disord 1996;6:247–53.
98. Frayha R. Muscle involvement in Behçet's disease. Arthritis Rheum 1981;24:636–63.
99. Abarbanel JM, Berginer VM, Osimani A, et al. Neurologic complications after gastric restriction surgery for morbid obesity. Neurology 1987;37:196–200.
100. Banerji NK, Hurwitz LJ. Nervous system manifestations after gastric surgery. Acta Neurol Scand 1971;47:485–513.
101. Hsia AW, Hattab EM, Katz JS. Malnutrition-induced myopathy following Roux-en-Y gastric bypass. Muscle Nerve 2001;24:1692–4.
102. McLoughlin DM, Spargo E, Wassif WS, et al. Structural and functional changes in skeletal muscle in anorexia nervosa. Acta Neuropathol 1998;95:632–40.
103. Guglieri M, Straub V, Bushby K, Lochmuruller H. Limb-girdle muscular dystrophies. Curr Opin Neurol 2008;21(5):576–84.
104. Brunoa C, DiMauro S. Lipid storage myopathies. Curr Opin Neurol 2008;21:601–6.

# Chapter 15
# Outcomes and Assessment for Inflammatory Muscle Disease

Lisa G. Rider

**Abstract** This chapter describes the development and preliminary validation of measures to evaluate myositis disease activity, damage, and health-related quality of life for the adult and juvenile idiopathic inflammatory myopathies. The focus is primarily on the core set measures that have been developed through consensus methods by multidisciplinary collaborative study groups as well as new definitions of improvement that provide a composite response measure that combines the core set tools. Additional approaches that are not as fully validated but may also be important in the evaluation of individual myositis patients or useful in certain myositis studies are also reviewed. The utilization of standardized, validated approaches to assess myositis disease activity, damage, and health-related quality of life is enhancing the conduct of myositis clinical studies and therapeutic trials.

**Keywords** Outcome assessment • Disease activity • Disease damage • Quality of life

## Introduction

The clinical assessment of the idiopathic inflammatory myopathies (IIMs) has been advanced by the development and partial validation of assessment tools and a movement toward standardization of outcome measures, particularly for therapeutic trials. Collaborative researchers working in this area have recognized that to understand fully myositis outcomes, it is useful to assess disease activity, damage, and patient self-assessment of quality of life (QOL) using validated and standardized approaches. *Disease activity* has been defined as the reversible illness manifestations resulting from inflammatory processes, whereas disease damage consists of persistent changes

L.G. Rider
Environmental Autoimmunity Group, Office of Clinical Research, National Institute
of Environmental Health Sciences, National Institutes of Health, Bethesda, MD, USA

L.J. Kagen (ed.), *The Inflammatory Myopathies*,
DOI 10.1007/978-1-60327-827-0_15,
© Humana Press, a part of Springer Science+Business Media, LLC 2009

secondary to previously active disease, including fibrosis and atrophy, as well as complications of therapy or other coexisting illnesses *(1)*.

The assessment of myositis is compounded by the fact that these are heterogeneous systemic connective tissue diseases. Dermatomyositis (DM), polymyositis (PM), and inclusion body myositis (IBM), the most common subgroups in adults and children, each have unique pathophysiologies, differences in disease expression, and varying rates of progression and responses to therapy. The assessment of myositis disease activity and damage is also frequently confounded by illness features that interfere with the accurate assessment of muscle strength and physical function, including steroid and other drug-induced myopathies, joint contractures, calcinosis, cardiopulmonary disease, and muscle pain. Patients also may adapt to their slowly progressive or chronic deficits, so objective assessment, including measurement of the compensatory maneuvers, is important. Many outcome measures, including muscle strength and physical function, do not distinguish between disease activity and prior damage, and many measures of disease activity are insensitive in detecting ongoing activity in the presence of accumulating damage *(2)*.

Collaborative research groups with expertise and special interest in myositis have developed and preliminarily validated tools to assess distinct aspects of disease activity and damage. These partially validated measures now place physicians in a much-improved position to assess adult and juvenile IIM patients comprehensively and to make informed therapeutic decisions. Despite extraordinary progress, the assessment of the IIMs remains in an early phase of development, with a need to further validate and refine existing tools, to define their performance characteristics in various IIM subgroups, to develop new response criteria that combine core set measures into a single composite end point for use in therapeutic trials, to develop improved and quantitative imaging techniques, and to develop and validate new surrogate biomarkers.

This chapter updates the progress in the assessment of the IIMs, highlighting the newly validated measures available to assess disease activity, damage, and health-related quality of life (HR-QOL) for the adult and juvenile IIMs as well as alternative or novel approaches that may be important in the assessment of certain IIM patients or as part of more focused clinical studies. Several reviews provide more in depth exploration of these topics *(2–4)*.

## Core Set Measures to Assess Disease Activity

The International Myositis Assessment and Clinical Studies Group (IMACS) and the Pediatric Rheumatology International Trials Organization (PRINTO) have both developed core set measures of disease activity that are recommended for use in all IIM therapeutic studies but may also be used in the clinical assessment of patients (Table 15.1). These core sets were derived through slightly differing consensus processes. IMACS reviewed therapeutic trial data and outcome measure validation studies. Core set domains and measures were selected based on their validity, availability, ease of use, and applicability to all forms of adult- and juvenile-onset myositis

Table 15.1 Proposed preliminary core sets measures for disease activity assessment for therapeutic trials in adult and juvenile idiopathic inflammatory myopathies

| Domain | International Myositis Assessment and Clinical Studies Group (IMACS)[1] | Pediatric Rheumatology International Trials Organization (PRINTO)[8] |
| --- | --- | --- |
| Applicable populations | Adult and juvenile patients with polymyositis (PM), dermatomyositis (DM), and inclusion body myositis | Juvenile dermatomyositis |
| *Domain* | *IMACS core set measure* | *PRINTO core set measure* |
| Physician global activity | Physician global disease activity assessment by Likert or visual analog scale | Physician global disease activity assessment by visual analog scale |
| Patient/parent global activity | Patient/parent global disease activity assessment by Likert or visual analog scale | Patient/parent global disease activity assessment by visual analog scale |
| Muscle strength | Manual muscle testing by a scale of 0–10 points or expanded 0–5 points to include proximal, distal, and axial muscles[a] | Childhood Myositis Assessment Scale (CMAS), manual muscle testing |
| Physical function | Validated patient/parent questionnaire of activities of daily living, such as the Health Assessment Questionnaire (HAQ)/Childhood Health Assessment Questionnaire (CHAQ)[b] Validated observational tool of function, strength and endurance, such as the CMAS[b] | CHAQ |
| Laboratory assessment | At least two serum muscle-associated enzyme activities from the following: creatine kinase (CK), aldolase, lactate dehydrogenase (LDH), aspartate aminotransferase (AST), or alanine aminotransferase (ALT) | Not included |
| Extraskeletal muscle disease | Assessment of constitutional, cutaneous, gastrointestinal, joint, cardiac, and pulmonary activity; the Myositis Disease Activity Assessment Tool has been partially validated in adult and juvenile DM and PM | Not included |
| Global disease activity tool | Not included | Disease Activity Score (DAS) Myositis Disease Activity Assessment Tool |
| Health-related quality of life | Not included as a disease activity core set measure; separate domain to be assessed in clinical trials | Child Health Questionnaire (CHQ) Physical Summary score |

[a] Not recommended for children less than 4 years of age
[b] One validated tool is recommended for adults and children more than 4 years of age and two tools for children less than 4 years of age

*(1, 5).* Consensus was reached on use of these domains and measures through face-to-face meetings using nominal group technique (NGT) and a Delphi process involving 80 specialists in adult and juvenile myositis (including rheumatologists, neurologists, dermatologists, physiatrists, and statisticians) *(1, 5).* IMACS has subsequently developed, using NGT to form consensus, a composite clinical end point for therapeutic trials that combines the core set measures *(6).*

Also, PRINTO, an international group of pediatric rheumatologists, reviewed validation studies but applied the more formal NGT consensus process to derive a preliminary set of activity domains and core set measures for juvenile DM trials *(7).* PRINTO then developed a provisional core set of outcome measures for therapeutic trials based on data from a large, multicenter prospective natural history study in recent-onset juvenile DM patients that examined each measure's responsiveness and, for selected measures, the construct validity, internal consistency, and discriminant validity *(8).* PRINTO has developed a composite end point for juvenile DM therapeutic trials *(9).* Despite some differences in these derivation processes and in the core set activity domains, the proposed core set activity measures are similar between IMACS and PRINTO *(see* Table 15.1).

## *Physician and Patient/Parent Global Assessment*

Physician and parent/patient global assessments of activity integrate the clinical history, physical examination, and laboratory testing to provide an overall impression of disease activity, using a visual analog scale (VAS) or a Likert scale, which highly correlate with each other *(10).* The physician global activity may also be derived as a composite score of the different organ systems assessed in the VAS portion of the Myositis Disease Activity Assessment Tool (MDAAT) *(11).* Physicians agree on inclusion of a core set of clinical parameters in formulating their global activity assessments, including strength, serum muscle enzymes, muscle biopsy findings, and the evaluation of extramuscular features, including dysphagia, dysphonia, gastrointestinal tract manifestations, and cardiac and pulmonary disease *(10).* Global disease activity assessments can discriminate between active disease and damage. Physician or patient global activity assessments have been used as secondary end points in approximately 20% of prospective adult and juvenile PM, DM, and IBM therapeutic trials *(1, 12).*

Global activity assessments have undergone preliminary validation in two large juvenile DM natural history studies and in adult DM/PM disease-modifying agent trials. They demonstrated excellent interrater reliability, face and content validity, and discriminant validity as well as moderate sensitivity to change *(5, 8, 10).* Physician and patient/parent global assessments also have good construct validity, correlating well with other measures of disease activity, including muscle strength and physical function in both adult and juvenile IIM and with muscle-associated enzymes in adult IIM and with extramuscular activity in juvenile IIM *(5, 8).* Physician global activity is the strongest predictor of response to therapy among the core set activity measures *(8).* Adult and pediatric specialists with expertise in myositis have defined, using NGT consensus, that 20% improvement in physician and patient/parent global activity is the minimum degree of clinically important change needed to define an IIM patient as clinically improved *(5)*.

## Muscle Strength

*Muscle strength*, defined as the capacity of a group of muscles to exert force, has been the primary clinical outcome used to assess muscle involvement in the IIMs. Muscle strength is commonly assessed using either manual muscle testing (MMT) or quantitative isometric strength testing using dynamometry, which correlate strongly with each other *(13)*. The patient's motivation, cooperation, and strength are important factors in the reliability of muscle strength testing, as are the patient's familiarity with the test, fatigue, and the testing position *(14)*. Due to normal developmental increases in strength throughout childhood, varied resistance must be applied by the tester in using MMT to assess children's strength, and strength testing cannot be objectively assessed in children younger than 5 or 6 years due to lack of cooperation with the exam *(14)*. Most myositis therapeutic trials conducted over the past two decades incorporated MMT as a primary outcome measure but differed widely in its use, utilizing MMT scores derived from 4 to 20 muscle groups and different MMT grading scales *(5, 12)*.

Manual muscle testing, in which the examiner applies resistance through movement with gravity eliminated or evaluates muscle force exerted at specified joint angles, is measured on an ordinal six-point 0-5 Medical Research Council scale or a twelve-point 0–10 ordinal scale that defines each grade and thus may improve sensitivity *(15)*. MMT of individual muscle groups has poor rater reliability, but a total score has relatively good inter- and intrarater reliability *(16)*. MMT has been partially validated in adult and juvenile DM/PM, and a total MMT score of 24 proximal, distal, and axial muscle groups demonstrates good interrater and intrarater reliability, moderate-to-excellent sensitivity to change, good internal consistency, and good construct validity with global activity and functional measures *(5, 16)*. A subset of eight proximal, distal, and axial muscles tested unilaterally performs similarly to the entire set of 24 muscles tested *(8, 17)*, and a subset of 8 axial and proximal muscles tested bilaterally has also been used as a primary end point in several adult PM/DM trials *(18)*. A gradient of weakness may exist between IIM subgroups, with PM patients weakest, DM intermediate, and juvenile DM strongest, using MMT to assess strength. Hip flexors, extensors, and abductors, as well as neck flexors and shoulder abductors, were the weakest muscle groups among all three clinical groups. However, neck flexors were weakest among juvenile DM patients, and hip girdle muscles were the weakest muscle groups for adult DM and PM *(19)*. Clinically significant improvement in muscle strength has been determined through NGT consensus to be a 15% improvement in MMT score in adult DM/PM patients and 18% improvement in juvenile DM *(5)*.

Handheld or fixed dynamometers, including modified sphygmomanometers, are more objective than MMT and quantitate muscle force in a linear range using a strain gauge while the patient generates a maximal isometric contraction *(20)*. Dynamometers, including isokinetic dynamometry, are sensitive in detecting mild degrees of weakness *(21)*. In adult PM/DM, selected muscle groups tested by cable tensiometry demonstrated good intra- and interrater reliability and good correlation with serum creatine kinase (CK) levels *(22)*. Dynamometry has been used to assess muscle strength in several adult and juvenile DM and IBM trials *(1, 12)*. While isometric dynamometry is more sensitive than MMT, specialized instruments are often required, normative data and clinically meaningful change in dynamometry are not available, and these instruments generally test only a limited number of extremity muscles.

## Physical Function

Functional assessment of IIM patients encompasses two distinct elements: physical function (which assesses performance of activities of daily living) and muscle function (which assesses the ability of muscles to perform work and evaluates muscle endurance and fatigue). Both of these areas of function can be assessed by observational tools or by patient-reported questionnaires. Functional assessment has been an important outcome measure in IIM therapeutic trials, with the majority of trials using physical function in conjunction with MMT or other measures as a primary end point, some using functional disability by itself as the primary end point, and a few incorporating functional disability into the secondary end point *(1, 5, 12)*. Like muscle strength, physical function does not discriminate between active disease and disease damage.

The (Childhood) Health Assessment Questionnaire [(C)HAQ], a parent/patient functional status questionnaire, has been the primary tool used to assess activities of daily living. In juvenile IIM patients, the CHAQ has moderate construct validity, correlating with measures of muscle strength and global activity better than muscle enzymes or skin activity *(23, 24)*. The CHAQ also has good internal reliability, excellent reliability, and high responsiveness and excellent discriminant validity *(8, 23)*. The CHAQ appears to have a large ceiling effect, with some patients achieving a normal score who have documented abnormalities in strength or function.

The Myositis Activity Profile (MAP) has been developed to assess daily life physical disability in adult myositis patients. The instrument consists of 31 items assessing such domains as movement, walking, and self-care as well as domestic and other activities *(25)*. The instrument's performance is moderately good in testing for content validity, internal consistency and redundancy, test–retest reliability in adult DM/PM, and construct validity with other daily life questionnaires such as the HAQ and the Arthritis Impact Measurement Scale 2 (AIMS2).

Other instruments assessing activities of daily living, including the modified Convery questionnaire, the Neuromuscular Symptom and Disability Functional Score (NSS), and the Barthel Index, have been used in therapeutic studies of adult IIM patients but have not been fully validated *(1, 5, 12)*. The modified Convery assessment (a questionnaire on activities of daily living that measures transfer, ambulation, dressing, and upper extremity reaching on a Likert scale) correlates well with MMT scores but not with serum muscle enzymes and has good discriminant validity *(5)*. A five-item Barthel Index, focused on transfers, bathing, toilet use, stairs, and mobility, has good performance characteristics and may be more pertinent to IIM patients than the ten-item version *(26)*.

Based on review of therapeutic trial and other clinical study data, a clinically meaningful degree of improvement in physical function has been determined through NGT consensus to be 15% for adult DM/PM as well as juvenile DM patients *(5)*.

Two observational instruments, the Childhood Myositis Assessment Scale (CMAS) and the Myositis Functional Index-2 (MFI-2), are observational tools that evaluate muscle strength, function, and endurance. In the CMAS, the pediatric patient is scored in the performance of 14 tasks that emphasize proximal and axial muscles more than distal involvement, and scores are assigned based on the relative ability to perform each maneuver or on endurance in holding a test position. The CMAS has demonstrated very good inter- and intrarater reliability as well as good construct validity, correlating highly with measures of strength, physical function, and physician global disease activity *(27)*. It has excellent responsiveness and good discriminant validity *(5, 8)*. Modeling of the CMAS and CHAQ has provided some clinical inter-pretation to the scores *(27)*, and healthy children of varying ages have also been studied to understand the impact of normal child development, including age and gender effects, on CMAS scores *(28)*.

With the MFI-2, the adult IIM patient is observed while performing a series of tasks testing repetition in movements of upper and lower proximal muscles, neck flexion, and distal lower extremities. The revised tool, which has eliminated ceiling and floor effects seen in the original version, had good content validity, excellent intra- and interrater reliability, and moderate construct validity with isokinetic dynamometry in a cohort of adult DM and PM patients. The tool exhibits good correlation between right- and left-sided tasks and so can be performed unilaterally to decrease the performance time to 20 min *(29)*.

Timed functional tests also provide observational information regarding muscle function and endurance and test both type I and II muscle fibers, which are both affected in IIM pathology. The 1-kg arm lift and chair stand tests, in which both tasks are performed repetitively over a 30-s interval, examine the endurance of proximal upper and lower muscles. These tests demonstrate good test-retest reliability in healthy subjects, IIM patients' scores correlate inversely with CK level, and patients with active disease exhibit lower scores than patients in remission or healthy subjects, demonstrating good construct validity *(30)*. These timed functional tests, however, have a floor effect. Very weak patients are unable to perform these tasks, and muscle or joint pain interferes with the assessment.

Aerobic and anaerobic exercise testing by cycle ergometry or a treadmill test using the Bruce protocol is a sensitive method of investigating muscle function and endurance in both adult and juvenile IIM patients *(31, 32)*. Peak oxygen uptake and work correlate well with global disease activity and damage, CMAS scores, and atrophy or fatty replacement present on T1 magnetic resonance imaging (MRI) *(33, 34)*. Aerobic exercise capacity is frequently decreased in children with mildly active or inactive disease, but these parameters are sensitive to change, being further impaired in patients with active disease *(33, 35)*.

## Core Set Activity Domain: Muscle-Associated Serum Enzyme Activities

The activity of muscle-derived enzymes released into the serum has been used as an indicator of myositis disease activity in the clinical care of IIM patients. Of the core set measures, this is one of the few assessments that discriminates active disease (in which abnormally high serum levels are detectable) from disease remission or disease damage (in which enzyme levels return to normal or subnormal levels) (reviewed in Ref. *36*).

Despite use of CK and other enzymes among the primary end point in a number of myositis therapeutic trials, there is often an inconsistent correlation of CK with muscle histopathology or myositis activity measures. This is due to a difference in the rate of improvement in CK and other muscle-derived enzymes compared to muscle strength, the presence of autoantibodies to CK that result in rapid clearance of the enzyme and normalization *(37)*, as well as long-standing disease, in which muscle atrophy results in a loss of measurable CK activity. CK correlates well with alanine aminotransferase (ALT) in adult DM/PM patients and is elevated approximately 1.5-fold more than ALT levels *(38)*. As many as 76% of JDM patients do not have an elevated serum CK level at the time of diagnosis *(39)*, and greater delay to diagnosis is associated with a trend to normalize muscle enzyme values *(40)*.

Current data suggests serum lactate dehydrogenase (LDH) activity may be the most clinically useful serum muscle enzyme in patients with juvenile DM. It has the best construct validity in correlating with global disease activity, physical dysfunction, and extramuscular activity *(5)*. LDH, in combination with aspartate aminotransferase (AST), may be best in predicting flares of juvenile DM activity *(41)*. Whereas CK level may have a low sensitivity to change in juvenile DM patients *(8)*, improvement in CK levels have ranged from 38 to 97% in published adult DM/PM therapeutic trials. The amount of clinically important change in muscle-associated enzymes has been derived through NGT consensus, based on published trial data in adults, to be at least 30% improvement *(5)*.

In adult DM/PM patients without evidence of cardiac involvement, myosin heavy chain is increased in approximately 60% of active patients, compared to CK-MB isoenzyme, serum myoglobin, or cardiac troponin T (cTnT), which are elevated in 40-50% of patients. In contrast, cardiac troponin I (cTnI) is rarely elevated in the absence of cardiac disease. These enzymes correlate with each other and with measures of muscle severity, except cTnI does not appear to correlate well with either *(42, 43)*. In muscular dystrophy patients, CK-MB and heart fatty acid-binding protein correlate well with total serum CK levels, whereas cTnI and brain naturietic factor are frequently elevated, but independent of the elevation in CK *(44)*. Measurement of muscle metabolites using proton spectroscopy also revealed creatine, choline, betaine, and trimethylamine oxide to be elevated in first morning void urine specimens of juvenile DM patients compared to healthy controls. Most of these metabolites correlate with global disease activity and muscle-associated enzymes, including aldolase and ALT, whereas creatine correlates strongly with global disease damage *(45)*.

## *Core Set Activity Domain: Extraskeletal Muscle Disease Activity*

Extraskeletal muscle organs frequently involved in DM and PM include skin, gastrointestinal tract, joints, pulmonary, and cardiac organs *(46)*. The MDAAT, developed by IMACS, combines a series of VASs that capture severity of activity in a particular organ system (Myositis Disease Activity Assessment Visual Analog Scales) and the Myositis Intention to Treat Activity Index (MITAX), which captures change in active manifestations in six extraskeletal muscle organ systems (constitutional, cutaneous, joints, gastrointestinal, pulmonary, and cardiac). Muscle disease activity is a separate domain in this instrument. In an exercise in which experts in adult and juvenile myositis assessed patients using the MDAAT, the interrater reliability was good to excellent, except for the gastrointestinal and muscle systems in adult patients and the skeletal system in juvenile DM patients. Reliability improved with additional training *(5, 11)*. In support of good content validity, anti-Jo-1 autoantibody titers correlate well with muscle, pulmonary, and skeletal activity in adult DM/PM patients when assessed with the MDAAT *(47)*. Responsiveness of both components of the instrument is excellent, and global extramuscular disease also shows good discriminant validity *(8)*. NGT consensus of myositis experts has determined that 20% improvement in extramuscular disease activity represents clinically meaningful improvement *(5)*.

Organ-specific measures to assess extraskeletal muscle involvement are being developed, with focus on a comprehensive assessment of the skin for patients with adult and juvenile DM. The Cutaneous Assessment Tool (CAT), developed by a multidisciplinary group of rheumatologists and dermatologists, is a 21-item tool that assesses the severity of activity and damage lesions in DM. It demonstrated good interrater reliability, construct validity, and responsiveness in a large population of individuals with juvenile DM *(48, 49)*. A shortened version of the CAT, which assesses the same 21 lesions but only for their presence or absence, performs as well as the full-length tool *(50)*. The Dermatomyositis Skin Severity Index (DSSI) assesses redness, induration, scaliness, and surface area of skin involvement but does not assess specific skin lesions. It appears to have good inter- and intrarater reliability and construct validity, but responsiveness has not been assessed *(51)*. The Cutaneous Dermatomyositis Disease Area and Severity Index (CDASI), also developed by a group of dermatologists, assesses 16 body areas, scoring each for erythema, thickness, scale, excoriation, and ulceration. Gottron's papules, periungual changes, and alopecia are scored separately. The performance characteristics of this tool have been evaluated in adults with DM by a group of dermatologists, and it has been shown to be reliable and exhibit good construct validity in a small study, but responsiveness has not yet been evaluated *(52)*.

In a small study that compared the performance of the CAT, DSSI, and CDASI, all three tools demonstrated good construct validity with physician and patient global activity, and the CAT and CDASI both exhibited good interrater reliability *(52)*. Skin symptoms, particularly pruritus contribute to QOL impairment in DM patients. QOL impairment, as assessed by the Dermatology Quality of Life Index and the

Skindex-16, is significantly higher in DM than other inflammatory skin diseases, including psoriasis and atopic dermatitis *(53)*.

Quantitative nailfold capillaroscopy, either via manual counting of capillary density or videocapillaroscopy, appears promising as a noninvasive measure. Capillary density is diminished in juvenile DM compared to healthy controls, and capillary loop area is increased. Dilation, tortuosity, and bushy loop formation are also often present in active disease. Nailfold capillary density strongly correlates with physician global and skin disease activity but less strongly with muscle strength and function *(54)*. A higher density of end-row nailfold capillary loops at 36 months is also associated with lower skin activity and a unicyclic illness course *(55)*. Using laser Doppler perfusion imaging, skin blood flow has been shown to be increased not only at sites of erythematous rashes and periungual capillary changes in DM patients but also at sites of uninvolved skin compared to healthy controls *(56)*. Skin blood flow correlates inversely with DSSI scores.

Dysphagia has been observed in 50–80% of patients with adult and juvenile IIMs *(57)*. The most frequent reported symptoms of dysphagia include "food sticking in the throat," coughing while eating, and difficulty with solid and dry foods, although aspiration pneumonia also occurs *(58)*. IIM patients may have swallowing abnormalities in each phase of swallowing. This includes tongue weakness, which may be manifest as difficulty moving the bolus of food to the pharynx or impaired tongue retraction; pharyngeal or laryngeal muscle weakness, resulting in pooling of the bolus in the pharynx or in coughing or hoarseness during swallowing; and cricopharyngeal muscle weakness, with resultant esophageal reflux or delayed emptying of the esophagus *(57, 58)*. Swallowing function may be evaluated by a combination of ultrasonography of the oropharyngeal swallow to examine tongue strength, bolus transfer, and swallowing duration as well as by modified barium swallow examination, which assesses esophageal mobility, pharyngeal pooling, laryngeal penetration, and the risk of aspiration *(57)*.

At least half of patients with PM or DM have pulmonary function impairment. Chest wall restrictive disease and involvement of the alveolar capillary interface is common *(59)*, and interstitial lung disease (ILD) occurs in 5–45% of adult PM/DM patients *(60)*. High-resolution computed tomography (HRCT) of the lungs is a sensitive imaging method for detecting ILD. In DM patients, the severity of ground glass appearance and reticular opacities and a lower degree of consolidation is associated with higher mortality from ILD *(61)*. In patients with anti-synthetase autoantibodies, the changes are often severe, diffuse, and consistent with an underlying pathology of nonspecific interstitial pneuomonitis (NSIP), including frequent reticular opacities, ground glass appearance, honeycombing, and interlobular septal thickening *(62)*. Pulmonary function tests are also important in following these patients as they can normalize even when radiologic signs persist *(63)*. In addition to repeated evaluation by pulmonary function testing and HRCT, several serum biomarkers appear promising aids in monitoring ILD progression. Serum levels of KL-6, a mucinlike high molecular weight glycoprotein expressed on regenerating alveolar type II pneumocytes, alveolar macrophages, and pulmonary endothelial cells, as well as E-selection, von Willebrand factor-related antigen, and surfactant protein D, are elevated in PM/DM and systemic sclerosis patients with ground glass opacities and pulmonary fibrosis *(64)*.

## Core Set Activity Domain: Comprehensive Measures

An additional activity domain specified by the PRINTO collaborative group as part of the core activity measures for juvenile DM is a composite assessment of activity, with two instruments currently specified as core set measures in this domain: the MDAAT and the Disease Activity Score (DAS) for juvenile DM *(7)*. The MDAAT was discussed in this chapter as primarily a measure of extraskeletal muscle activity as the majority of the instrument assesses extraskeletal muscle activity. This measure, however, which includes muscle as one of seven evaluated organ systems, could potentially be used as a composite index to assess adult and juvenile myositis.

The Juvenile DM Disease Activity Score is a composite activity index that assesses the extent and distribution of cutaneous involvement, muscle weakness, functional status, and vasculopathic manifestations. In preliminary validation, the DAS has good interrater reliability, as well as internal consistency, in that muscle strength measured by the DAS correlates well with muscle strength assessed independently by a physical therapist *(65)*. The DAS has moderate construct validity, correlating well with physician global activity and moderately with nailfold capillary density; physical dysfunction assessed by the CMAS, CHAQ, and the Child Health Questionnaire; muscle enzyme levels (LDH, AST); and von Willebrand factor VIII-related antigen, an endothelial activation marker *(8, 54)*. The DAS also has excellent responsiveness and good discriminant validity in differentiating patients who clinically improved from those who did not *(8)*.

## Composite Response Indices

Preliminary work has been undertaken by IMACS to combine the core set measures into a composite response index that could be used as a clinical end point for therapeutic trials. To derive this composite end point, myositis experts first rated paper patient profiles of adult and juvenile DM/PM patients, developed from therapeutic trials and natural history studies, as clinically improved or not improved. Candidate definitions of improvement that combined clinically meaningful change in various core set measures were tested for sensitivity and specificity, based on the expert ratings as a gold standard. In addition classification and regression tree (CART) and logistic regression modeling were used to examine additional combinations of the core set measures. A number of definitions of improvement performed satisfactorily, but in a second consensus conference, the experts ranked their top-choice definitions and came to agreement on several definitions of improvement using an NGT

**Table 15.2** Performance characteristics of the top three preliminary definitions of improvement for adult and juvenile myositis developed by the International Myositis Assessment and Clinical Studies (IMACS) group *(6)*\*

| Definition of improvement | Sensitivity (%) | Specificity (%) | Sensitivity × Specificity | Final score[a] (0–60) |
|---|---|---|---|---|
| *Adult definitions of improvement* | | | | |
| **A1.** Three of any six measures improved by 20% or more, with no more than two worse by 25% or more, which cannot be MMT | 86 | 88 | 0.76 | 49 |
| **A2.** MD global activity improved by greater than 30% and MMT improved by 1–15%, *or* MMT improved by greater than 15% and MD global activity improved by greater than 10%, *and* no more than two worse by 25% or more | 92 | 91 | 0.84 | 47 |
| **A3a.** MMT improved by at least 15%, *or* MD global activity improved by greater than 30% and MMT improved by 1–15%, *and* no more than two worse by 25% or more | 97 | 80 | 0.78 | 23 |
| **A3b.** Three of any six measures improved by 20% or more, with no more than two worse by 25% or more | 86 | 88 | 0.76 | 23 |
| *Pediatric definitions of improvement* | | | | |
| **P1.** Three of any six measures improved by 20% or more, with no more than two worse by 25% or more, which cannot be MMT | 83 | 98 | 0.82 | 57 |
| **P2.** Three of any six measures improved by 20% or more, with no more than two worse by 25% or more | 83 | 98 | 0.82 | 53 |
| **P3.** Three of any six measures improved by 20% or more | 83 | 98 | 0.82 | 34 |

*Note*: A1 is the same as P1; A3b is the same as P2. *MD* physician; *MMT* manual muscle testing
\*From Rider LG, Giannini EH, Brunner HI et al, International consensus on preliminary definitions of improvement in adult and juvenile myositis. Arthritits Rheum. 2004; 50: 2281–2290.
[a]Definitions were ranked 5–1 by 12 adult or juvenile myositis experts using a score of 5 for each physician's top choice and a score of 1 for their lowest-choice definition

consensus process (Table 15.2). The top-ranking definition of improvement common to both adult and juvenile myositis is flexible in requiring improvement by at least 20% in three of any six core set measures, with no more than two worsening, which cannot be MMT *(6)*. This top definition of improvement is currently in use as a composite clinical end point in a number of myositis therapeutic trials. PRINTO used a modification of this consensus formation process to derive their preliminary definition of improvement for juvenile myositis, which, similar to the IMACS definition, requires three of any six core set measures improved by at least 20%, with no more than one worse, which cannot be the CMAS *(9)*.

Also IMACS developed, through delphi and NGT consensus methods, standardized guidelines for the conduct of myositis therapeutic trials *(12)*. These include such issues as trial inclusion or exclusion criteria, allowable concomitant therapy, withdrawal criteria, placebo and trial duration, and suggestions for post hoc stratification. IMACS also developed preliminary criteria for worsening, as well as definitions of remission and complete clinical response.

These newly developed definitions of improvement, as well as the proposed criteria for worsening and remission, are in need of prospective validation. Newer methods of developing composite end points also need to be applied, including use of continuous end points and defining patients with a large degree of response short of remission *(66, 67)*. IMACS is undertaking a project to assemble data from a number of therapeutic trials to develop further composite clinical end points for adult and juvenile myositis.

## Ancillary Measures to Assess Disease Activity

### *Imaging*

Magnetic resonance imaging of the thigh muscles is the imaging method currently most valuable in the assessment of and discrimination between myositis disease activity and damage (Fig. 15.1) *(68)*. Muscle edema on short tau inversion recovery (STIR) or T2 fat-suppressed images is indicative of inflammation, necrosis, or myophagocytosis, whereas T1-weighted images demonstrate muscle atrophy and fatty infiltration in the presence of damage, which increases with longer disease duration (Fig. 15.2) *(69)*. In PM, edema of the muscles is usually symmetric,

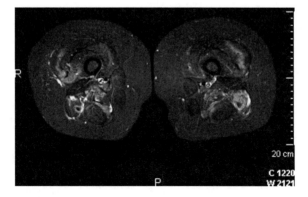

**Fig. 15.1**  Widespread muscle edema, demonstrated as bright signal intensity on a short tau inversion recovery (STIR) axial magnetic resonance image of the thigh muscles from a patient with active, refractory polymyositis.

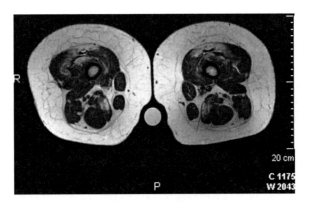

**Fig. 15.2** Diffuse muscle atrophy and moderate fatty infiltration of quadriceps and hamstring muscles, demonstrated as white signal within the musculature, on T1-weighted axial magnetic resonance image of the thigh muscles from the same patient as in Fig. 15.1.

involving proximal more than distal muscles, and may include the vasti, glutei, adductors, hamstrings, tibialis anterior, gastrocnemius, and soleus muscles *(70)*. In adult and juvenile DM, muscle edema is often present in the gluteus maximus, adductors, quadriceps, and hamstrings, whereas atrophy is greater in the gluteus maximus and quadriceps *(71, 72)*. The distribution in DM is most often symmetric but can be patchy and asymmetric *(70)*. In adult and juvenile DM, edema is also often frequently present in the myofascia and subcutaneous tissues *(69, 71)* and does not correlate with edema in the muscle or with other myositis disease activity measures *(73)*. Edema in the subcutaneous tissues may precede the deposition of calcinosis in juvenile DM *(73)*.

Magnetic resonance imaging is useful in selecting a site to perform a muscle biopsy, with more inflammatory cells present at sites of thigh muscle edema *(74)*. MRI is also valuable in clinically monitoring responses to therapy as the intensity and extent of muscle edema on STIR images correlate with measures of myositis activity, including physician global activity, serum CK level, and muscle histopathology *(74)*. T2 relaxation time from T2 mapping, a quantitative method of examining MRI edema signal intensity, is increased in the thigh muscles of active juvenile DM patients compared to patients with inactive disease or healthy controls. T2 relaxation times also correlate moderately with measures of disease activity, including physician global activity, muscle strength, and CMAS, but not with serum muscle enzymes *(75)*. A small study of diffusion-weighted MRI in PM/DM revealed elevated intra- and extracellular diffusion in inflamed muscles, whereas fatty infiltration results in lower diffusion coefficients than control muscle *(76)*.

Ultrasound, a less-costly imaging modality, also assesses muscle and other structural abnormalities, and with the advent of power Doppler technology, resolution has improved, as has the ability to assess muscle function and blood vessel flow and vascularity. In the IIMs, as well as in other myopathies, increased echo intensity of muscles and increased muscle thickness have been observed in disease of short duration due to inflammation, whereas with long-standing disease increased echogenicity may relate to fatty replacement, and muscle atrophy is also frequently present *(77–79)*. PM patients have lower rectus femoris muscle diameters in the contracted state compared with healthy controls, and muscle contraction correlates with muscle strength by MMT *(80)*. Power Doppler sonography appears promising in examining muscle vascularity; peak muscle vascularity is increased in PM/DM patients with shorter duration of disease *(77, 81)*. The newer technique of contrast-enhanced microbubble ultrasound examines blood vessel perfusion down to the capillary level and demonstrates higher blood flow, blood flow velocity, and blood volume in the biceps femoris of patients with DM or PM compared to healthy control subjects *(82)*. The sensitivity, specificity, and predictive value of microbubble ultrasound findings are good, but not as high as T2-weighted MRI *(83)*.

At rest and during exercise, P-31 magnetic resonance spectroscopy (MRS) detects and quantitates high-energy phosphate compounds and magnesium (free or bound to adenosine triphosphate [ATP]) in muscle *(84, 85)*. In DM and PM patients, the phosphocreatine, adenosine diphosphate, and magnesium are lower than in healthy controls at rest and following exercise, their recovery times are prolonged following exercise, and the maximal rate of ATP production is lower than in healthy individuals *(84–86)*. Proton efflux detected by proton spectroscopy is also reduced in DM more than PM patients, suggesting an effect resulting from impaired blood supply *(86)*. Although this technique provides an elegant method to quantitate muscle fatigue and mitochondrial oxidative phosphorylation, it is only available at a few specialized centers. In amyopathic DM patients, P-31 MRS may have clinical utility in that MRS demonstrates diminished production of phosphocreatine and ATP generation at submaximal voluntary contraction, even when MRI of the thighs is normal *(85)*. There is no correlation between MRS abnormalities and the degree of muscle edema or fatty infiltration on MRI *(86)*.

## *Biomarkers*

Potential biomarkers of disease activity, including activation markers on peripheral blood mononuclear cells assessed by flow cytometry, soluble markers of immune activation, cytokines and their receptors, and measures of endothelial cell activation, have been studied in adult and juvenile DM/PM and have been reviewed previously *(2)*. In most cases, the studies have been small and unconfirmed, and their relationship to standardized measures of disease activity has not been carefully assessed. Immunophenotypic analysis of peripheral blood mononuclear cells using flow cytometry, as well as a few commercially available soluble immunologic or endothelial activation markers such as von Willebrand factor VIII-related antigen, has been partially validated as a measure of disease activity. This type of analysis may have potential clinical utility in the assessment of selected patients, particularly those with long-standing disease for whom there is a question whether the myositis remains active or with certain illness complications, such as ulcerations or ILD.

A central role for interferon-α pathways and plasmacytoid dendritic cells in the pathogenesis of adult and juvenile DM has become evident. Patients with active DM, more so than active PM, have upregulation of a number of interferon-α/β-inducible genes in their peripheral blood in the setting of active myositis as compared to inactive patients, patients with IBM, and healthy controls *(87, 88)*. The messenger RNA (mRNA) of myxovirus resistance protein A (MxA), a type I interferon-inducible gene, is highly upregulated in the peripheral blood mononuclear cells of juvenile DM patients compared to healthy controls, and this correlates well with the DAS muscle activity score (not the DAS skin score) *(89)*. The protein levels of several interferon-regulated chemokines, including monocyte chemoattractant protein (MCP) 1, MCP-2, and Human interferon-inducible protein *10 (IP-10)*, are upregulated in the peripheral blood of patients with adult and juvenile DM, and these also correlate with myositis disease activity *(88)*. Interleukin 17 (IL-17), which is produced through Th17 pathway activation, is also increased in the serum of adult and juvenile DM and PM patients and correlates well with these interferon-regulated chemokines *(90)*.

## Assessment of Disease Damage

Although it is critically important in therapeutic decision making to discriminate myositis damage (which does not respond to anti-inflammatory therapy) from active disease (which often requires such therapy), less attention has been focused on the development of measures to assess myositis damage. *Disease damage* has been defined as persistent pathologic changes, such as fibrosis, scarring or atrophy, or persistent changes in physiology or function present for at least 6 months that are the result of prior active disease, drug toxicity, or unrelated coexisting disease processes *(1)*. Assessment of disease damage is also important in understanding the natural history and prognosis of these disorders, as well as in therapeutic trials, with a secondary goal of reducing the rate of damage accumulation.

A comprehensive instrument to assess damage has been developed by IMACS and is currently undergoing retrospective and prospective validation by two international collaborative groups. This measure, the Myositis Damage Index, combines a modification of the Systemic Lupus International Collaborative Clinics (SLICC)/American College of Rheumatology (ACR) Damage Index (which assesses the extent of damage in different organ systems) with a series of VASs to capture severity of damage in each system. Organ systems assessed by the Myositis Damage Index include muscle, skeletal (joints and bones), cutaneous, gastrointestinal, pulmonary, cardiac, peripheral vascular, endocrine (including linear growth and sexual development in pediatric patients), ocular, infectious, malignancy, and other systems *(11)*. The interrater reliability of the Myositis Damage Index in a real patient exercise was good, except for the gastrointestinal and skeletal systems, which showed fair interrater reliability. Reliability improved with training in the instrument *(11)*. Preliminary studies using the Myositis Damage Index in large populations of adult and juvenile

**Table 15.3** Proposed preliminary core set measures for disease damage assessment in juvenile dermatomyositis as recommended by the Pediatric Rheumatology International Trials Organization (PRINTO) *(7)*

| Domain | Core set measure |
|---|---|
| Physician global damage | Physician global disease damage assessment by visual analog scale |
| Physical function | Childhood Health Assessment Questionnaire (CHAQ) |
| Growth and development | Linear growth and sexual development |
| Health-related quality of life | Child Health Questionnaire (CHQ) |
| Global disease damage tool | Myositis damage index |
| Muscle strength | Childhood Myositis Assessment Scale (CMAS) |

In assessment of myositis damage, IMACS has proposed including physician global damage, the Myositis Damage Index, and physical function.

myositis suggested that the vast majority of patients do develop myositis damage. In juvenile DM, cutaneous scarring or atrophy was present in approximately 30–40% of the patients in these cohorts, joint contractures in 17–30%, and persistent muscle dysfunction or weakness in 11–30% of patients with long-term follow-up. Persistent dysphagia and dysphonia were also reported in 5–20% of patients in these cohorts examined for long-term damage *(91, 92)*. In adult DM/PM patients, muscles, followed by gastrointestinal and pulmonary, were the target organs with greatest severity of damage, whereas damage in skeletal, cutaneous, cardiac, endocrine, and ocular systems was detectable but mild *(91)*.

As a core element to be assessed in all adult and juvenile IIM therapeutic trials and natural history studies, IMACS has recommended inclusion of disease damage. The Myositis Damage Index, physician global assessments of disease damage, and physical function measured by the HAQ/CHAQ are potential candidates as core set measures, but further validation of these as damage measures for the IIMs has been suggested before a core set for damage is developed *(1)*. PRINTO has recommended six elements for a core set of disease damage for juvenile DM trials (Table 15.3). These include physician global assessment of damage, functional assessment measured by the CHAQ, an assessment of linear growth and sexual development, Health Related Quality of Life (HR-QOL, assessed by the Child Health Assessment Questionnaire (CHQ)), a comprehensive damage tool assessed by the Myositis Damage Index, and muscle strength measured by the CMAS *(7)*.

## Patient Self-Assessment: Health-Related Quality of Life

For IIM patients, IMACS has recommended HR-QOL as an important domain to include in therapeutic trials and observational studies *(1)*. For adult patients, the Medical Outcomes Study 36-Item Short Form (SF-36) has been proposed for use in adult myositis patients as a generic QOL measure that has been widely adapted across diseases and is available in many languages. The SF-36 has not been validated for use in IIMs, but in two natural history studies in which the SF-36 was administered at long-term follow-up, SF-36 scores differed between IIM patients and controls in all subdomains of the instrument, although there was no difference in the scores among clinical subgroups (DM, PM, or overlap myositis) or a correlation with disease activity. MMT scores did correlate with physical functioning, role functioning, and bodily pain. Patients with chronic progressive disease course had higher pain scores than patients with a relapsing-remitting illness course *(93, 94)*. The Nottingham Health Profile, another generic QOL instrument, demonstrated increased scores in all six subdomains (energy, pain, emotion, sleep, social, and physical) in adult PM/DM patients compared to healthy controls *(95)*. PM patients had more physical disability than DM patients. Both physical disability and emotional status significantly predicted energy level and social isolation in IIM patients, with pain as another subdomain that significantly predicted energy level *(95)*.

A disease-specific QOL measure has been developed, the Individualized Neuro-muscular Quality of Life Questionnaire (INQoL), for adult patients with myositis, dystrophies, and congenital myopathies *(96)*. The INQoL consists of 45 questions, including a focus on the impact of key muscle disease symptoms (weakness, myotonia, fatigue, and pain) and the impact of neuromuscular disease on particularly areas of life, including daily life activities, relationships, and emotions. Content of the questionnaire was validated based on interviews with patients, with a high prevalence of abnormalities in these domains and patients' indicating a great importance of these areas to their overall HR-QOL. Portions of the instrument have good construct validity with other validated instruments for neuromuscular disease, such as timed functional tests, the SF-36, the Barthel Index, and fatigue questionnaires. Little change in the INQoL was seen in 3- or 6-month follow-up; however, it is unclear if the patients experienced clinical improvement in other measures at follow-up evaluation.

For juvenile IIM patients, two generic HR-QOL instruments are available to assess pediatric patients. The CHQ is modeled more closely to the SF-36 and has been adapted and validated for juvenile idiopathic arthritis in 32 countries in Europe, Asia, and South America, enabling cross-cultural use in international studies *(97)*. The physical summary score of the CHQ, as expected, correlates well with measures of physical dysfunction (such as the CHAQ and CMAS) and moderately well with measures of disease activity (global activity, DAS). It has excellent responsiveness (in contrast to the psychosocial summary score of the CHQ, which has moderate responsiveness), but the CHQ does not have good discriminant validity, with a great deal of overlap in scores between patients who clinically improved and those who did not *(8)*.

The Pediatric Quality of Life Inventory (PedsQL) has been validated in childhood rheumatic disease patients for internal consistency, reliability, construct validity, and responsiveness, with rheumatic disease patients exhibiting scores different from healthy control subjects. Although juvenile DM patients did not demonstrate differences in their overall score from healthy children, it appears that the subdomains of physical health as well as emotional and social functioning trended toward a difference in juvenile DM compared with healthy controls *(98)*.

# Conclusions

Through the efforts of multicenter collaborative groups, measures to assess myositis to assess disease activity, disease damage, and HR-QOL have been developed and partially validated. Preliminary core set domains and core set measures of activity and damage, as well as preliminary definitions of improvement as a composite end point of the core set activity measures for use in therapeutic trials, have been developed for adult and juvenile myositis. Initial guidelines for the conduct of therapeutic trials should also begin to bring much-needed standardization to myositis therapeutic and clinical research studies. Despite this substantial progress, there is a need to develop more sensitive measures to assess IIM disease activity and damage, particularly to validate and refine these approaches further, to develop more sensitive and quantitative imaging methods, and to validate biomarkers as surrogate measures of disease activity. The continued collaboration of multiple specialists with expertise in these disorders in combination with novel technologies should continue to improve the assessment of myositis and result in enhanced clinical care and novel therapies for myositis patients.

**Acknowledgment** This work was supported by the intramural research program of the National Institute of Environmental Health Sciences, National Institutes of Health.

# References

1. Miller FW, Rider LG, Chung YL, et al. Proposed preliminary core set measures for disease outcome assessment in adult and juvenile idiopathic inflammatory myopathies. Rheumatology 2001;40:1262–73.
2. Rider LG. Outcome assessment in the adult and juvenile idiopathic inflammatory myopathies. Rheum Dis Clin North Am 2002;28(4):935–77.
3. Lundberg IE, Alexanderson H. Technology insight: tools for research, diagnosis and clinical assessment of treatment in idiopathic inflammatory myopathies. Nat Clin Pract Rheumatol 2007;3(5):282–90.
4. Ravelli A, Ruperto N, Trail L, Felici E, Sala E, Martini A. Clinical assessment in juvenile dermatomyositis. Autoimmunity 2006;39(3):197–203.
5. Rider LG, Giannini EH, Harris-Love M, et al. Defining clinical improvement in adult and juvenile myositis. J Rheumatol 2003;30(3):603–17.
6. Rider LG, Giannini EH, Brunner HI, et al. International consensus on preliminary definitions of improvement in adult and juvenile myositis. Arthritis Rheum 2004;50(7):2281–90.
7. Ruperto N, Ravelli A, Murray KJ, et al. Preliminary core sets of measures for disease activity and damage assessment in juvenile systemic lupus erythematosus and juvenile dermatomyositis. Rheumatology (Oxford) 2003;42(12):1452–9.
8. Ruperto N, Ravelli A, Pistorio A, et al. The provisional Paediatric Rheumatology International Trials Organisation/American College of Rheumatology/European League Against Rheumatism Disease activity core set for the evaluation of response to therapy in juvenile dermatomyositis: a prospective validation study. Arthritis Rheum 2008;59(1):4–13.
9. Ruperto N, Woo P, Cuttica R, et al. The validated PRINTO core set and definition of improvement for juvenile myositis. Arthritis Rheum 2004;50:S534.

10. Rider LG, Feldman BM, Perez MD, et al. Development of validated disease activity and damage indices for the juvenile idiopathic inflammatory myopathies: I. Physician, parent, and patient global assessments. Juvenile Dermatomyositis Disease Activity Collaborative Study Group. Arthritis Rheum 1997;40(11):1976–83.
11. Isenberg DA, Allen E, Farewell V, et al. International consensus outcome measures for patients with idiopathic inflammatory myopathies. Development and initial validation of myositis activity and damage indices in patients with adult onset disease. Rheumatology (Oxford) 2004;43(1):49–54.
12. Oddis CV, Rider LG, Reed AM, et al. International consensus guidelines for trials of therapies in the idiopathic inflammatory myopathies. Arthritis Rheum 2005;52(9):2607–15.
13. Bohannon RW. Measuring knee extensor muscle strength. Am J Phys Med Rehabil 2001; 80:13–8.
14. Hinderer KA, Hinderer SR. Muscle strength development and assessment in children and adolescents. In: Harms-Ringdahl K, ed. Muscle strength. Edinburgh: Churchill Livingstone, 1993:93–140.
15. Kendall FP, McCreary EK, Provance PG. Muscles: testing and function. 4th ed. Baltimore: Williams and Wilkins; 1993.
16. Jain M, Smith M, Cintas H, et al. Intra-rater and inter-rater reliability of the 10-point Manual Muscle Test (MMT) of strength in children with juvenile idiopathic inflammatory myopathies (JIIM). Phys Occup Ther Pediatr 2006;26(3):5–17.
17. Hicks J, Wesley R, Koziol D, et al. Preliminary validation of abbreviated manual muscle testing in the assessment of juvenile dermatomyositis. Arthritis Rheum 2000;43(Suppl):S195.
18. Cherin P, Pelletier A, Teixeria A, et al. Results and long-term follow-up of intravenous immunoglobulin infusions in chronic, refractory polymyositis: an open study with thirty-five adult patients. Arthritis Rheum 2002;46:467–74.
19. Harris-Love M, Shrader JA, Koziol D, et al. Distribution and severity of weakness among patients with polymyositis, dermatomyositis and juvenile dermatomyositis. Rheumatology 2009;48(2):134–9.
20. Watkins MP, Harris BA. Evaluation of skeletal muscle performance. In: Harms-Ringdahl K, ed. Muscle strength. Edinburgh: Churchill Livingstone, 1993:19–36.
21. Neri R, Mosca M, Stampacchia G, et al. Functional and isokinetic assessment of muscle strength in patients with idiopathic inflammatory myopathies. Autoimmunity 2006;39(3): 255–9.
22. Stoll T, Bruhlmann P, Stucki G, Seifert B, Michel BA. Muscle strength assessment in polymyositis and dermatomyositis evaluation of the reliability and clinical use of a new, quantitative, easily applicable method. J Rheumatol 1995;22:473–7.
23. Huber AM, Hicks JE, Lachenbruch PA, et al. Validation of the Childhood Health Assessment Questionnaire in the juvenile idiopathic myopathies. J Rheumatol 2001;28:1106–11.
24. Feldman BM, Ayling-Campos A, Luy L, Stevens D, Silverman ED, Laxer RM. Measuring disability in juvenile dermatomyositis: validity of the Childhood Health Assessment Questionnaire. J Rheumatol 1995;22:326–31.
25. Alexanderson H, Lundberg IE, Stenstrom CH. Development of the Myositis Activities Profile—validity and reliability of a self-administered questionnaire to assess activity limitations in patients with polymyositis/dermatomyositis. J Rheumatol 2002;29(11):2386–92.
26. Hobart JC, Thompson AJ. The five item Barthel index. J Neurol Neurosurg Psychiatry 2001;71:225–30.
27. Huber AM, Feldman BM, Rennebohm RM, et al. Validation and clinical significance of the Childhood Myositis Assessment Scale for assessment of muscle function in the juvenile idiopathic inflammatory myopathies. Arthritis Rheum 2004;50(5):1595–603.
28. Rennebohm RM, Jones K, Huber AM, et al. Normal scores for nine maneuvers of the Childhood Myositis Assessment Scale. Arthritis Rheum 2004;51(3):365–70.
29. Alexanderson H, Broman L, Tollback A, Josefson A, Lundberg IE, Stenstrom CH. Functional Index-2: validity and reliability of a disease-specific measure of impairment in patients with polymyositis and dermatomyositis. Arthritis Rheum 2006;55(1):114–22.

30. Agarwal S, Kiely PD. Two simple, reliable and valid tests of proximal muscle function, and their application to the management of idiopathic inflammatory myositis. Rheumatology (Oxford) 2006;45(7):874–9.

31. Wiesinger GF, Quittan M, Nuhr M, et al. Aerobic capacity in adult dermatomyositis/polymyositis patients and healthy controls. Arch Phys Med Rehabil 2000;81:1–5.

32. Takken T, van der Net J, Helders PJ. Anaerobic exercise capacity in patients with juvenile-onset idiopathic inflammatory myopathies. Arthritis Rheum 2005;53(2):173–7.

33. Hicks JE, Drinkard B, Summers RM, Rider LG. Decreased aerobic capacity in children with juvenile dermatomyositis. Arthritis Rheum 2002;47(2):118–23.

34. Takken T, Spermon N, Helders PJ, Prakken AB, van der Net J. Aerobic exercise capacity in patients with juvenile dermatomyositis. J Rheumatol 2003;30(5):1075–80.

35. Takken T, van der Net J, Engelbert RH, Pater S, Helders PJ. Responsiveness of exercise parameters in children with inflammatory myositis. Arthritis Rheum 2008;59(1):59–64.

36. Rider LG, Miller FW. Laboratory evaluation of the inflammatory myopathies. Clin Diagn Lab Immunol 1995;2:1–9.

37. Warren GL, O'Farrell L, Rogers KR, Billings KM, Sayers SP, Clarkson PM. CK-MM autoantibodies: prevalence, immune complexes, and effect on CK clearance. Muscle Nerve 2006;34(3): 335–46.

38. Edge K, Chinoy H, Cooper RG. Serum alanine aminotransferase elevations correlate with serum creatine phosphokinase levels in myositis. Rheumatology (Oxford) 2006;45(4): 487–8.

39. Pachman LM, Hayford JR, Chung A, et al. Juvenile dermatomyositis at diagnosis: clinical characteristics of 79 children. J Rheumatol 1998;25:1198–204.

40. Pachman LM, Abbott K, Sinacore JM, et al. Duration of illness is an important variable for untreated children with juvenile dermatomyositis. J Pediatr 2006;148(2):247–53.

41. Guzman J, Petty RE, Malleson PN. Monitoring disease activity in juvenile dermatomyositis: the role of von Willebrand factor and muscle enzymes. J Rheumatol 1994;21:739–43.

42. Erlacher P, Lercher A, Falkensammer J, et al. Cardiac troponin and B-type myosin heavy chain concentrations in patients with polymyositis or dermatomyositis. Clin Chim Acta 2001;306: 27–33.

43. Lindberg C, Klintberg L, Oldfors A. Raised troponin T in inclusion body myositis is common and serum levels are persistent over time. Neuromuscul Disord 2006;16(8):495–7.

44. Matsumura T, Saito T, Fujimura H, Shinno S. Cardiac troponin I for accurate evaluation of cardiac status in myopathic patients. Brain Dev 2007;29(8):496–501.

45. Chung YL, Rider LG, Bell JD, et al. Muscle metabolites, detected in urine by proton spectroscopy, correlate with disease damage in juvenile idiopathic inflammatory myopathies. Arthritis Rheum 2005;53(4):565–70.

46. Spiera R, Kagen L. Extramuscular manifestations in idiopathic inflammatory myopathies. Curr Opin Rheumatol 1998;10:556–61.

47. Stone KB, Oddis CV, Fertig N, et al. Anti-Jo-1 antibody levels correlate with disease activity in idiopathic inflammatory myopathy. Arthritis Rheum 2007;56(9):3125–31.

48. Huber AM, Dugan EM, Lachenbruch PA, et al. The Cutaneous Assessment Tool: development and reliability in juvenile idiopathic inflammatory myopathy. Rheumatology (Oxford) 2007;46(10): 1606–11.

49. Huber AM, Dugan EM, Lachenbruch PA, et al. Preliminary validation and clinical meaning of the Cutaneous Assessment Tool in juvenile dermatomyositis. Arthritis Rheum 2008;59(2): 214–21.

50. Huber AM, Lachenbruch PA, Dugan EM, Miller FW, Rider LG. Alternative scoring of the Cutaneous Assessment Tool in juvenile dermatomyositis: results using abbreviated formats. Arthritis Rheum 2008;59(3):352–6.

51. Carroll CL, Lang W, Snively B, Feldman SR, Callen J, Jorizzo JL. Development and validation of the Dermatomyositis Skin Severity Index. Br J Dermatol 2008;158(2):345–50.

52. Klein RQ, Bangert CA, Costner M, et al. Comparison of the reliability and validity of outcome instruments for cutaneous dermatomyositis. Br J Dermatol 2008;159 (4): 887–94.

53. Hundley JL, Carroll CL, Lang W, et al. Cutaneous symptoms of dermatomyositis significantly impact patients' quality of life. J Am Acad Dermatol 2006;54(2):217–20.

54. Smith RL, Sundberg J, Shamiyah E, Dyer A, Pachman LM. Skin involvement in juvenile dermatomyositis is associated with loss of end row nailfold capillary loops. J Rheumatol 2004;31(8):1644–9.

55. Christen-Zaech S, Seshadri R, Sundberg J, Paller AS, Pachman LM. Persistent association of nailfold capillaroscopy changes and skin involvement over thirty-six months with duration of untreated disease in patients with juvenile dermatomyositis. Arthritis Rheum 2008;58(2):571–6.

56. Dawn A, Thevarajah S, Cayce KA, et al. Cutaneous blood flow in dermatomyositis and its association with disease severity. Skin Res Technol 2007;13(3):285–92.

57. Sonies BC. Evaluation and treatment of speech and swallowing disorders associated with myopathies. Curr Opin Rheumatol 1997;9:486–95.

58. Oh TH, Brumfield KA, Hoskin TL, Stolp KA, Murray JA, Bassford JR. Dysphagia in inflammatory myopathy: clinical characteristics, treatment strategies, and outcome in 62 patients. Mayo Clin Proc 2007;82(4):441–7.

59. Trapani S, Camiciottoli G, Vierucci A, Pistolesi M, Falcini F. Pulmonary involvement in juvenile dermatomyositis: a two-year longitudinal study. Rheumatology 2001;40:216–20.

60. Fathi M, Lundberg IE, Tornling G. Pulmonary complications of polymyositis and dermatomyositis. Semin Respir Crit Care Med 2007;28(4):451–8.

61. Hayashi S, Tanaka M, Kobayashi H, et al. High-resolution computed tomography characterization of interstitial lung diseases in polymyositis/dermatomyositis. J Rheumatol 2008;35(2): 260–9.

62. Karadimitrakis S, Plastiras SC, Zormpala A, et al. Chest CT findings in patients with inflammatory myopathy and Jo1 antibodies. Eur J Radiol 2008;66(1):27–30.

63. Fathi M, Vikgren J, Boijsen M, et al. Interstitial lung disease in polymyositis and dermatomyositis: longitudinal evaluation by pulmonary function and radiology. Arthritis Rheum 2008;59(5): 677–85.

64. Kumanovics G, Minier T, Radics J, Palinkas L, Berki T, Czirjak L. Comprehensive investigation of novel serum markers of pulmonary fibrosis associated with systemic sclerosis and dermato/polymyositis. Clin Exp Rheumatol 2008;26(3):414–20.

65. Bode RK, Klein-Gitelman MS, Miller ML, Lechman TS, Pachman LM. Disease Activity Score for children with juvenile dermatomyositis: reliability and validity evidence. Arthritis Rheum 2003;49(1):7–15.

66. Felson DT, Furst DE, Boers M. Rationale and strategies for reevaluating the ACR20. J Rheumatol 2007;34(5):1184–7.

67. Aletaha D, Landewe R, Karonitsch T, et al. Reporting disease activity in clinical trials of patients with rheumatoid arthritis: EULAR/ACR collaborative recommendations. Arthritis Rheum 2008;59(10):1371–7.

68. Park JH, Olsen NJ. Utility of magnetic resonance imaging in the evaluation of patients with inflammatory myopathies. Curr Rheum Rep 2001;3:334–45.

69. Adams EM, Chow CK, Premkumar A, Plotz PH. The idiopathic inflammatory myopathies: spectrum of MR imaging findings. Radiographics 1995;15:563–74.

70. Reimers CD, Schedel H, Fleckenstein JL, et al. Magnetic resonance imaging of skeletal muscles in idiopathic inflammatory myopathies of adults. J Neurol 1994;241:306–14.

71. Hernandez RJ, Sullivan DB, Chenevert TL, Keim DR. MR imaging in children with dermatomyositis: musculoskeletal findings and correlation with clinical and laboratory findings. Am J Roentgenol 1993;161:359–66.

72. Hilario MO, Yamashita H, Lutti D, Len C, Terreri MT, Lederman H. Juvenile idiopathic inflammatory myopathies: the value of magnetic resonance imaging in the detection of muscle involvement. Sao Paulo Med J 2000;118:35–40.

73. Kimball AB, Summers RM, Turner M, et al. Magnetic resonance imaging detection of occult skin and subcutaneous abnormalities in juvenile dermatomyositis: implications for diagnosis and therapy. Arthritis Rheum 2000;43:1866–73.

74. Tomasova SJ, Charvat F, Jarosova K, Vencovsky J. The role of MRI in the assessment of polymyositis and dermatomyositis. Rheumatology (Oxford) 2007;46(7):1174–9.
75. Maillard SM, Jones R, Owens C, et al. Quantitative assessment of MRI T2 relaxation time of thigh muscles in juvenile dermatomyositis. Rheumatology (Oxford) 2004;43(5):603–8.
76. Qi J, Olsen NJ, Price RR, Winston JA, Park JH. Diffusion-weighted imaging of inflammatory myopathies: polymyositis and dermatomyositis. J Magn Reson Imaging 2008;27(1):212–7.
77. Meng C, Adler R, Peterson M, Kagen L. Combined use of power Doppler and gray-scale sonography: a new technique for the assessment of inflammatory myopathy. J Rheumatol 2001;28:1271–82.
78. Pillen S, Verrips A, van Alfen N, Arts IM, Sie LT, Zwarts MJ. Quantitative skeletal muscle ultrasound: diagnostic value in childhood neuromuscular disease. Neuromuscul Disord 2007 ; 17(7):509–16.
79. Reimers CD, Fleckenstein JL, Witt TN, Muller-Felber W, Pongratz DE. Muscular ultrasound in idiopathic inflammatory myopathies of adults. J Neurol Sci 1993;116:82–92.
80. Chi-Fishman G, Hicks JE, Cintas HM, Sonies BC, Gerber LH. Ultrasound imaging distinguishes between normal and weak muscle. Arch Phys Med Rehabil 2004;85(6):980–6.
81. Pilkington C, Owen NJ, Bose S, Machado C, Owens CM, Murray K. A preliminary comparative study of high frequency muscle ultrasound and magnetic resonance imaging in 7 patients with juvenile dermatomyositis. Ann Rheum Dis 2000;59:727–728.
82. Weber MA, Krix M, Jappe U, et al. Pathologic skeletal muscle perfusion in patients with myositis: detection with quantitative contrast-enhanced US—initial results. Radiology 2006; 238(2):640–9.
83. Weber MA, Jappe U, Essig M, et al. Contrast-enhanced ultrasound in dermatomyositis- and polymyositis. J Neurol 2006;253(12):1625–32.
84. Niermann KJ, Olsen NJ, Park JH. Magnesium abnormalities of skeletal muscle in dermatomyositis and juvenile dermatomyositis. Arthritis Rheum 2002;46:475–88.
85. Park JH, Olsen NJ, King L Jr, et al. Use of magnetic resonance imaging and P-31 magnetic resonance spectroscopy to detect and quantify muscle dysfunction in the amyopathic and myopathic variants of dermatomyositis. Arthritis Rheum 1995;38:68–77.
86. Cea G, Bendahan D, Manners D, et al. Reduced oxidative phosphorylation and proton efflux suggest reduced capillary blood supply in skeletal muscle of patients with dermatomyositis and polymyositis: a quantitative 31P-magnetic resonance spectroscopy and MRI study. Brain 2002;125(Pt 7):1635–45.
87. Walsh RJ, Kong SW, Yao Y, et al. Type I interferon-inducible gene expression in blood is present and reflects disease activity in dermatomyositis and polymyositis. Arthritis Rheum 2007;56(11):3784–92.
88. Baechler EC, Bauer JW, Slattery CA, et al. An interferon signature in the peripheral blood of dermatomyositis patients is associated with disease activity. Mol Med 2007;13(1-2):59–68.
89. O'Connor KA, Abbott KA, Sabin B, Kuroda M, Pachman LM. MxA gene expression in juvenile dermatomyositis peripheral blood mononuclear cells: association with muscle involvement. Clin Immunol 2006;120(3):319–25.
90. Bilgic H, Ytterberg SR, McNallan KT, et al. IL-17 and IFN-regulated genes and chemokines as biomarkers of disease activity in inflammatory myopathies. Arthritis Rheum 2008; 58:S922.
91. Rider L, Reed A, James-Newton L, et al. Assessing the extent and severity of damage in adult and juvenile myositis by the Myositis Damage Index (MDI). Arthritis Rheum 2003;48:S307.
92. Traill L, Ruperto N, Pilkington C, et al. The long-term outcome of juvenile idiopathic inflammatory myopathies: a multicenter, multinational study of 557 patients. Arthritis Rheum 2007;52:S830.
93. Ponyi A, Borgulya G, Constantin T, Vancsa A, Gergely L, Danko K. Functional outcome and quality of life in adult patients with idiopathic inflammatory myositis. Rheumatology (Oxford) 2005;44(1):83–8.
94. Sultan SM, Ioannou Y, Moss K, Isenberg DA. Outcome in patients with idiopathic inflammatory myositis: morbidity and mortality. Rheumatology 2002;41:22–6.

95. Chung YL, Mitchell HL, Houssien DA, Al-Mahrouki H, Carr AJ, Scott DL. A comparative study of outcome in myositis and other musculoskeletal disorders assessed using the Nottingham Health Profile. Clin Exp Rheumatol 2001;19:447–50.

96. Vincent KA, Carr AJ, Walburn J, Scott DL, Rose MR. Construction and validation of a quality of life questionnaire for neuromuscular disease (INQoL). Neurology 2007;68(13):1051–7.

97. Ruperto N, Ravelli A, Pistorio A, et al. Cross-cultural adaptation and psychometric evaluation of the Childhood Health Assessment Questionnaire (CHAQ) and the Child Health Questionnaire (CHQ) in 32 countries. Review of the general methodology. Clin Exp Rheumatol 2001;19(Suppl 23):S1–9.

98. Varni JW, Seid M, Knight TS, Burwinkle T, Brown J, Szer IS. The PedsQL in pediatric rheumatology: reliability, validity, and responsiveness of the Pediatric Quality of Life Inventory Generic Core Scales and Rheumatology Module. Arthritis Rheum 2002;46:714–25.

# Chapter 16
# Muscle Strength and Exercise in Patients with Inflammatory Myopathies

**Helene Alexanderson and Ingrid E. Lundberg**

**Abstract** Muscle weakness and low muscle endurance are the primary clinical features of the inflammatory myopathies, myositis. Most patients with polymyositis and dermatomyositis respond to medical treatment, but few recover former muscle function. Patients with inclusion body myositis respond poorly to immunosuppressive treatment, and most patients develop progressive muscle weakness. Different mechanisms that cause impaired muscle performance are involved in different subsets of myositis and in different phases of disease. Muscle fiber degeneration and muscle atrophy, as well as an acquired metabolic myopathy, are likely to contribute. In this context, physical exercise is of importance; however, historically patients with myositis have been discouraged from exercising due to the notion that it might be harmful and cause increased muscle inflammation, but importantly, there are no studies or reports supporting this notion. On the contrary, since 1993, a number of studies have reported both efficacy and safety of different kinds of exercise regimens in patients with chronic as well as recent-onset adult polymyositis and dermatomyositis. In addition, exercise may even reduce muscle inflammation. For inclusion body myositis, exercise data are scarce and the effects less convincing on muscle performance. Children with juvenile dermatomyositis, with chronic as well as active disease, tolerate maximal oxygen uptake tests and exercise tolerance tests, supporting the use of exercise also in children with inflammatory myopathies, although there are no studies evaluating effects of exercise employed over weeks or months in children. Overall, physical exercise is beneficial, and there is a clear role for adapted physical exercise as additional therapy in the rehabilitation of patients with inflammatory myopathies.

**Keywords** Polymyositis • Dermatomyositis • Juvenile dermatomyositis • Inclusion body myositis • Exercise • Training

H. Alexanderson
Department of Physical Therapy, Orthopedic and Rheumatology Unit, Karolinska University Hospital,

I.E. Lundberg
Rheumatology Unit, Department of Medicine, Karolinska University Hospital, Solna, Karolinska Institutet, Stockholm, Sweden

L.J. Kagen (ed.), *The Inflammatory Myopathies*,
DOI 10.1007/978-1-60327-827-0_16,

# Muscle Impairment in Patients with Adult Polymyositis and Dermatomyositis

Patients with adult idiopathic inflammatory myopathies (IIMs) have impaired muscle function, in both muscle strength and muscle endurance. Patients with polymyositis and dermatomyositis characteristically have symmetrical muscle weakness and low endurance of proximal muscles. Most of these patients improve with conventional immunosuppressive treatment, but few recover former strength and muscle endurance. Most patients with polymyositis or dermatomyositis have persisting impairment that affects functional abilities in daily life. Muscle endurance (referring to repetitive movements and exemplified by walking, climbing stairs, or working with the arms above the head) is more affected than single movements with comparable loads. A group of patients with chronic disease (24 with dermatomyositis, 20 with polymyositis, and 5 with inclusion body myositis) achieved 23% of the maximal score on the muscle endurance measure Functional Index (FI) 2, compared to 96% of the maximal score of the eight-muscle group manual muscle test (MMT) *(1)*.

In addition to the reported proximal muscle weakness, there are some reports that also suggested involvement of distal muscles in polymyositis and dermatomyositis. Unpublished data from Malin Regardh, occupational therapist indicated 50% decreased grip strength was found in patients with chronic polymyositis and dermatomyositis compared to normal values assessed by the Grippit instrument. Decreased muscle function in dorsi and plantar flexors of the ankle was reported in another study *(2)*. There are also data suggesting that patients with chronic polymyositis and dermatomyositis have low aerobic capacity compared to healthy controls *(3)*.

The mechanisms that cause impaired performance vary and could be different in various phases of disease. Loss of muscle due to inflammatory cell-induced fiber necrosis is one mechanism. However, the lack of association between the degree of inflammatory cell infiltrates and the degree of muscle weakness suggests that factors other than cell-mediated muscle fiber necrosis may contribute to the muscle weakness. General muscle atrophy is one such factor but is not always present, particularly not in early phases of disease. In the chronic phase of disease, after conventional immunosuppressive treatment, some degree of impaired muscle performance is often present despite absence of inflammation in muscle tissue or muscle atrophy. In muscle tissue from polymyositis and dermatomyositis patients with muscle weakness, there are some consistent molecular findings that are present in different phases of disease: increased expression of major histocompatibility complex (MHC) class 1 on muscle fibers and signs of activated endothelial cells in microvessels of muscles and capillary loss in some patients *(4, 5)*. The loss of capillaries and the activated, thick, high endothelium-like endothelial cells of the microvessels may affect the circulation to muscle tissue and impair supply of oxygen and other nutrients and thus cause signs of metabolic myopathy. An acquired metabolic myopathy is also suggested by the low levels of adenosine triphosphate (ATP) and phosphocreatine, found by magnetic resonance spectroscopy *(6)*. A low frequency of oxidative type I fibers in thigh muscles was recorded, indicating an adaptation of the muscle tissue to a hypoxic environment. Tissue hypoxia was further suggested by the improved clinical effect and increased frequency of type I fibers after intervention with physical exercise *(7)*. Proinflammatory cytokines, like interferon alpha and gamma, tumor necrosis factor (TNF), and interleukin (IL) 1, which have all been detected in muscle tissue of polymyositis or dermatomyositis, may induce upregulation of MHC class I in muscle fibers *(8)*. The MHC class I expression may negatively affect the muscle contractility by the endoplasmic reticulum (ER) stress mechanism *(9)*.

Taken together, these data suggest that polymyositis and dermatomyositis patients may develop muscle fiber loss, muscle fiber atrophy, and an acquired metabolic myopathy that might contribute to the clinical muscle symptoms.

## Muscle Impairment in Patients with Inclusion Body Myositis

Patients with sporadic inclusion body myositis (s-IBM) typically have pronounced weakness and atrophy of thigh muscles as well as weakness of distal muscles, particularly of finger flexors. These patients do not respond favorably to medical treatment, leaving them with a slowly progressing muscle weakness. The reason for this is not clear; however, a review questioned the role of inflammatory infiltrates as a confounding mechanism, causing muscle weakness due to the poor treatment response. This instead suggests that s-IBM is more of a multifactorial muscle disorder with myodegeneration and protein alterations *(10)*. In late disease course, many patients are wheelchair bound and in need of assistance in activities of daily living (ADL).

## Exercise in a Historical Perspective

The persisting impaired muscle performance after conventional immunosuppressive treatment and the signs of an acquired metabolic myopathy make physical exercise interesting as a treatment modality, combined with immunosuppressive drugs in patients with polymyositis or dermatomyositis. Exercise in the inflammatory myopathies has been controversial for many years due to fear that active exercise would aggravate the disease. This caution was based on studies describing increased serum levels of creatine phosphokinase (CPK) as well as inflammatory cells in muscle biopsies following strenuous exercise, such as a marathon race *(11, 12)*. However, there are (to our knowledge) no published studies describing aggravated disease following physical exercise or physical activity in patients with inflammatory myopathies. Textbooks from the 1990s and early 2000s stated that patients with inflammatory myopathies with active disease should be recommended bed rest, with only passive range-of-motion exercise to preserve mobility. After some clinical improvement, active range-of-motion exercises and careful isometric strength training could be introduced *(13)*. Textbooks from 2004, 2005, and 2008 were of the same opinion, adding that active exercise such as cycling without resistance, aerobic exercise, or pool exercise can be employed in a chronic phase *(14-16)*.

Until now, exercise in inflammatory myopathies has not been a prioritized topic in textbooks due to lack of scientific evidence for efficacy and safety of physical exercise in these patients. Since 1993, a number of studies have described safety and the positive effects of different kinds of exercise regimens in patients with polymyositis and dermatomyositis; these regimens are discussed in this chapter. A few studies have been performed in patients with inclusion body myositis, but they are less conclusive. The resistance to conventional immunosuppressive drugs in patients with inclusion body myositis, as well as other features of this entity, suggests that other disease mechanisms may be predominant in this subset of inflammatory myopathy. In children with juvenile dermatomyositis, the experience of exercise training is scarce. There are only a few studies validating exercise tests and one study describing effects of a single exercise session. Thus, strength and effects of exercise in inclusion body myositis and juvenile dermatomyositis are discussed separately.

# Exercise in Adult Polymyositis and Dermatomyositis

The pioneer studies evaluating exercise in patients with polymyositis and dermatomyositis were published in the same issue of *Journal of Rheumatology* in 1993. One of them reported positive effects of 6 weeks of isometric strength training of the quadriceps on the right side, with the left leg serving as a control in one patient with chronic polymyositis *(17)*. Isometric quadriceps strength, assessed in a Cybex device, improved significantly in the trained leg compared to the control leg, without sustained increases of serum levels of CPK. The other study included five patients with active polymyositis or dermatomyositis *(18)*. They performed active strength training for 2 weeks, rested with passive range-of-motion exercises for 2 weeks, and then went on to active exercise again. Most patients performed between three and four periods of active exercise, four of them improving isometric quadriceps strength significantly (as assessed by a Cybex device), and one patient had unchanged muscle strength. Sustained increases of serum CPK levels were not seen in any of these patients. Together, these two studies included only six patients, but they have a significant importance since they were the first to contradict the long-standing notion that active exercise aggravates disease activity in patients with inflammatory myopathies and for inspiring others to evaluate other exercise regimens in these patients. Since then, 11 studies have been published on exercise in adult polymyositis and dermatomyositis (Table 16.1).

In a controlled study, 14 patients with chronic polymyositis or dermatomyositis were randomized to a training group or a control group *(19)*. The training group performed an aerobic 1-h stationary cycle and step-up exercise program at 60% of their maximal heart rate for 6 weeks. They exercised twice a week for the first 2 weeks and then three times a week for the remaining 4 weeks; the control group did

**Table 16.1** Summary of published exercise studies in adult patients with inflammatory myopathies

| Study/design | Patients (n) | Diagnosis | Disease activity | Exercise duration | Load/intensity (% of max) | Outcome safety | Results safety | Outcome benefits | Results benefits |
|---|---|---|---|---|---|---|---|---|---|
| Spector et al. (39), open study, 1997 | 5 | IBM | Chronic | 12 weeks | 10–20 VRM | CPK Muscle Biopsy | 0 | Isometric peak torque 3 VRM | 0 + |
| Alexanderson et al. (22), open study, 1999 | 10 | PM/DM | Chronic | 12 weeks | NR | CPK Muscle Biopsy MRI | 0 0 0 | Muscle endurance (FI) SF-36 | + + |
| Alexanderson et al. (33), open study, 2000 | 11 | PM/DM | Active | 12 weeks | NR | CPK Muscle Biopsy MRI | 0 0 0 | Muscle endurance (FI) SF-36 | + + |
| Heikkila et al. (24), open study, 2001 | 22 | PM/DM/ IBM | Chronic | 3 weeks | NR | CPK | 0 | Muscle endurance (FI) Activity limitation (HAQ) | + 0 |
| Varju et al. (25), open study, 2003 | 19 | PM/DM | Active | 3 weeks | NR | CPK | 0 | Isometric peak torque Forced vital capacity Activity limitation (HAQ) | + + + |
| Arnardottir et al. (42), open study, 2003 | 7 | IBM | Chronic | 12 weeks | NR | CPK Muscle Biopsy | 0 0 | Isokinetic peak torque Muscle endurance (FI) | 0 0 |
| Harris-Love et al. (32), case report, controlled, 2005 | 1 | PM | Chronic | 12 weeks | 70 | CPK Pain (VAS) ROM | 0 0 0 | Isometric peak torque | + |
| Chung et al. (35), randomized, controlled, double blind, 2007 | 37 | PM/DM | Chronic | 20 weeks | NR | CPK MRS Pain | 0 + 0 | Functional capacity (AFPT) Muscle endurance (FI) Muscle strength (MMT) Perceived health (NHP) Depression/anxiety | + + + 0 0 |

(continued)

**Table 16.1** (continued)

| Study/design | Patients (n) | Diagnosis | Disease activity | Exercise duration | Load/intensity (% of max) | Outcome safety | Results safety | Outcome benefits | Results benefits |
|---|---|---|---|---|---|---|---|---|---|
| Alexanderson et al. (26), open study, repeated measures, 2007 | 8 | PM/DM | Chronic | 7 weeks | 70 | CPK | 0 | Muscle strength (10 VRM) | + |
| | | | | | | Muscle Biopsy | 0 | Muscle endurance (FI-2) | + |
| | | | | | | 6 Item Core set | + (+)[b] | Activity limitation (MAP) | 0(±)[a] |
| | | | | | | | | Participation restriction (VAS) | 0 |
| *Aerobic exercise* | | | | | | | | | |
| Wiesinger et al. (19), randomized, controlled, 1998 | 14 | PM/DM | Chronic | 6 Weeks | 60 | CPK | 0 | $VO_{2peak}$ | + |
| | | | | | | | | Isometric peak torque | + |
| | | | | | | | | Activity limitation (FASQ) | + |
| Wiesinger et al. (20), controlled, 1998 | 13 | PM/DM | Chronic | 24 Weeks | 60 | CPK | 0 | $VO_{2peak}$ | + |
| | | | | | | | | Isometric peak torque | + |
| | | | | | | | | Activity limitation (FASQ) | + |

*PM* polymyositis; *DM* dermatomyositis; *IBM* inclusion body myositis; + statistically significant improvement on group level; *0* unchanged group level;; *VRM* voluntary repetition maximum; *SF-36* Medical Outcomes Study 36-Item Short Form questionnaire; *FI* Functional Index in myositis; *HAQ* Stanford Health Assessment Questionnaire; *ROM* range of motion; *AFPT* aggregate functional performance time is a total score of measures; *timed up and go* walking 15 ft, ascending and descending nine stairsteps; *MMT* manual muscle test; *NHP* Nottingham Health Profile; *MAP* Myositis Activities Profile; *VAS* visual analogue scale; *VO2peak* maximal oxygen uptake; *FASQ* Functional Assessment Screening Questionnaire. NR = not registered

[a]Unchanged group level with individual improvement and deterioration according to minimal clinically relevant criteria for improvement and deterioration according to Paulus et al. (*30*)

[b]Statistically significant improvement on group level as well as responders with decreased disease activity according to minimal clinically important criteria suggested by IMACS (*29*)

not engage in any intervention. A maximal oxygen uptake stationary bike test, which was well tolerated by the patients, was performed before and after the exercise period. Maximal peak isometric torque (PIT) was assessed in hip flexors and knee extensors using a Cybex 6000 isokinetic dynamometer, and ADL were assessed by a questionnaire. The training group improved in maximal oxygen uptake by a mean of 12%, isometric quadriceps strength by a mean of 29.4%, as well as activity limitation (measured by the Functional Assessment Screening Questionnaire) by a mean of 20%. These improvements were statistically significant compared to the control group. After completing this study, patients from the exercise group and the control group were invited to take part in an extended 6-month program with similar exercise regimen (20). Four patients from the exercise group and four from the control group volunteered to exercise. Five of the remaining patients served as controls, not exercising but visiting the clinic regularly. Patients exercised on a cycle and did step-up exercises at 60% of their earlier established maximal heart rate for 1 h twice a week during the first 2 weeks, three times a week during the following 4 weeks, and then once a week during the following 18 weeks. Patients were also encouraged to do additional exercises, such as walking or cycling three times a week. The intervention group improved statistically significantly in maximal oxygen uptake by 28%, compared to the nonexercising group, and improved their ADL and isometric muscle strength. Serum CPK levels remained unchanged during the exercise periods in both these studies.

There is a lack of correlation among serum CPK levels, disease activity, and muscle impairment in many patients (21). Therefore, a more careful approach was undertaken to evaluate safety of exercise in patients with chronic, stable, as well as recent-onset, active polymyositis and dermatomyositis. Ten patients with chronic polymyositis and dermatomyositis, with low disease activity and long-standing muscle impairment, were evaluated regarding muscle inflammation using repeated muscle biopsies of the vastus lateralis, magnetic resonance imaging (MRI) of the thighs, and analysis of serum CPK levels during an exercise program (22). This was a 12-week resistance home exercise program, at approximately 50% of their maximal muscle function, with additional walks 5 days a week (Figs. 16.1–16.14). Exercise resistance was adjusted according to changes in muscle function during the study. Muscle performance was measured by the FI, which measures the number of repetitions in several proximal and distal muscle groups (2). After 12 weeks of exercise, a repeated muscle biopsy was performed from the contralateral side as well as follow-up MRI and analysis of CPK levels. No patient had signs of increased muscle inflammation in any of these assessments, and the group improved significantly in muscle endurance, with 17% improvement of the FI and in perceived health in the Physical Functioning domain of the Medical Outcomes Study 36-Item Short Form (SF-36) (23).

A home exercise regimen consisting of passive and active training individually or in a group as well as pool exercises and walks was performed by 22 patients, 19 with chronic polymyositis or dermatomyositis and 3 with inclusion body myositis (24). They performed various amounts of exercise regimens approximately 3 days a week for 3 weeks. Although the exercise period was only 3 weeks, the group

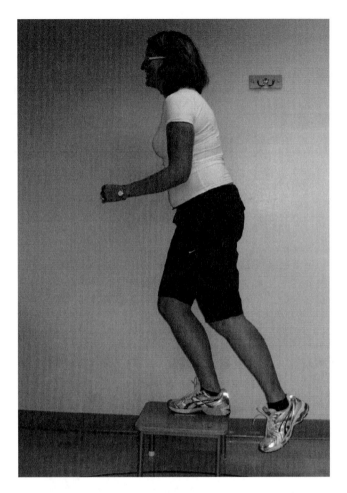

**Fig. 16.1** The resistance home exercise program employed in patients with adult inflammatory myopathies *(22, 33, 42)*. Warming up: using a stool 20 cm high, step up with the right leg for 1 min, then change legs. Move your arms as if you were walking. If necessary, hold on to something to keep your balance. (Adapted from **Ref. *50***)

showed minor, but statistically significant, 11% improvement in muscle endurance assessed by the FI. Another study evaluated a similar 3-week course of stretching, relaxation, hot baths, isotonic muscular training, and respiratory exercises *(25)*. Twenty-one patients, 10 with active disease and 11 with chronic disease, performed these exercises 5 days a week. Patients with active disease improved their isometric muscle strength (measured by a manual dynamometer) by an average of 17–37%, and patients with chronic disease improved by an average of 34–46% in different muscle groups. Due to the study design, the two last studies could not conclude which type of exercise regimen was beneficial, and information on exercise intensity is lacking.

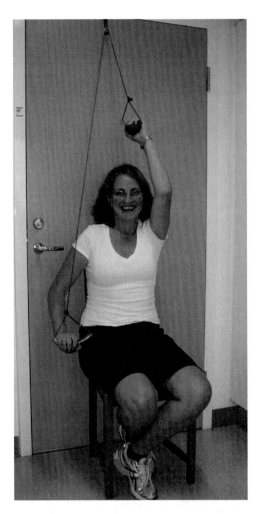

**Fig. 16.2** Shoulder flexion: for mobility in the upper extremities, use a pulley apparatus. Push one arm down to help the other up. Work with your elbows pointed forward and up. Ten repetitions each arm. (Adapted from **Ref. 50**)

However, both studies contributed to the evidence of the safety of short-term rehabilitation programs since no patients reported increased muscle pain or developed increased CPK levels.

Because only easy-to-moderate muscular exercise programs had been evaluated, a study attempted to employ an intensive resistance training program in patients with chronic polymyositis or dermatomyositis (26). Eight patients were included, and they performed isotonic training on an intensity of ten voluntary repetition maximum (VRM) in five muscle groups. They exercised every muscle group in

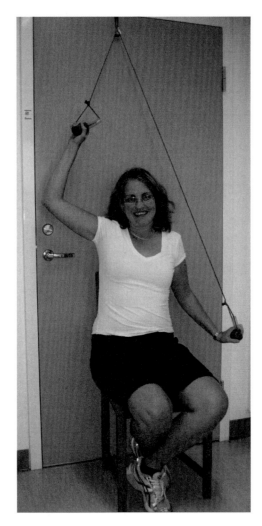

**Fig. 16.3** Shoulder abduction: use the pulley apparatus as in Fig. 16.3. Point your elbows out to the side. Ten repetitions each arm. (Adapted from **Ref. 50**)

three sets with a 90-s rest in between, and they exercised in this manner 3 days a week for 7 weeks (Figs. 16.15–16.19). For further validity of the study, clinical measures of disability were performed at 4 weeks prior to exercise start, at baseline, and after 7 weeks of exercise. All patients had unchanged medication for 3 months prior to entering the study. Measures of disease activity using the six-item core set *(27)*, as well as muscle biopsies from vastus lateralis, and analysis of muscle enzymes were performed at baseline and after 7 weeks of exercise. The group had unchanged disability during the 4 weeks prior to exercise start but improved statistically significantly with increased muscle strength by an average of 20–900% as

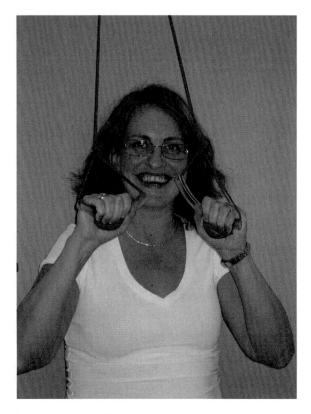

**Fig. 16.4**  Grip: for grip strength hold on to the handles of the pulley apparatus and squeeze tightly with one hand at a time. Ten repetitions per hand. (Adapted from **Ref. 50**)

assessed by ten VRM in four of five muscle groups. The group also improved significantly in muscle endurance of shoulder flexion, assessed by the FI 2 *(28)*, by an average of 29–49%. Other muscle groups of the FI 2, measures of activity limitation, and participation restriction remained unchanged. The group also improved significantly in the extramuscular disease activity score Myositis Intention to Treat Activity Index (MITAX), mostly due to decreased dyspnea in several patients after 7 weeks of exercise, compared to baseline. All patients were also analyzed individually according to proposed criteria for minimal clinically relevant improvement of disease activity and disability. The proposed criteria presented by the International Myositis Assessment Clinical Study Group (IMACS) were used to assess disease activity *(29)*. Two patients were responders with decreased disease activity, and no patient worsened according to the IMACS criteria.

Criteria proposed by Paulus et al. *(30)* were used to analyze muscle impairment, activity limitation, and participation restriction. All patients were responders, improving more than 20% in at least one muscle group in muscle strength and muscle endurance.

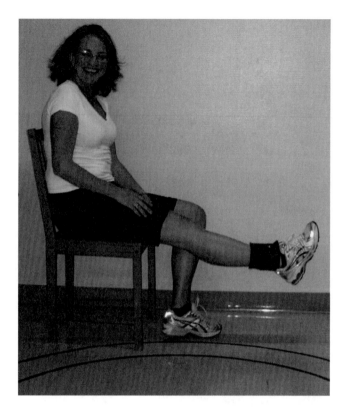

**Fig. 16.5** Quadriceps: for strength in the quadriceps, sit on a chair or a bed with the thighs supported. If needed, put a weight cuff round the ankle. Tense the quadriceps and extend the knee. Hold for 5 s and then relax. Ten repetitions each leg. (Adapted from **Ref.** *50*)

Two patients were responders with improvements in two or more scale steps in three subscales, and one patient deteriorated two or more scale steps in one single item of the activity limitation questionnaire Myositis Activities Profile *(31)*. No patient was a responder or deteriorated according to criteria for participation restriction assessed by patients' global disease impact on general well-being on a visual analog scale *(26)*. Immunohistochemistry analysis of muscle biopsies initially revealed several inflammatory infiltrates in one patient and a few, scattered infiltrates in two patients; the remaining five patients had no inflammatory infiltrates at all. After the exercise program, one of the patients with a few infiltrates had no signs of inflammation, while the other two were unchanged, and serum CPK levels remained unchanged.

Another type of exercise, a submaximal eccentric exercise, was used in a case report, which described 40–50% increases in knee extensor isometric muscle strength in the exercised leg, compared to the nonexercised leg, following a submaximal 12-week eccentric exercise program in a patient with a diagnosis of polymyositis; there was no increase in CPK levels, muscle pain, or muscle stiffness *(32)*.

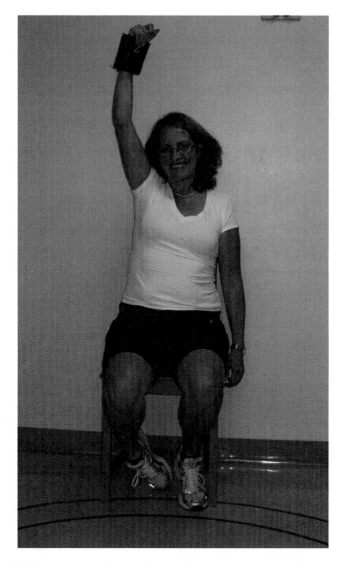

**Fig. 16.6** Deltoids: to strengthen the shoulder muscles, sit on a chair. If needed, use a weight cuff around the wrist. Raise one arm above your head as high as you can. Ten repetitions per arm. (Adapted from **Ref.** *50*)

There were some questions concerning the diagnosis. Muscle biopsy findings suggested polymyositis, but due to the lack of treatment response, the diagnosis of inclusion body myositis could not be ruled out. However, this report suggests that submaximal eccentric exercise could be feasible for patients with adult IIMs. Further studies are required to ensure the safety and efficacy of this type of exercise in myositis patients.

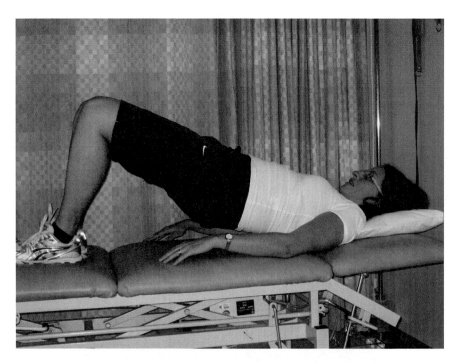

**Fig. 16.7** Hip extensors: for strength in the lower extremities, lay down on the floor or a bed. Bend your knees and push your pelvis up. Hold for 5 s, then relax. Ten repetitions. (Adapted from **Ref. 50**)

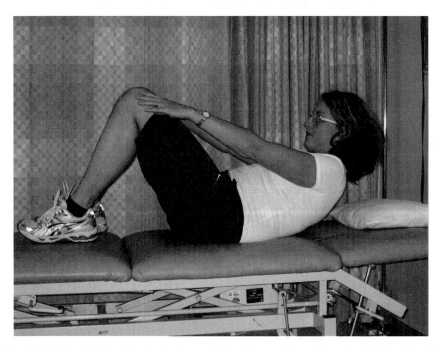

**Fig. 16.8** Situps: to strengthen the trunk muscles, lay down with your knees bent. Lift your head, tighten the trunk muscles, and do a situp. Put your hand up against the knees. Ten repetitions. (Adapted from **Ref. 50**)

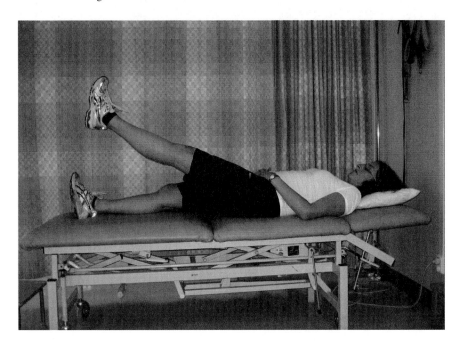

**Fig. 16.9** Hip flexors: for strength in the hip muscles, lay down on your back and lift one leg at a time about 30 cm. Ten repetitions each leg. (Adapted from **Ref. 50**)

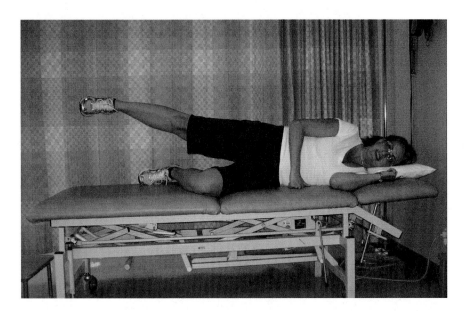

**Fig. 16.10** Hip abductors: to strengthen the hip muscles, lay down on one side. Bend one knee and raise the other leg up about 30 cm with a straight knee. Ten repetitions each leg. (Adapted from **Ref. 50**)

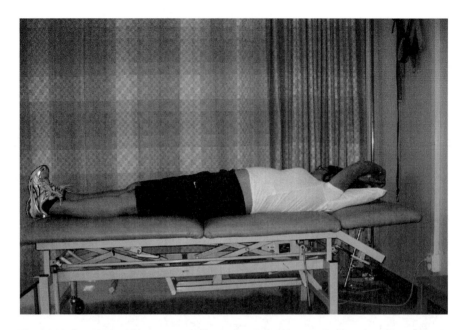

**Fig. 16.11** Stretch shoulders: to stretch the trunk and shoulder muscles, lay down on your back. Put your arms above your head and stretch out one side at a time. Hold the position for 20 s. (Adapted from **Ref. 50**)

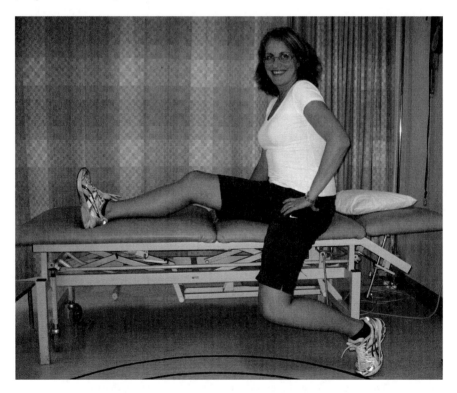

**Fig. 16.12** Stretch hamstrings: sit on a bed. Put one leg up on the bed and put the opposite foot on the floor. Keep your back straight and hold for 20 s. Repeat on other side. (Adapted from **Ref. 50**)

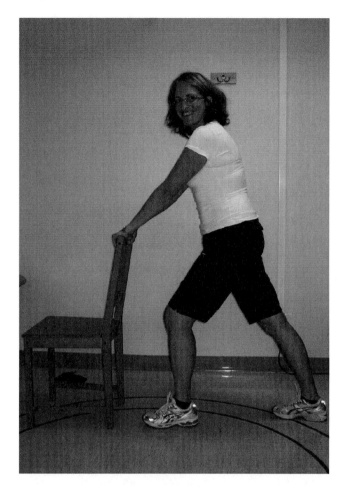

**Fig. 16.13** Gastrocnemius stretch: to stretch the gastrocnemius, stand and put both hands on the back of a chair. Put one foot behind the other, bend the knee in front, and lean forward against the chair, keeping your heel on the floor. Hold the position for 20 s. Switch leg positions and repeat. (Adapted from **Ref. 50**)

Encouraged by these results, 11 patients with recent-onset, active polymyositis and dermatomyositis performed the same home exercise program as the chronic myositis patients described *(33)*. At baseline, patients had median diagnosis duration of 1 (1–3) month and were on a median of 40 (35–60) mg of oral corticosteroids. All patients (except one with dermatomyositis) had inflammatory infiltrates or increased T2-weighted MRI signals, indicating ongoing inflammation and elevated CPK levels. Although patients performed resistance exercise 5 days a week for 12 weeks, their muscle biopsies, MRI scans, and CPK levels indicated unchanged or decreased signs of inflammation. There was no evidence of increased muscle inflammation in any of the variables in any of the patients. The group improved significantly in FI-assessed muscle endurance by 13–18% and in domains Physical Functioning, Bodily Pain, and Vitality of the SF-36 questionnaire *(33)*.

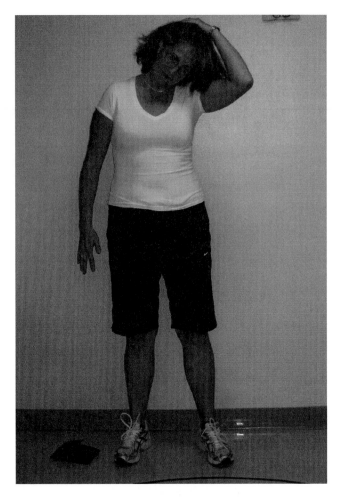

**Fig. 16.14** Stretch neck: to stretch the neck muscles, in a standing position, lay your ear against your shoulder. Stretch the opposite arm to the floor. Hold for 20 s. Repeat on the other side. (Adapted from **Ref. 50**)

## Exercise and Creatine Supplements

Because studies have reported metabolic changes in muscle tissue (such as lower levels of ATP and phosphocreatine) at rest, during, and after exercise in patients with dermatomyositis and polymyositis *(6, 34)*, there could be a role for creatine supplements in this group of patients. This was confirmed in a randomized, double-blind, placebo-controlled, multicenter trial, in which the effects of creatine supplements, together with exercise, were compared to exercise alone in patients with chronic polymyositis and dermatomyositis *(35)*. All 37 patients included in the study performed the same resistance home exercise program used in some earlier studies *(22, 33)* 5 days a week for 5 months. Before starting the exercise program, patients were

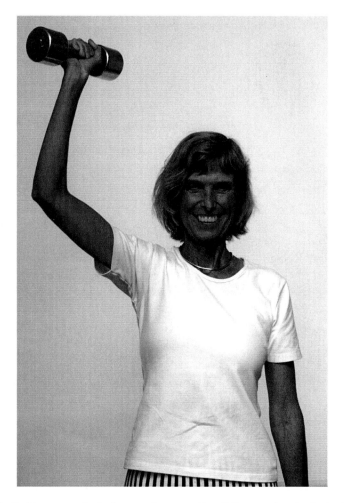

**Fig. 16.15** Resistance exercise in five muscle groups. For all five exercises, loads should be used to allow a maximum of ten repetitions, and all exercises should be performed at a calm pace through both the concentric and eccentric phases. Deltoids: raise one arm above the head through range of motion in a position of shoulder flexion/abduction

randomized to a creatine supplement group or a placebo group. Completer analysis showed that the creatine group improved its functional capacity significantly (measured by the Aggregate Functional Performance Time score *(36)*), by a median of 13% compared to 3.7% in the placebo group. Improvement was also seen in muscle endurance, using the FI, with a median improvement of 18%, compared to 11% improvement in the placebo group. Minor, but statistically significant, changes in isometric muscle strength of two muscle groups assessed by MMT were also revealed *(35)*. Magnetic resonance spectroscopy showed increased phosphocreatine/β-nucleoside ratio in the creatine group compared to the placebo group. No significant adverse effects occurred in the creatine supplement group during the study.

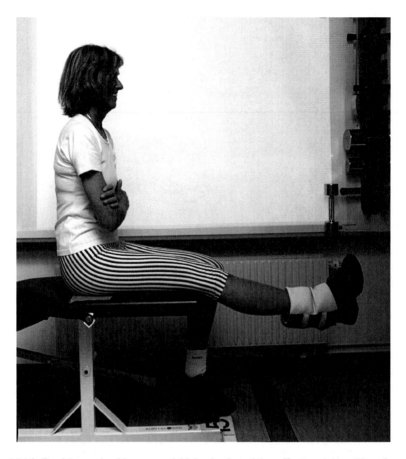

**Fig. 16.16** Quadriceps: sit with supported thighs. Apply weight cuffs around the ankle and extend the knee through range of motion

Thus, creatine supplements in addition to resistance exercise have added value compared to exercise alone and could be combined with conventional immunosuppressive treatment.

## Molecular Effects of Exercise in Polymyositis or Dermatomyositis

Clinical beneficial effects of physical exercise in adult polymyositis or dermatomyositis have been consistent using various types of exercise. A relevant question is whether the types of exercise used could have molecular effects on muscle tissue that could explain some of the beneficial achievements. In an at-home exercise study in which a 12-week, moderate resistance program was employed with beneficial effects as reported here, patients were investigated by repeat muscle biopsies. In patients with

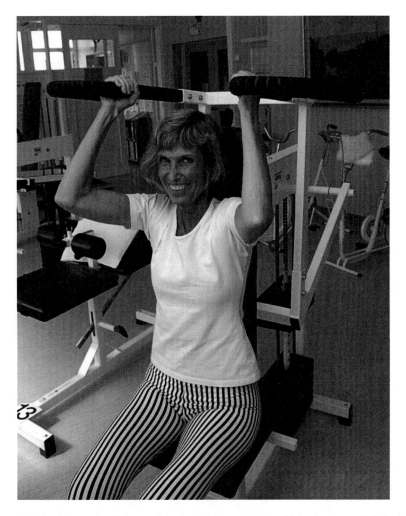

**Fig. 16.17** Latissimus dorsi/biceps: sit in the training apparatus with back support. Pull the handles down and back up again

polymyositis or dermatomyositis with chronic disease and low degree of inflammation, a low percentage of type I oxidative muscle fibers and a high percentage of intermediate type IIC fibers were recorded at baseline compared to healthy controls. After the 12-week home exercise program, a significant increased percentage of type I fibers, together with a significantly decreased percentage of type IIC fibers, was recorded, as was increased type II fiber cross-sectional area (Fig. 16.20) *(7)*. In the more recent intensive resistance exercise study reported *(26)*, repeated muscle biopsies were analyzed using a microarray technique, exploring gene expressions in muscle tissue. Interestingly, our unpublished data (Dr. Gustavo Nader) suggest that intensive resistant exercise can reduce the expression of genes involved in

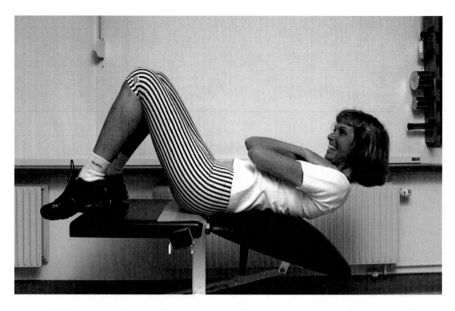

**Fig. 16.18** Trunk muscles: lay with bent knees and arms crossed in front of you or hands supporting the head. Lift the head and trunk

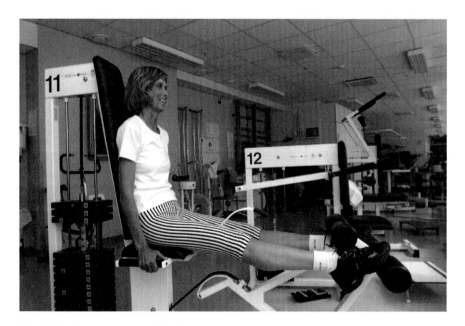

**Fig. 16.19** Gastrocnemius: sit in the training apparatus with extended knees and metatarsal phalangeal joints against the foot pad. Begin with the ankle dorsi flexed and push down toward plantar flexion

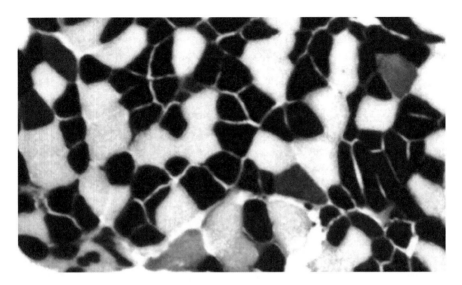

**Fig. 16.20**   Fiber-type pattern in a cross-sectional area of muscle tissue from a woman with poly-myositis. Adenosine triphosphatase (ATPase) staining at pH 10.3 was used to distinguish type I (oxidative) as *white*, type IIA and IIB (glycolytic) as *black,* and type IIC (intermediate) as *gray* fibers. (Courtesy Mona Esbjörnsson)

inflammation and fibrosis in patients with myositis. These findings are in line with the observations of a local anti-inflammatory response, with a reduction in the expression of TNF, IL-6, IL-1β, and inducible nitric oxide synthase in subjects with chronic heart failure, who often develop a myopathy with low muscle endurance *(37)*, and observations that exercise can increase muscle mass, thereby reducing cachexia and overproduction of TNF in patients with rheumatoid arthritis *(38)*. Taken together, the molecular studies in polymyositis and dermatomyositis suggest that myositis-affected muscle retains the ability to respond to exercise in a similar fashion as muscle from healthy individuals.

## Exercise in Inclusion Body Myositis

Including the Haikkilaa et al. *(24)* study mentioned, to date there are only three studies evaluating exercise in patients with inclusion body myositis. Haikkilaa et al. reported that all three patients with inclusion body myositis improved; however, no specific results were reported for these patients. Another study employed a resist-ance strength exercise program in which five patients with inclusion body myositis performed three sets of 10, 15, and 20 repetitions in six muscle groups 3 days a week for 12 weeks *(39)*. Exercised muscle groups were knee extensors, flexors on each side, right elbow flexors, and wrist extensors. Exercise load was determined by using 5 VRM and then decreasing loads a little to allow more repetitions. The group improved significantly in 3-VRM strength, with an average of 20–120%, showing the largest improvements in knee flexors, which had been considered as the muscle group least affected by the disease. However, there were no significant improvements in measures of MMT, PIT established on a Cin/Com dynamometer, fatigue assessed by the fatigue Severity Scale *(40)*, or activity limitation of the Barthel Index *(41)*. An open biopsy of either biceps or vastus lateralis was performed 4 weeks prior to exercise start and after the 12-week exercise program. There were no signs of increased muscle inflammation as assessed by analysis of muscle biopsies and muscle enzymes (see Table 16.1).

A third study employed the described resistance home exercise program *(22, 33)* used in polymyositis and dermatomyositis *(42)*. Seven patients with inclusion body myositis performed the home exercise program 5 days a week for 12 weeks in an open study. No significant improvements were recorded for measures of muscle impairment (e.g., MMT, PIT, or muscle endurance) using the FI. Muscle biopsies were taken before and after exercise from either vastus lateralis or tibialis anterior, and CPK levels were analyzed. Most patients had inflammatory infiltrates and elevated serum CPK levels when starting the exercise program. After 12 weeks, there were no signs of increased muscle inflammation in the biopsies, and the CPK levels were unchanged (see Table 16.1).

Another study suggested that exercise might have a role in patients with inclusion body myositis since 15 patients had statistically significant decreased muscle strength and developed more muscle atrophy of the nondominant forearm and hand compared to the dominant side *(43)*. Data on the role of exercise in the treatment of inclusion body myositis are still insufficient, but no signs of harmful effects on the muscles have been recorded to date. More studies are needed with training protocols aimed to improve the specific functional deficits that predominate in inclusion body myositis. Furthermore, measures that are relevant for the clinical problem of inclusion body myositis need to be developed and validated.

## Exercise in Juvenile Dermatomyositis

The role of exercise in patients with juvenile dermatomyositis or polymyositis has been equally controversial as that for the adult patients. To date, a few studies have investigated validity and effects of maximal exercise tests or a single exercise session (Table 16.2). Although children often are physically active during play every day for long periods of time, no studies have been carried out to evaluate more long-term effects of physical activity or resistance exercise in these patients.

Children with an inactive to moderately inflammatory active disease had significantly poorer maximal oxygen uptake ($VO_{2peak}$), with 63% of values of healthy controls *(44)*. Lower $VO_{2peak}$ and shorter exercise test duration correlated well with measures of disease activity and muscle impairment. Another study included 13 children with dermatomyositis who performed maximal exercise tests, both during

**Table 16.2** Summary of studies evaluating exercise tests and single exercise session in patients with juvenile dermatomyositis

| Author | Patients/healthy subjects | Disease activity | Outcome measure | Results |
|---|---|---|---|---|
| Hicks et al. (*44*), 2002 | 14/14 | Low to moderate | $VO_{2peak}$ $W_{peak}$ (Stationary bike) | Patients with JDM had significantly reduced $VO_{2peak}$ and $W_{peak}$ compared to healthy controls |
| Takken et al. (*45*), 2008 | 13 | Active and in remission | $VO_{2peak}$ $W_{peak}$ (Stationary bike) | Patients with active disease had significantly reduced $VO_{2peak}$ and $W_{peak}$ compared to patients in remission; test well tolerated by all patients |
| Takken et al. (*46*), 2003 | 15 | Active Remission | $VO_{2peak}$ Relative $VO_{2peak}$ Exercise time (treadmill) | Patients with JDM had significantly reduced $VO_{2peak}$, relative $VO_{2peak}$, and exercise time compared to reference values from age-matched healthy Dutch population; test was feasible; exercise time can be used as indicator for $VO_{2peak}$ |
| Takken et al. (*47*), 2005 | 16 | Low | WAnT $VO_{2peak}$, $W_{peak}$ (Stationary bike) | Acceptable reliability for the WAnT test and very good reliability for the aerobic exercise test |
| Maillard et al. (*48*), 2005 | 20/20 | Low–active | PAG disease activity VAS MRI CPK, LDH, isometric strength (handheld dynamometer) | A single submaximal exercise session did not cause any changes in disease activity or muscle function |

*VO2peak* maximal oxygen uptake; *Wpeak* maximal work; *JDM* juvenile dermatomyositis; *WAnT* Wingate Anaerobic exercise Test; *PAG* physician's global assessment; *VAS* visual analog scale; *MRI* magnetic resonance imaging; *CPK* creatine phosphokinase; *LDH* lactate dehydrogenase

an active phase of disease and during remission. During active disease, $VO_{2peak}$ in milliliters as well as milliliters per kilogram per minute, peak power ($W_{peak}$), and $VO_{2peak}$ per heart rate was significantly lower than in remission phase (*45*). After 1 min of unloaded cycling, the workload was increased by 10, 15, or 20 W/min, depending on actual disease activity and height. Patients maintained a pedal cadence of 60–80 rpm until exhaustion. This protocol was well tolerated by patients in both remission and active disease (*45*).

Takken et al. (*46, 47*) also reported on feasibility and validity of another maximal aerobic exercise test on a treadmill as well as an anaerobic all-out cycle test. One study evaluated a submaximal single exercise session consisting of dynamic 20 repetitions against gravity in different muscle groups of the lower limbs in 10 children with active disease, 10 with inactive disease, and 20 healthy controls. Physician's Global Assessment of disease activity and analysis of muscle enzymes were performed before and after the exercise session. Muscle strength was assessed with a myometer, and muscle inflammation was assessed by MRI T2-weighted imaging before and at 30 and 60 min after completed exercise. There were no changes in parameters of disease activity or muscle impairment, leading to the conclusion that patients with inactive as well as active juvenile dermatomyositis safely can perform a single submaximal exercise session (*48*).

Children with juvenile dermatomyositis experience low aerobic capacity compared with healthy controls (*44*), low exercise capacity (*47*), as well as low muscle strength and walking ability (*49*), indicating the need for further research on efficacy and safety of various types of exercise to further reduce disability for these patients.

## Exercise Recommendations

The body of evidence to date on exercise effects suggests that physical exercise is beneficial to patients with adult polymyositis or dermatomyositis and should be included in the treatment regimen of these patients. Available data support that this could be recommended to the patients in the early phase of treatment as a combination therapy with pharmacological treatment. The role of exercise in inclusion body myositis and juvenile dermatomyositis is still uncertain. Available data suggest that adapted exercise does not impose a risk for increased disease activity in these patients. Also, for adult polymyositis or dermatomyositis, data are still too scarce to outline general recommendations regarding load and intensity. Furthermore, the terms *polymyositis* and *dermatomyositis* encompass heterogeneous groups of patients presenting with various clinical symptoms, disease activity, levels of disability, and grade of response to medical treatment. From clinical experience, it is likely that a good response to adequate medical treatment is a foundation for successful exercise treatment in patients with IIMs, both adults and children. Therefore, exercise should always be employed as adapted to disease activity, medical treatment response, and level of disability and should always be performed with guidance of a trained physical therapist in close collaboration with the patient's physician. To ensure that appropriate exercise intensity is used, follow-up measures of disease activity as well as disability should be employed in addition to baseline measures. From our experience, we recommend assessment every third month during the first year of disease and thereafter less often, depending on the response to treatment. In this way, it is possible to increase or decrease loads or intensity depending on how the patient is performing. In the chronic phase of disease, patients can perform exercise outside hospitals or physical therapy practices, such as in home exercise programs. In the case of a disease flare, however, it is important to adjust exercise regimens according to the increased disease activity and changed level of disability. It is also important to set goals for exercise treatment and, if possible, prescribe exercise regimens targeted to reach goals of choice.

As patients with inflammatory myopathies could be at higher risk of cardio-vascular disease, the recommendations for the general population of 30 min of physical activity most days of the week could also be employed in patients with myositis. It is also likely that common side effects of corticosteroid treatment, like osteoporosis and muscle atrophy, could be reduced using adapted exercise and physical activity from beginning of disease course in these patients.

## Conclusion

In summary, although the exercise studies are relatively few and include a limited number of patients, accumulating evidence suggests that physical exercise has beneficial effects on muscle impairment, activity limitation, and perceived health in adult patients with polymyositis or dermatomyositis without exacerbating disease progression. In addition, training seems to have beneficial effects on certain molecular processes in skeletal muscle. However, large controlled, randomized studies are needed to increase the body of evidence and to increase our knowledge of which exercise regimens are most efficient for patients with different myositis subsets. More studies are also needed to increase our knowledge of disease mechanisms, and the effects of exercise on muscle tissue, and to answer the question whether exercise could have a role as an anti-inflammatory intervention. For patients with inclusion body myositis, data are less conclusive, and for patients with juvenile dermatomyositis, there are no data on safety and efficacy of short-term and long-term exercise, but available data suggest that these patients tolerate physical exercise well. More investigations are needed concerning the efficacy and potential molecular effects of exercise in these patients.

## References

1. Alexanderson H, Dastmalchi M, Lundberg IE. Patients with chronic inflammatory myopathies have reduced muscle endurance rather than reduced muscle strength. Arthritis Rheum 2006;54(Suppl)1639:S658.
2. Josefson A, Romanus E, Carlsson J. A functional index in myositis. J Rheumatol 1996;23(8): 1380–4.

3. Wiesinger GF, Quittan M, Nuhr M, et al. Aerobic capacity in adult dermatomyositis/polymyositis patients and healthy controls. Arch Phys Med Rehabil 2000;81(1):1–5.
4. Nyberg P, Wikman AL, Nennesmo I, Lundberg I. Increased expression of interleukin 1alpha and MHC class I in muscle tissue of patients with chronic, inactive polymyositis and dermatomyositis. J Rheumatol 2000;27(4):940–8.
5. Englund P, Nennesmo I, Klareskog L, Lundberg IE. Interleukin-1alpha expression in capillaries and major histocompatibility complex class I expression in type II muscle fibers from polymyositis and dermatomyositis patients: important pathogenic features independent of inflammatory cell clusters in muscle tissue. Arthritis Rheum 2002;46(4):1044–55.
6. Park JH, Phothimat P, Oates CT, Hernanz-Schulman M, Olsen NJ. Use of P-31 magnetic resonance spectroscopy to detect metabolic abnormalities in muscles of patients with fibromyalgia. Arthritis Rheum 1998;41(3):406–13.
7. Dastmalchi M, Alexanderson H, Loell I, et al. Effect of physical training on the proportion of slow-twitch type I muscle fibers, a novel nonimmune-mediated mechanism for muscle impairment in polymyositis or dermatomyositis. Arthritis Rheum 2007;57(7):1303–10.
8. Nagaraju K, Raben N, Merritt G, Loeffler L, Kirk K, Plotz P. A variety of cytokines and immunologically relevant surface molecules are expressed by normal human skeletal muscle cells under proinflammatory stimuli. Clin Exp Immunol 1998;113(3):407–14.
9. Nagaraju K, Casciola-Rosen L, Lundberg I, et al. Activation of the endoplasmic reticulum stress response in autoimmune myositis: potential role in muscle fiber damage and dysfunction. Arthritis Rheum 2005;52(6):1824–35.
10. Askanas V, Engel WK. Inclusion-body myositis, a multifactorial muscle disease associated with aging: current concepts of pathogenesis. Curr Opin Rheumatol 2007;19(6):550–9.
11. Warhol MJ, Siegel AJ, Evans WJ, Silverman LM. Skeletal muscle injury and repair in marathon runners after competition. Am J Pathol 1985;118(2):331–9.
12. Brown JA, Elliott MJ, Sray WA. Exercise-induced upper extremity rhabdomyolysis and myoglobinuria in shipboard military personnel. Mil Med 1994;159(7):473–5.
13. Ruddy S, Harris ED, Sledge CB, Kelley WN. Kelley's textbook in rheumatology. 6th ed. Philadelphia: Saunders, 2001.
14. Hochberg M. Rheumatology. 3rd ed. Edinburgh: Mosby, 2003.
15. Koopman WJ, Moreland LW. Arthritis and allied conditions; a textbook of rheumatology. 15th ed. Philadelphia: Lippincott Williams & Wilkins, 2005.
16. Hochberg MC. Rheumatology. 4th ed. Philadelphia: Mosby/Elsevier, 2008.
17. Hicks JE, Miller F, Plotz P, Chen TH, Gerber L. Isometric exercise increases strength and does not produce sustained creatinine phosphokinase increases in a patient with polymyositis. J Rheumatol 1993;20(8):1399–401.
18. Escalante A, Miller L, Beardmore TD. Resistive exercise in the rehabilitation of polymyositis/dermatomyositis. J Rheumatol 1993;20(8):1340-4.
19. Wiesinger GF, Quittan M, Aringer M, et al. Improvement of physical fitness and muscle strength in polymyositis/dermatomyositis patients by a training programme. Br J Rheumatol 1998;37(2):196–200.
20. Wiesinger GF, Quittan M, Graninger M, et al. Benefit of 6 months long-term physical training in polymyositis/dermatomyositis patients. Br J Rheumatol 1998;37(12):1338–42.
21. Plotz PH, Dalakas M, Leff RL, Love LA, Miller FW, Cronin ME. Current concepts in the idiopathic inflammatory myopathies: polymyositis, dermatomyositis, and related disorders. Ann Intern Med 1989;111(2):143–57.
22. Alexanderson H, Stenstrom CH, Lundberg I. Safety of a home exercise programme in patients with polymyositis and dermatomyositis: a pilot study. Rheumatology (Oxford) 1999;38(7):608–11.
23. Sullivan M, Karlsson J, Ware JE Jr. The Swedish SF-36 Health Survey—I. Evaluation of data quality, scaling assumptions, reliability and construct validity across general populations in Sweden. Soc Sci Med 1995;41(10):1349–58.
24. Heikkila S, Viitanen JV, Kautiainen H, et al. Rehabilitation in myositis: preliminary study. Physiotherapy 2001;87(6):301–9.

25. Varju C, Petho E, Kutas R, Czirjak L. The effect of physical exercise following acute disease exacerbation in patients with dermato/polymyositis. Clin Rehabil 2003;17(1):83–7.
26. Alexanderson H, Dastmalchi M, Esbjornsson-Liljedahl M, Opava CH, Lundberg IE. Benefits of intensive resistance training in patients with chronic polymyositis or dermatomyositis. Arthritis Rheum 2007;57(5):768–77.
27. Miller FW, Rider LG, Chung YL, et al. Proposed preliminary core set measures for disease outcome assessment in adult and juvenile idiopathic inflammatory myopathies. Rheumatology (Oxford) 2001;40(11):1262–73.
28. Alexanderson H, Broman L, Tollback A, et al. Functional index-2: validity and reliability of a disease-specific measure of impairment in patients with polymyositis and dermatomyositis. Arthritis Rheum 2006;55(1):114–22.
29. Rider LG, Giannini EH, Brunner HI, et al. International consensus on preliminary definitions of improvement in adult and juvenile myositis. Arthritis Rheum 2004;50(7):2281–90.
30. Paulus HE, Egger MJ, Ward JR, Williams HJ. Analysis of improvement in individual rheumatoid arthritis patients treated with disease-modifying antirheumatic drugs, based on the findings in patients treated with placebo. The Cooperative Systematic Studies of Rheumatic Diseases Group. Arthritis Rheum 1990;33(4):477–84.
31. Alexanderson H, Lundberg IE, Stenstrom CH. Development of the myositis activities profile— validity and reliability of a self-administered questionnaire to assess activity limitations in patients with polymyositis/dermatomyositis. J Rheumatol 2002;29(11):2386–92.
32. Harris-Love MO. Safety and efficacy of submaximal eccentric strength training for a subject with polymyositis. Arthritis Rheum 2005;53(3):471–4.
33. Alexanderson H, Stenstrom CH, Jenner G, Lundberg I. The safety of a resistive home exercise program in patients with recent onset active polymyositis or dermatomyositis. Scand J Rheumatol 2000;29(5):295–301.
34. Cea G, Bendahan D, Manners D, et al. Reduced oxidative phosphorylation and proton efflux suggest reduced capillary blood supply in skeletal muscle of patients with dermatomyositis and polymyositis: a quantitative 31P-magnetic resonance spectroscopy and MRI study. Brain 2002;125(Pt 7):1635–45.
35. Chung YL, Alexanderson H, Pipitone N, et al. Creatine supplements in patients with idiopathic inflammatory myopathies who are clinically weak after conventional pharmacologic treatment: six-month, double-blind, randomized, placebo-controlled trial. Arthritis Rheum 2007;57(4):694–702.
36. Hurley MV, Scott DL, Rees J, Newham DJ. Sensorimotor changes and functional performance in patients with knee osteoarthritis. Ann Rheum Dis 1997;56(11):641–8.
37. Gielen S, Adams V, Mobius-Winkler S, et al. Anti-inflammatory effects of exercise training in the skeletal muscle of patients with chronic heart failure. J Am Coll Cardiol 2003;42(5):861–8.
38. Marcora SM, Lemmey AB, Maddison PJ. Can progressive resistance training reverse cachexia in patients with rheumatoid arthritis? Results of a pilot study. J Rheumatol 2005;32(6):1031–9.
39. Spector SA, Lemmer JT, Koffman BM, et al. Safety and efficacy of strength training in patients with sporadic inclusion body myositis. Muscle Nerve 1997;20(10):1242–8.
40. Krupp LB, LaRocca NG, Muir-Nash J, Steinberg AD. The fatigue severity scale. Application to patients with multiple sclerosis and systemic lupus erythematosus. Arch Neurol 1989;46(10):1121–3.
41. Mahoney FI, Barthel DW. Functional evaluation: the Barthel Index. Md State Med J 1965;14:61–5.
42. Arnardottir S, Alexanderson H, Lundberg IE, Borg K. Sporadic inclusion body myositis: pilot study on the effects of a home exercise program on muscle function, histopathology and inflammatory reaction. J Rehabil Med 2003;35(1):31–5.
43. Felice KJ, Relva GM, Conway SR. Further observations on forearm flexor weakness in inclusion body myositis. Muscle Nerve 1998;21(5):659–61.
44. Hicks JE, Drinkard B, Summers RM, Rider LG. Decreased aerobic capacity in children with juvenile dermatomyositis. Arthritis Rheum 2002;47(2):118–23.

45. Takken T, van der Net J, Engelbert RH, Pater S, Helders PJ. Responsiveness of exercise parameters in children with inflammatory myositis. Arthritis Rheum 2008;59(1):59–64.

46. Takken T, Spermon N, Helders PJ, Prakken AB, Van Der Net J. Aerobic exercise capacity in patients with juvenile dermatomyositis. J Rheumatol 2003;30(5):1075–80.

47. Takken T, van der Net J, Helders PJ. Anaerobic exercise capacity in patients with juvenile-onset idiopathic inflammatory myopathies. Arthritis Rheum 2005;53(2):173–7.

48. Maillard SM, Jones R, Owens CM, et al. Quantitative assessments of the effects of a single exercise session on muscles in juvenile dermatomyositis. Arthritis Rheum 2005;53(4):558–64.

49. Lohmann Siegel K, Hicks JE, Koziol DE, Gerber LH, Rider LG. Walking ability and its relationship to lower-extremity muscle strength in children with idiopathic inflammatory myopathies. Arch Phys Med Rehabil 2004;85(5):767–71.

50. Alexanderson H. Exercise: an important component of treatment in the idiopathic inflammatory myopathies. Curr Rheum Rep 2005;7:115–24.

# Chapter 17
# The Risk of Malignancy in Patients with Dermatomyositis and Polymyositis

Alan N. Baer and Robert L. Wortmann

**Abstract** Dermatomyositis is associated with an underlying malignancy in approximately 25% of patients. A weaker association is evident for polymyositis. The underlying malignancy is usually an adenocarcinoma of the ovary, lung, or gastrointestinal tract. Patients with dermatomyositis or polymyositis need to be evaluated uniformly for an underlying malignancy at the time of initial diagnosis and, in some cases, in the event of a subsequent recurrence. This apparent paraneoplastic syndrome may stem from an immune reaction to antigens expressed in cancer cells that crosses over to the same antigens expressed by regenerating fibers in damaged or diseased muscle.

**Keywords** Dermatomyositis • Polymyositis • Malignancy • Paraneoplastic syndrome

Dermatomyositis (DM) was first reported to be associated with an underlying malignancy in 1916 *(1,2)*. This association has only recently been confirmed with large population-based retrospective cohort studies *(3)*. Patients with DM have a significantly increased risk of a malignancy identified at the time of or within 1 year of diagnosis. The risk of an underlying malignancy is much lower for polymyositis (PM) but remained statistically significant in these population-based studies. A variety of malignancies have been associated with DM, but the most common are carcinomas of the ovary, lung, and gastrointestinal tract. In PM, the association is strongest for non-Hodgkin's lymphoma. Two aspects of this association remain a source of ongoing study and debate. The first relates to the type of evaluation that should be performed for underlying malignancy in a patient presenting with DM or PM. The second relates to the potential pathogenetic mechanism that might underlie this association. In this chapter, the evidence supporting this association,

A.N. Baer (✉) and R.L. Wortmann
Division of Rheumatology, Johns Hopkins University School of Medicine, Baltimore, MD, USA

L.J. Kagen (ed.), *The Inflammatory Myopathies*,
DOI 10.1007/978-1-60327-827-0_17,
© Humana Press, a part of Springer Science+Business Media, LLC 2009

the types of associated malignancies, and the factors predictive of underlying malignancy are reviewed. Mechanisms that might relate DM or PM with an underlying malignancy are also discussed.

# Epidemiology

In 1975, Barnes *(4)* summarized the 258 cases of malignancy-associated DM that had been reported in the medical literature since 1916. Published in the same year as Barnes's study, the Bohan and Peter criteria for the diagnosis of PM and DM ensured that subsequent reports of this association would differentiate the subtypes of inflammatory myopathies with greater rigor *(5)*. A total of 36 retrospective case series of inflammatory myopathy, as defined by the Bohan and Peter criteria, were published between 1975 and 2008 and reported the occurrence of malignancy in these patients (Table 17.1). These series included 1,495 patients with DM, of whom 405 (27%) had an associated malignancy, and 941 patients with PM, of whom 97 (10%) had an associated malignancy. Carcinomas of the breast (21%), lung (14%), nasopharynx (12%), colon (6%), ovary (6%), and stomach (6%) were the most common associated malignancies in the patients with DM *(6–27)*. There was no predominant tumor type among the reported cases associated with PM.

These case series did not provide scientific proof of the association between malignancy and either DM or PM *(28)*. They were subject to referral bias, almost all having been conducted using patients seen in tertiary hospitals or specialty clinics. In addition, a patient with an occult malignancy and associated PM or DM is more likely to be hospitalized than a patient with a similar occult malignancy without DM, PM, or another associated condition (Berkson's bias). The bias of increased suspicion and scrutiny for malignancy in DM/PM patients also exists. The case series lacked uniformity in defining a positive temporal association between the two diseases. On the other hand, they demonstrated that the association was much stronger for DM than for PM. They also highlighted the influence of ethnicity on the types of associated malignancy, the temporal association between the myositis and the malignancy, and the type of evaluation used to recognize the malignancy (discussed below).

Five population-based, retrospective cohort studies have been published since 1992 and have examined the association of malignancy with DM and PM (Table 17.2). The methodology and results of these studies were reviewed critically by Buchbinder and Hill *(3)*. Each of these studies identified a population-based cohort of PM and DM patients and compared their risk of malignancy with the normal population. This study design served to reduce biases related to referral and diagnostic suspicion of malignancy. In four of the studies, all patients with PM and DM hospitalized during a defined period were identified from national hospital discharge databases *(29–32)*. These studies were performed in Sweden, Denmark, Finland, and Scotland and were thus ethnically homogeneous. The fifth study identified all cases of biopsy-proven idiopathic inflammatory myopathies in

**Table 17.1** Frequency of malignancy in retrospective case series of adult men and women with dermatomyositis or polymyositis defined by the Bohan and Peter criteria (5)

| References | Malignancy in DM (%) | Malignancy in PM (%) | Source of patients |
|---|---|---|---|
| *(15)* | 1/12 (8) | 1/15 (7) | One medical center (United States) |
| *(75)* | 5/11 (45) | 2/11 (18) | One medical center (Canada); 73% fulfilled Bohan and Peter criteria |
| *(18)* | 15/40 (38) | 2/35 (6) | Cases referred to three EMG laboratories (Singapore) |
| *(7)* | 30/103 (29) | 7/206 (3) | One medical center (Hungary) |
| *(24)* | 10/28 (36) | 2/64 (3) | One medical center (Japan) |
| *(11)* | 7/27 (26) | 1/31 (3) | One medical center (United States) |
| *(21)* | 9/20 (45) | 4/15 (27) | One medical center (Israel) |
| *(9)* | 8/53 (15) | 5/57 (9) | One medical center (United States) |
| *(76)* | 10/39 (26) | 3/21 (14) | All general hospitals in Israel; overlap myositis excluded |
| *(38)* | 12/56 (21) | 12/84 (14) | One medical center (France) |
| *(35)* | 16/91 (18) | 2/14 (14) | One medical center (Taiwan) |
| *(48)* | 9/31 (29) | 8/40 (20) | One inpatient rheumatic disease unit (Canada) |
| *(49)* | 11/50 (22) | 18/65 (28) | One medical center (United States) |
| *(77)* | 7/36 (19) | 9/69 (13) | One medical center (Australia) |
| *(78)* | 3/19 (16) | 4/51 (8) | Multiple medical centers (Sweden) |
| *(27)* | 4/10 (40) | 0/18 | Muscle biopsy cases in one laboratory (Canada) |
| *(79)* | 7/39 (18) | 2/20 (10) | One medical center (France) |
| *(20)* | 5/16 (31) | 6/25 (24) | One medical center (Korea) |
| *(65)* | 13/33 (39) | 3/7 (43) | One medical center (France) |
| *(80)* | 3/24 (13) | 3/34 (9) | One inpatient rheumatic disease unit (United States) |
| *(81)* | 25/62 (40) | 3/59 (5) | One medical center (United States) |
| *(14)* | 12/50 (24) | | One medical center (Bulgaria) |
| *(16)* | 9/32 (28) | | One medical center (France) |
| *(10)* | 13/32 (41) | | One medical center (France) |
| *(13)* | 23/53 (43) | | Two medical centers (United Kingdom) |
| *(17)* | 6/10 (60) | | One medical center (Singapore) |
| *(19)* | 12/38 (32) | | One medical center (Singapore) |
| *(6)* | 34/118 (28) | | All dermatological university medical centers in France |
| *(8)* | 12/28 (43) | | One medical center (Singapore) |
| *(57)* | 9/18 (50) | | One medical center (Norway) |
| *(22)* | 20/130 (15) | | All university hospitals of Tunisia |
| *(12)* | 5/12 (41) | | One medical center (Singapore) |
| *(25)* | 9/18 (50) | | One medical center (Denmark) |
| *(54)* | 16/84 (19) | | One medical center (Hungary) |
| *(23)* | 10/29 (35) | | One medical center (France) |
| *(26)* | 5/43 (12) | | One medical center (United States) |

**Table 17.2** Population-based cohort studies of the association of malignancy with dermatomyositis and polymyositis

| References | Frequency of malignancy in DM (%) | Dermatomyositis SIR[a] | Frequency of malignancy in PM (%) | Polymyositis SIR[a] |
|---|---|---|---|---|
| *(33)* | 36/85 (42) | 6.2 (3.9–10) | 58/321 (18) | 2.0 (1.4–2.7) |
| *(30)* | 19/71 (27) | 6.5 (3.9–10) | 12/175 (7) | 1.0 (0.5–1.8) |
| *(31)* | 77/286 (27) | 7.7 (5.7–10.1) | 71/419 (17) | 2.1 (1.5–2.9) |
| *(29)* | 31/203 (15) | 3.8 (2.6–5.4) | 26/336 (8) | 1.7 (1.1–2.4) |
| *(32)* | 59/392 (15) | 2.4 (1.6–3.6), male 3.4 (2.4–4.7), female | 37/396 (9) | 1.8 (1.1–2.7), male 1.7 (1.0–2.5), female |

[a]*SIR* standardized incidence ratio; numbers in parentheses are the 95% confidence intervals

the state of Victoria, Australia, during a defined period, utilizing the records of the state reference neuropathology laboratory in which all muscle biopsies are reviewed *(33)*. The occurrence of malignancy (excluding nonmelanoma skin cancers) in these patients was determined from national cancer registries and, in one study, from death records for the same period. Malignancies that were identified at the same time or after the diagnosis of myositis were included in the calculation of risk. In some studies, malignancies that were identified during the first 3–12 months after the myositis diagnosis were excluded in separate analyses to eliminate diagnostic suspicion bias *(31–33)*.

Each of these five studies identified an increased risk of malignancy in patients with DM compared with the general population *(see* Table 17.2). The overall standardized incidence ratios ranged from 3.8 to 7.7. In addition, two of the studies identified an increased but lesser risk in patients with PM, with overall standardized incidence ratios of 1.7-2.0 *(29, 31, 33)*. These risks were determined for malignancies that were identified at the same time or after the myositis diagnosis. The cancer risk was increased approximately sixfold during the first year but was lower during the second year, with no significant excesses in subsequent years of follow-up *(29)*. The increased risk of malignancy in DM remained evident when malignancies identified during the first 3 months or the first year following the diagnosis of myositis were excluded to eliminate diagnosis suspicion bias *(31,33)*. Inclusion body myositis, myositis associated with connective tissue disease, and childhood myositis were also each associated with an apparently increased risk of malignancy, although the small number of patients in these subsets made these statistical associations less certain *(33)*.

These population-based cohort studies had limitations. Four of the studies relied on the accuracy of discharge coding to identify patients with myositis. Airio et al. *(30)* attempted to review the medical records of all identified patients and subsequently excluded 226 of 627 patients. Sigurgeirsson et al. *(32)* reviewed every tenth record and found that 7% probably had neither DM nor PM. There was no medical record review in the other three studies. With the exception of the study of Buchbinder et al. *(33)*, the diagnoses of PM and DM were based on the 1975 criteria of Bohan and Peter *(5)* and thus did not always require histologic confirmation. This may have led to misclassification of myositis types and inclusion of cases of inclusion body myositis among the PM subtype.

# Types of Malignancies Associated with DM and PM

A broad range of malignancies is associated with DM. Hill et al. *(34)* performed a pooled analysis of the three population-based cohort studies performed in Sweden, Denmark, and Finland and included more recent follow-up data from Denmark and Finland. This study provided the most comprehensive analysis of the cancer types associated with DM and PM. Among a total of 618 cases of DM, 115 developed cancer after the diagnosis of myositis. The overall standardized incidence ratio (SIR) was 3.0 (95% confidence interval [CI] 2.5–3.6). The types of cancer with the greatest increased relative risk were ovary (SIR 10.5, 95% CI 6.1–18.1), lung (5.9, 3.7–9.2), pancreatic (3.8, 1.6–9.0), stomach (3.5, 1.7–7.3), colorectal (2.5, 1.4–4.4.), and non-Hodgkin's lymphoma (3.6, 1.2–11.1). Among 914 cases of PM, 95 developed cancer after the diagnosis of myositis. The relative risks were raised for non-Hodgkin's lymphoma (3.7, 1.7–8.2), lung cancer (2.8, 1.8–4.4), and bladder cancer (2.4, 1.3–4.7). The most common cancer type was adenocarcinoma, accounting for 70% of all associated tumors in both DM and PM patients.

The study of Hill et al. *(34)* was based on data from three Nordic countries with little ethnic diversity and is thus applicable only to Scandinavian populations. Among Asian populations, nasopharyngeal carcinoma and hepatocellular carcinoma have each been strongly associated with DM in a number of case series *(8, 12, 19, 35, 36)*. In their series of 143 patients with DM/PM in Taiwan, Chen et al. *(35)* observed that 18 patients (13%) had an identified malignancy, the most common being nasopharyngeal carcinoma (4 cases, 22.2% compared with 2.8% expected in normal population). Similarly, gastric carcinoma may be the most common associated cancer in Japanese populations *(37)*.

The histologic type and stage of certain cancers that are associated with DM have been characterized. These studies relied on case reports and case series since the population-based cohort studies do not provide such detailed clinical information. Ovarian cancer was almost always epithelial in origin (adenocarcinoma or cystadenocarcinoma) and in stage III or IV when recognized in the context of DM. The ovarian cancer was most often diagnosed during the first year following the diagnosis of DM *(38–40)*. In a review of the literature, Fujita et al. *(41)* identified 24 patients (5 women and 19 men) with primary lung cancer associated with DM or PM. The most common cell types were small-cell carcinoma (29%), squamous cell carcinoma (21%), and adenocarcinoma (8%). In five of these patients, the onset of myositis preceded the diagnosis of cancer by more than a year.

## Clinical Course of Malignancy and Myositis

A parallel course between the DM and the underlying malignancy has been highlighted in isolated case reports of patients in whom the DM improved after successful treatment of the tumor or worsened with evidence of tumor recurrence *(42–45)*. This parallel course has been described in only a minority of case reports *(4,6, 46)*. It was observed in only 8 of 45 patients with cancer-associated DM reported by Bonnetblanc et al. *(6)*. In contrast, Andras et al. *(7)* reported remission of the myositis in 16 of 22 patients with cancer-associated DM who received effective antitumor therapy. The failure to demonstrate this parallel course may reflect the advanced stage of the malignancy when it is ultimately diagnosed *(47)*. While this parallel clinical course suggests a paraneoplastic syndrome, it does not explain the excess risk of malignancy that remains as long as 5 years after the diagnosis of myositis *(33)*.

## Risk Factors for Malignancy in DM and PM

A variety of factors influences the risk of an associated malignancy in DM/PM. The risk of malignancy is higher in older patients presenting with DM or PM *(82)*. In the Finnish and Danish population-based cohort studies of Chow et al. and Airio et al. *(29, 30)*, an increased risk of malignancy was only evident in patients over the age of 45–50 years at the time of myositis diagnosis. An increased risk was evident for DM patients aged 45–74 and PM patients aged 15–44 in the study of Stockton et al. *(31)*. This increased risk of malignancy in older DM patients was also evident in the pooled analysis of Hill et al. *(34)*. This observation has been confirmed in two case-control studies *(35, 48)* but not in two others *(49, 50)*.

Gender is not a consistent risk factor for malignancy in DM patients. Standardized incidence ratios were higher for men in the studies of Airio et al. and Stockton et al. but not in that of Sigurgeirsson et al. *(30–32)*. An increased risk of malignancy in PM patients was evident for women but not for men in the study of Stockton et al. *(31)*.

Several features of the rash of DM have been associated with underlying malignancy, including the presence of leukocytoclastic vasculitis *(51)*, cutaneous necrosis *(10, 52, 53)*, and ulceration *(7, 16)*. The rash has been cited as more refractory to treatment *(19, 54)*. *Malignant erythema* refers to a fiery red suffusion on the face, scalp, neck, and shoulders that blanches with pressure and may overlie areas of chronic erythema *(55)*. It has been reported to be more common in DM patients with an underlying malignancy. Erythroderma may be a presenting feature of DM but is not necessarily an indication of an underlying malignancy *(56)*.

More severe myositis has been reported in the setting of an underlying malignancy, with a higher frequency of distal muscle weakness *(7, 54)*, dysphagia *(7, 57)*, respiratory muscle involvement *(7)*, and resistance to immunosuppressive treatment *(7)*. These findings have not been confirmed by other authors *(49)*. In addition, amyopathic DM has also been observed in this setting *(8, 58, 59)*.

The presence of clinical or laboratory features that overlap with other connective tissue diseases diminishes the risk of an underlying malignancy. These include the presence of interstitial lung disease *(7, 35, 54)*, arthritis *(7)*, Raynaud's pheno-menon *(7)*, fever *(7)*, and a high titer of antinuclear antibodies *(7, 54)*. Myositis-specific anti-bodies, such as those directed against Jo-1 (histidyl t-RNA synthetase), are markers of specific subsets of the idiopathic inflammatory myopathies but can also be seen in up to 13% of cases of cancer-associated myositis (Table 17.3). Their presence thus does

**Table 17.3** Myositis-specific antibodies (MSAs) in cancer-associated myositis (CAM) and idiopathic myositis (IM)

| References | Number of patients | MSAs in CAM | MSAs in IM |
|---|---|---|---|
| *(62)* | 282 | 3/16 | 92/266 |
| *(83)* | 97 | 1/3 | 38/94 |
| *(84)* | 86 | 2/8 | 26/78 |
| *(85)* | 556 | 4/51 | 195/505 |
| Total | 842 | 10/78 (13%) | 351/943 (37%) |

not preclude the diagnosis of cancer-related myositis *(60)*. Kaji et al. *(61)*identified a novel autoantibody reactive with 155- and 140-kDa nuclear proteins in patients with DM. This autoantibody was present in 71% of DM patients with an underlying malignancy and in only 11% of those without one. In a study of Chinoy et al. *(62)*, this 155/140 autoantibody had 50% sensitivity and 96% specificity for cancer-associated myositis. When combined with negative results of hospital-based routine testing for Jo-1, Ku (p70/p80 antigen), PM-Scl PM/Scl (polymyositis/scleroderma complex), U1-RNP (U1-ribonucleoprotein), and U3-RNP antibodies, a positive 155/140 antibody result had 94% sensitivity and 99% negative predictive value.

Certain laboratory markers in patients with DM or PM may also serve as predictors of an underlying malignancy. The erythrocyte sedimentation rate and C-reactive protein are typically higher in the setting of an underlying malignancy *(10, 25, 63)*. The maximal level of creatine kinase has been reported to be lower in DM/PM patients with an underlying malignancy when compared to those with DM/PM without an underlying malignancy *(7, 20, 54, 64)*. This is not a uniform observation *(49, 65)*. Not surprisingly, tumor marker elevation is associated with an increased risk of developing an underlying malignancy *(7,66–68)*. However, the sensitivity of CA-125 elevation for detecting ovarian cancer in DM patients was only 50% in the study of Whitmore et al. *(68)*.

## Evaluation for Malignancy

The extent to which a new patient with DM or PM should be evaluated for an underlying malignancy is controversial. Good clinical practice mandates that all patients presenting with an inflammatory myopathy, regardless of age of patient or type of myositis, undergo a careful history and physical examination as well as routine laboratory tests to screen for a possible underlying malignancy *(11, 13, 69)*. This evaluation should include a testicular examination in men, breast and pelvic examinations in women, and rectal examinations in all patients *(70)*. Additional periodic screening tests for malignancy, such as colonoscopy and mammography, should be up-to-date as recommended for particular demographic groups. Any abnormalities detected on this initial screening evaluation should be pursued carefully. Since the risk of an underlying malignancy is much higher in patients with DM, a more extensive evaluation for malignancy is advisable in specific subsets of these patients. Women with a new diagnosis of DM should undergo thorough gynecologic examinations to screen for an ovarian carcinoma. This evaluation should include pelvic and transvaginal ultrasonography and measurement of CA-125, and if necessary, pelvic computed tomography (CT) *(38, 40, 47)*. A repeat evaluation at 3 and 6 months has also been recommended in women presenting with DM whose initial evaluation for ovarian cancer is negative *(38)*. This recommendation is predicated on the fact that ovarian malignancies have a strong association with DM and may not be detected with a routine pelvic examination. The type of malignancy evaluation performed in DM should be modified for specific ethnic groups in which specific types of cancers are overrepresented. DM patients of Chinese descent need to be evaluated for carcinomas of the nasopharynx and liver *(8, 12, 19, 35, 36)*. Similarly, gastric carcinoma needs to be sought carefully in patients of Japanese descent *(37)*.

The vigor with which the search for an underlying malignancy is pursued in patients with DM has been contested, particularly as the diagnostic tools, such as positron emission tomography, have become more sensitive, yet also unacceptably expensive when used indiscriminately *(71)*. Although most malignancies can be identified with the screening evaluation detailed, some are missed and do not become clinically apparent until later in the patient's clinical course *(72)*. The malignancies that are most likely to be missed with screening examinations include those of the ovarian, pancreatic, lung, and lymphoma. Accordingly, CT imaging of the chest, abdomen, and pelvis is prudent in the subset of new-onset DM patients who are older or who have risk factors for specific types of malignancy (family history of ovarian cancer, smokers). The use of diagnostic tools for malignancy that go beyond the screening measures described should be considered in patients with DM with a more severe rash that is associated with cutaneous necrosis *(10, 52, 53)* or severe muscle disease that is refractory to steroid therapy *(7, 33, 54)*. In addition, a recurrence of the rash or muscle weakness after initial successful treatment should prompt a second look for malignancy. This type of evaluation may not be necessary in patients whose myositis is clearly associated with another connective tissue disease, such as lupus or scleroderma.

## Pathogenesis

The association between DM/PM and a malignancy has several potential explanations. These include biases inherent in the methodologies used to report the association as well as biological factors that may underlie a true association. The potential methodologic biases have been reviewed by Masi and Hochberg *(28)* and were highlighted in the preceding discussion. These biases have been addressed partially with case-control series *(48, 49)* and large population-based cohort studies *(29–32)*. At a biologic level, the association may reflect the presence of common host predispositions, infectious triggers, toxic exposures, or the presence of a paraneoplastic syndrome. Genetic traits underlying the association have been sought unsuccessfully *(7, 17)*. Influences of age and sex as common host predispositions have been addressed in epidemiologic studies. Finally, the immunosuppressive and occasionally cytotoxic therapies used to treat myositis may predispose to the development of a malignancy. However, this possibility has not been substantiated in several of the population-based cohort studies.

The confluence of DM and cancer, with both diagnoses often established within 1 year of each other, may indicate the presence of a paraneoplastic syndrome. The leading hypothesis to explain this relationship is an immune reaction to the tumor that cross-reacts with antigens in skin and muscle, leading to DM. Such an immune reaction occurs in the autoimmune paraneoplastic neurologic disorders, in which immune-mediated neuronal damage develops in the setting of solid tumors of the breast, ovary, and lung *(73)*. Casciola-Rosen et al. observed that the myositis autoantigens, Mi-2 (a component of the nuclesome remodeling-deacetylase complex) and Jo-1, are expressed at high levels in myositis muscle, particularly in regenerating muscle fibers, as well as in adenocarcinomas of the lung and breast, but not in the corresponding normal tissues *(74)*. These observations thus identify regenerating muscle cells and certain tumors as the source of ongoing myositis autoantigen expression in myositis. These authors have proposed a model of "crossover" immunity in which an initial cellular immune response is directed at tumor cells overexpressing antigens commonly targeted in myositis. In the setting of muscle injury and regeneration, myositis-specific autoantigens are expressed. An immune reaction initially directed at these autoantigens expressed in tumor cells crosses over and leads to the development of myositis.

## Conclusion

Dermatomyositis has been associated with an underlying malignancy for close to 100 years. Modern epidemiologic studies have provided strong support for this association and evidence that it may also be true for PM. It has not yet been established that this relationship is paraneoplastic in origin, although individual case reports have provided compelling examples of such a relationship. The majority of underlying malignancies are adenocarcinomas, particularly of the ovary, lung, pancreas, stomach, and colon. A search for an underlying malignancy is important in patients presenting with DM or PM, although the scope and vigor of this evaluation needs to be tailored to the individual patient, taking into account the presence of factors that may increase or diminish the likelihood of an associated malignancy.

## References

1. Stertz G. Polymyositis. Berl Klin Wochenschr 1916;53:489.
2. Kankeleit H. Uber primare nichteirige Polymyositis. Dtsch Arch Klin Med 1916;120:335–349.
3. Buchbinder R, Hill CL. Malignancy in patients with inflammatory myopathy. Curr Rheumatol Rep 2002;4:415–26.
4. Barnes BE, Mawr B. Dermatomyositis and malignancy. A review of the literature. Ann Intern Med 1976;84:68–76.
5. Bohan A, Peter JB. Polymyositis and dermatomyositis (first of two parts). N Engl J Med 1975;292:344–7.
6. Bonnetblanc JM, Bernard P, Fayol J. Dermatomyositis and malignancy. A multicenter cooperative study. Dermatologica 1990;180:212–6.
7. Andras C, Ponyi A, Constantin T, et al. Dermatomyositis and polymyositis associated with malignancy: a 21-year retrospective study. J Rheumatol 2008;35:438–44.
8. Ang P, Sugeng MW, Chua SH. Classical and amyopathic dermatomyositis seen at the National Skin Centre of Singapore: a 3-year retrospective review of their clinical characteristics and association with malignancy. Ann Acad Med Singapore 2000;29:219–23.
9. Bohan A, Peter JB, Bowman RL, Pearson CM. Computer-assisted analysis of 153 patients with polymyositis and dermatomyositis. Medicine (Baltimore) 1977;56:255–86.
10. Basset-Seguin N, Roujeau JC, Gherardi R, Guillaume JC, Revuz J, Touraine R. Prognostic factors and predictive signs of malignancy in adult dermatomyositis. A study of 32 cases. Arch Dermatol 1990;126:633–7.

11. Callen JP, Hyla, JF, Bole GG, Jr, Kay DR. The relationship of dermatomyositis and polymyositis to internal malignancy. Arch Dermatol 1980;116:295–8.

12. Chan HL. Dermatomyositis and cancer in Singapore. Int J Dermatol 1985;24:447–50.

13. Cox NH, Lawrence CM, Langtry JA, Ive FA. Dermatomyositis. Disease associations and an evaluation of screening investigations for malignancy. Arch Dermatol 1990;126:61–5.

14. Dourmishev LA. Dermatomyositis associated with malignancy. 12 case reports. Adv Exp Med Biol 1999;455:193–9.

15. Hoffman GS, Franck WA, Raddatz DA, Stallones L. Presentation, treatment, and prognosis of idiopathic inflammatory muscle disease in a rural hospital. Am J Med 1983;75:433–8.

16. Gallais V, Crickx B, Belaich S. Prognostic factors and predictive signs of malignancy in adult dermatomyositis. Ann Dermatol Venereol 1996;123:722–6.

17. Goh CL, Rajan VS. Dermatomyositis in a skin clinic. Ann Acad Med Singapore 1983;12:6–12.

18. Koh ET, Seow A, Ong B, Ratnagopal P, Tjia H, Chng HH. Adult onset polymyositis/dermatomyositis: clinical and laboratory features and treatment response in 75 patients. Ann Rheum Dis 1993;52:857–61.

19. Leow YH, Goh CL. Malignancy in adult dermatomyositis. Int J Dermatol 1997;36:904–7.

20. Lee SW, Jung SY, Park MC, Park YB, Lee SK. Malignancies in Korean patients with inflammatory myopathy. Yonsei Med J 2006;47:519–23.

21. Maoz CR, Langevitz P, Livneh A, et al. High incidence of malignancies in patients with dermatomyositis and polymyositis: an 11-year analysis. Semin Arthritis Rheum 1998;27:319–24.

22. Mebazaa A, Boussen H, Nouira R, et al. Dermatomyositis and malignancy in Tunisia: a multicenter national retrospective study of 20 cases. J Am Acad Dermatol 2003;48:530–4.

23. Rose C, Hatron PY, Brouillard M, et al. Predictive signs of cancers in dermatomyositis. Study of 29 cases. Rev Med Interne 1994;15:19–24.

24. Wakata N, Kurihara T, Saito E, Kinoshita M. Polymyositis and dermatomyositis associated with malignancy: a 30-year retrospective study. Int J Dermatol 2002;41:729–34.

25. Vesterager L, Worm AM, Thomsen K. Dermatomyositis and malignancy. Clin Exp Dermatol 1980;5:31–5.

26. Dawkins MA, Jorizzo JL, Walker FO, Albertson D, Sinal SH, Hinds A. Dermatomyositis: a dermatology-based case series. J Am Acad Dermatol 1998;38:397–404.

27. Holden DJ, Brownell AK, Fritzler MJ. Clinical and serologic features of patients with polymyositis or dermatomyositis. Can Med Assoc J 1985;132:649–53.

28. Masi AT, Hochberg MC. Temporal association of polymyositis-dermatomyositis with malignancy: methodologic and clinical considerations. Mt Sinai J Med 1988;55:471–8.

29. Chow WH, Gridley G, Mellemkjaer L, McLaughlin JK, Olsen JH, Fraumeni JF Jr. Cancer risk following polymyositis and dermatomyositis: a nationwide cohort study in Denmark. Cancer Causes Control 1995;6:9–13.

30. Airio A, Pukkala E, Isomaki H. Elevated cancer incidence in patients with dermatomyositis: a population based study. J Rheumatol 1995;22:1300–3.

31. Stockton D, Doherty VR, Brewster DH. Risk of cancer in patients with dermatomyositis or polymyositis, and follow-up implications: a Scottish population-based cohort study. Br J Cancer 2001;85:41–5.

32. Sigurgeirsson B, Lindelof B, Edhag O, Allander E. Risk of cancer in patients with dermatomyositis or polymyositis. A population-based study. N Engl J Med 1992;326:363–7.

33. Buchbinder R, Forbes A, Hall S, Dennett X, Giles G. Incidence of malignant disease in biopsy-proven inflammatory myopathy. A population-based cohort study. Ann Intern Med 2001;134:1087–95.

34. Hill CL, Zhang Y, Sigurgeirsson B, et al. Frequency of specific cancer types in dermatomyositis and polymyositis: a population-based study. Lancet 2001;357:96–100.

35. Chen YJ, Wu CY, Shen JL. Predicting factors of malignancy in dermatomyositis and polymyositis: a case-control study. Br J Dermatol 2001;144:825–31.

36. Peng JC, Sheen TS, Hsu MM. Nasopharyngeal carcinoma with dermatomyositis. Analysis of 12 cases. Arch Otolaryngol Head Neck Surg 1995;121:1298–301.

37. Hatada T, Aoki I, Ikeda H, et al. Dermatomyositis and malignancy: case report and review of the Japanese literature. Tumori 1996;82:273–5.

38. Cherin P, Piette JC, Herson S, et al. Dermatomyositis and ovarian cancer: a report of 7 cases and literature review. J Rheumatol 1993;20:1897–9.
39. Davis MD, Ahmed I. Ovarian malignancy in patients with dermatomyositis and polymyositis: a retrospective analysis of fourteen cases. J Am Acad Dermatol 1997;37:730–3.
40. Mordel N, Margalioth EJ, Harats N, Ben-Baruch N, Schenker JG. Concurrence of ovarian cancer and dermatomyositis. A report of two cases and literature review. J Reprod Med 1988; 33:649–55.
41. Fujita J, Tokuda M, Bandoh S, et al. Primary lung cancer associated with polymyositis/dermatomyositis, with a review of the literature. Rheumatol Int 2001;20:81–4.
42. Masuda H, Urushibara M, Kihara K. Successful treatment of dermatomyositis associated with adenocarcinoma of the prostate after radical prostatectomy. J Urol 2003;169:1084.
43. Tallai B, Flasko T, Gyorgy T, et al. Prostate cancer underlying acute, definitive dermatomyositis: successful treatment with radical perineal prostatectomy. Clin Rheumatol 2006;25:119–20.
44. Yoshinaga A, Hayashi T, Ishii N, Ohno R, Watanabe T, Yamada T. Successful cure of dermatomyositis after treatment of nonseminomatous testicular cancer. Int J Urol 2005;12:593–5.
45. Solomon SD, Maurer KH. Association of dermatomyositis and dysgerminoma in a 16-year-old patient. Arthritis Rheum 1983;26:572–3.
46. Callen JP. Dermatomyositis and female malignancy. J Surg Oncol 1986;32:121–4.
47. Whitmore SE, Rosenshein NB, Provost TT. Ovarian cancer in patients with dermatomyositis. Medicine (Baltimore) 1994;73:153–60.
48. Manchul LA, Jin A, Pritchard KI, et al. The frequency of malignant neoplasms in patients with polymyositis-dermatomyositis. A controlled study. Arch Intern Med 1985;145:1835–9.
49. Lakhanpal S, Bunch TW, Ilstrup DM, Melton LJ, III. Polymyositis-dermatomyositis and malignant lesions: does an association exist? Mayo Clin Proc 1986;61:645–53.
50. Pautas E, Cherin P, Piette JC, et al. Features of polymyositis and dermatomyositis in the elderly: a case-control study. Clin Exp Rheumatol 2000;18:241–4.
51. Hunger RE, Durr C, Brand CU. Cutaneous leukocytoclastic vasculitis in dermatomyositis suggests malignancy. Dermatology 2001;202:123–6.
52. Mahe E, Descamps V, Burnouf M, Crickx B. A helpful clinical sign predictive of cancer in adult dermatomyositis: cutaneous necrosis. Arch Dermatol 2003;139:539.
53. Mautner GH, Grossman ME, Silvers DN, Rabinowitz A, Mowad CM, Johnson BL, Jr. Epidermal necrosis as a predictive sign of malignancy in adult dermatomyositis. Cutis 1998;61:190–4.
54. Ponyi A, Constantin T, Garami M, et al. Cancer-associated myositis: clinical features and prognostic signs. Ann N Y Acad Sci 2005;1051:64–71.
55. Winkelmann RK. The cutaneous diagnosis of dermatomyositis, lupus erythematosus, and scleroderma. N Y State J Med 1963;63:3080–3086.
56. Nousari HC, Kimyai-Asadi A, Spegman DJ. Paraneoplastic dermatomyositis presenting as erythroderma. J Am Acad Dermatol 1998;39:653–4.
57. Selvaag E, Thune P, Austad J. Dermatomyositis and cancer. A retrospective study. Tidsskr Nor Laegeforen 1994;114:2378–80.
58. Whitmore SE, Watson R, Rosenshein NB, Provost TT. Dermatomyositis sine myositis: association with malignancy. J Rheumatol 1996;23:101–5.
59. Fung WK, Chan HL, Lam WM. Amyopathic dermatomyositis in Hong Kong—association with nasopharyngeal carcinoma. Int J Dermatol 1998;37:659–63.
60. Legault D, McDermott J, Crous-Tsanaclis AM, Boire G. Cancer-associated myositis in the presence of anti-Jo1 autoantibodies and the antisynthetase syndrome. J Rheumatol 2008; 35:169–71.
61. Kaji K, Fujimoto M, Hasegawa M, et al. Identification of a novel autoantibody reactive with 155 and 140 kDa nuclear proteins in patients with dermatomyositis: an association with malignancy. Rheumatology (Oxford) 2007;46:25–8.
62. Chinoy H, Fertig N, Oddis CV, Ollier WE, Cooper RG. The diagnostic utility of myositis autoantibody testing for predicting the risk of cancer-associated myositis. Ann Rheum Dis 2007;66:1345–9.
63. Amerio P, Girardelli CR, Proietto G, et al. Usefulness of erythrocyte sedimentation rate as tumor marker in cancer associated dermatomyositis. Eur J Dermatol 2002;12:165–9.

64. Fudman EJ, Schnitzer TJ. Dermatomyositis without creatine kinase elevation. A poor prognostic sign. Am J Med 1986;80:329–32.
65. Sparsa A, Liozon E, Herrmann F, et al. Routine vs extensive malignancy search for adult dermatomyositis and polymyositis: a study of 40 patients. Arch Dermatol 2002;138:885–90.
66. Amoura Z, Duhaut P, Huong DL, et al. Tumor antigen markers for the detection of solid cancers in inflammatory myopathies. Cancer Epidemiol Biomarkers Prev 2005;14:1279–82.
67. O'Gradaigh D, Merry P. Tumour markers in dermatomyositis: useful or useless? Br J Rheumatol 1998;37:914.
68. Whitmore SE, Anhalt GJ, Provost TT, et al. Serum CA-125 screening for ovarian cancer in patients with dermatomyositis. Gynecol Oncol 1997;65:241–4.
69. Callen JP. The value of malignancy evaluation in patients with dermatomyositis. J Am Acad Dermatol 1982;6:253–9.
70. Pautas E, Cherin P. Investigation of polymyositis-dermatomyositis in older people should include rectal examination. J Am Geriatr Soc 1998;46:1584.
71. Callen JP. When and how should the patient with dermatomyositis or amyopathic dermatomyositis be assessed for possible cancer? Arch Dermatol 2002;138:969–71.
72. Schulman P, Kerr LD, Spiera H. A reexamination of the relationship between myositis and malignancy. J Rheumatol 1991;18:1689–92.
73. Levine SM. Cancer and myositis: new insights into an old association. Curr Opin Rheumatol 2006;18:620–4.
74. Casciola-Rosen L, Nagaraju K, Plotz P, et al. Enhanced autoantigen expression in regenerating muscle cells in idiopathic inflammatory myopathy. J Exp Med 2005;201:591–601.
75. Baron M, Small P. Polymyositis/dermatomyositis: clinical features and outcome in 22 patients. J Rheumatol 1985;12:283–6.
76. Benbassat J, Gefel D, Larholt K, Sukenik S, Morgenstern V, Zlotnick A. Prognostic factors in polymyositis/dermatomyositis. A computer-assisted analysis of ninety-two cases. Arthritis Rheum 1985;28:249–55.
77. Tymms KE, Webb J. Dermatopolymyositis and other connective tissue diseases: a review of 105 cases. J Rheumatol 1985;12:1140–8.
78. Henriksson KG, Sandstedt P. Polymyositis—treatment and prognosis. A study of 107 patients. Acta Neurol Scand 1982;65:280–300.
79. Ponge A, Mussini JM, Ponge T, Maugars Y, Cottin S. Paraneoplastic dermatopolymyositis. Rev Med Interne 1987;8:251–6.
80. Hochberg MC, Feldman D, Stevens MB. Adult onset polymyositis/dermatomyositis: an analysis of clinical and laboratory features and survival in 76 patients with a review of the literature. Semin Arthritis Rheum 1986;15:168–78.
81. Antiochos BB, Brown LA, Wortmann RL, Rigby WF. Malignancy is associated with dermatomyositis, but not polymyositis in northern New England. Arthritis Rheum 2008;58:S230–1.
82. Marie I, Hatron PY, Levesque H, et al. Influence of age on characteristics of polymyositis and dermatomyositis in adults. Medicine (Baltimore) 1999;78:139–47.
83. Hengstman GJ, Brouwer R, Egberts WT, et al. Clinical and serological characteristics of 125 Dutch myositis patients. Myositis specific autoantibodies aid in the differential diagnosis of the idiopathic inflammatory myopathies. J Neurol 2002;249:69–75.
84. Selva-O'Callaghan A, Labrador-Horrillo M, Solans-Laque R, Simeon-Aznar CP, Martinez-Gomez X, Vilardell-Tarres M. Myositis-specific and myositis-associated antibodies in a series of eighty-eight Mediterranean patients with idiopathic inflammatory myopathy. Arthritis Rheum 2006;55:791–8.
85. O'Hanlon TP, Carrick DM, Targoff IN, et al. Immunogenetic risk and protective factors for the idiopathic inflammatory myopathies: distinct HLA-A, -B, -Cw, -DRB1, and -DQA1 allelic profiles distinguish European American patients with different myositis autoantibodies. Medicine (Baltimore) 2006;85:111–27.

# Chapter 18
# Treatment

Stephen J. DiMartino

**Abstract** Idiopathic inflammatory myopathy (IIM) comprises a group of rare autoimmune diseases in which the immune system targets skeletal muscle; the consequence is damage to the muscles and weakness in the patient. As in other autoimmune conditions, the general approach to therapy is to use immunosuppressive agents. While many options exist for the treatment of IIM, therapeutic approaches are largely based on empirical evidence and small studies, many of which were uncontrolled. New medications have been designed that target specific components of the immune response; these agents offer hope for more effective and safer therapy of IIM.

## Introduction

Idiopathic inflammatory myopathy (IIM) is comprised of the following diseases: polymyositis (PM), dermatomyositis (DM), inclusion body myositis (IBM), juvenile DM, myositis associated with malignancy, and myositis associated with systemic inflammatory disease (overlap syndromes). For academic reasons, these conditions are grouped together; however, they differ significantly in their individual clinical and histological features. For example, in the muscle biopsy of a patient with DM, one may observe atrophic muscle fibers at the periphery of the fascicle and cellular infiltrates composed of B lymphocytes and CD4-positive T lymphocytes in both a perifascicular and perivascular distribution. Complement components and immunoglobulins line the capillary walls, as seen by immunohistochemistry (*1*). In contrast, the muscle biopsies of PM patients may show cellular infiltrates composed mainly of CD8-positive T lymphocytes surrounding and invading normal muscle fibers. By immunohistochemistry, myofibers can be seen to express major histocompatibility

S.J. DiMartino
Division of Rheumatology, Hospital for Special Surgery, Weill Medical College
of Cornell University, New York, NY, USA

L.J. Kagen (ed.), *The Inflammatory Myopathies*,
DOI 10.1007/978-1-60327-827-0_18,
© Humana Press. a part of Springer Science + Business Media, LLC 2009

complex (MHC) class I on their surface *(1)*. Furthermore, while DM and PM are autoimmune conditions, IBM appears to be a degenerative process *(2)*. Despite the differences listed, the IIMs share a common theme: immune-mediated attack on skeletal muscle that causes weakness in the patient. Thus, because the trigger for the autoimmune attack on muscle is unknown, as in other inflammatory diseases, the general approach to therapy is the use of medications that suppress the immune system.

Several issues should be considered before treating a patient with presumed IIM. The first issue is to determine whether the diagnosis is correct. Many noninflammatory myopathies and neurological conditions can mimic IIM, such as central and peripheral nervous system disorders, neuromuscular junction disorders, adult-onset muscular dystrophies, metabolic myopathies, endocrine myopathies, viral myopathies, or toxic myopathies. Because statins are commonly used in clinical practice today *(3)*, statin myopathy often must be considered in the differential diagnosis of weakness or myalgia. Usually, the different diagnoses can be distinguished using a combination of clinical features, serological studies, electromyography (EMG), magnetic resonance imaging (MRI), and muscle biopsy. Because all of these studies have their own limitations, however, even a thorough workup may yield an equivocal conclusion, and if the patient is deteriorating quickly, time is an important factor; the physician may be pressed to make a treatment decision despite an unclear diagnosis. In these situations, a good response to therapy retroactively supports the diagnosis of a treatable IIM, whereas a poor response to therapy suggests a noninflammatory myopathy, IBM, myositis associated with malignancy, or anti-SRP (signal recognition particle) syndrome. When IIM is associated with the presence of a malignancy, the symptoms attributable to myositis may precede the discovery of the malignancy. Often, these patients will respond poorly to therapy for the myositis but will respond to treatment of the malignancy *(4)*.

Another issue to consider is the choice and management of the therapy itself. Because IIM is rare, few randomized controlled trials (RCTs) with placebo have been performed. Most studies of therapies for IIM (including the RCTs) use a small number of patients, have varied outcome criteria, or include heterogeneous populations; these features make it difficult to draw conclusions about the studies and apply the results to individual patients. Indeed, treatment approaches remain empirical. Today, high doses of corticosteroids (maintained for many months) are the first line of therapy; at these doses, corticosteroids will cause many serious side effects or worsen preexisting medical problems (e.g., diabetes, hypertension, glaucoma, loss of bone density, infections). Therefore, numerous medical issues, in addition to the myositis itself, become active simultaneously. This requires coordination of care and good communication between several health care providers. Furthermore, treatment of the inflammatory myopathy with steroids can cause a toxic myopathy, a paradox unique to the treatment of IIM.

Another challenging issue is managing patients who respond partially or are refractory to therapy. Unfortunately, there is no clear definition of when a patient is refractory. Usually, a patient's response to therapy is measured by serial strength testing and serial muscle enzymes (creatine kinase [CK], aldolase, aspartate aminotransferase [AST], alanine aminotransferase [ALT], myoglobin, lactate dehydrogenase [LDH]).

A patient with little or no improvement of strength, little or no decrease in serum muscle enzymes, or both is considered refractory. A minimal response or lack of a response after 4–6 weeks should prompt several questions: Is the diagnosis correct? Was the patient compliant with the medications? Was the steroid dose appropriate? Were the steroids tapered too quickly? Was the immunosuppressive agent at a high enough dose for a sufficient period of time?

In patients with long-standing disease, it may be difficult to determine how much of the patient's weakness is due to active inflammation and how much is due to atrophy or irreversible muscle damage. Serum muscle enzymes, MRI, or repeat muscle biopsy can help determine whether inflammation is active.

## General Approach to Therapy

If there is no major contraindication to the use of corticosteroids, the patient is started on a high dose of corticosteroid; the individual is maintained on this dose until there is improvement of strength and there is a decrease in the serum levels of muscle enzymes (approximately 4-6 weeks), and then the dose is slowly reduced over many months. Because some with IIM may have a monocyclic disease course, patients who respond well to this therapy may eventually be tapered off steroids completely or may be maintained on a low dose. However, if patients do not respond well or if they flare during the taper, the addition of second-line therapies and possibly third-line therapies is then considered. During treatment, patients are usually followed closely using a combination of serum muscle enzyme evaluations, muscle strength testing, and attention to extramuscular manifestations of the disease. Of note, the muscle enzymes may return to normal before the patient has either subjective or objective improvement in strength. Moreover, a rise in muscle enzymes may predict subsequent worsening of clinical status (5).

The approach to IBM is controversial. IBM tends to respond poorly to all therapies. In a retrospective study, although no one with IBM had a complete response to steroid therapy, about one-half of patients had a partial response (6). However, in a small natural history study of 11 patients with IBM followed for 6 months, one-third of patients showed either stability of disease or even slight improvement (7). Therefore, some investigators believe that a trial of therapy, especially early in the disease course, may result in some improvement.

## Corticosteroids

In 1948, corticosteroids were first employed for the treatment of another autoimmune condition, rheumatoid arthritis (RA; reviewed in (8)). Since the 1950s, corticosteroids have been the first line of therapy for PM and DM. Prednisone (which is given orally) or methylprednisone (which is given orally or intravenously) are commonly used corticosteroids. Although there have not been adequate trials comparing different steroid treatment protocols, the recommendations of physicians who have treated a large number of IIM patients are similar. The following are three examples of specific approaches to steroid therapy.

1. In 1989, Oddis and Medsger *(5)* suggested the following: Start the patient on approximately 1 mg/kg/day or 60 mg prednisone (or equivalent steroid dose) daily in a divided dose and continue for at least 1 month and until the CK value has become normal. Then, decrease the dose by about 25% each month, with a goal of a once-daily maintenance dose of 5–10 mg per day (4–6 months).
2. Also in 1989, Dalakas *(9)* suggested the following: Start 80-100 mg once daily for 3–4 weeks, then taper over 10 weeks to 80–100 mg every other day. This can be achieved by reducing the "off-day" dose by 10 mg per week (side effects of the steroids may make a faster taper necessary) until the dose is zero. Assuming a clinical response, continue to reduce the dose by 5–10 mg every 3–4 weeks until down to approximately 50 mg every other day. At this point, the rate of taper is slowed even further to a decrease of 2.5 mg every few months.
3. In 2003, Amato and Griggs *(10)* suggested the following: Start the patient at 1–1.5 mg/kg/day of prednisone (maximum of 100 mg/day), changing to every-other-day dosing in 2–4 weeks (or 2–3 months in patients with more severe disease). This is continued until the patient has regained normal strength or until strength has plateaued (approximately 4–5 months). Then, taper by 5 mg every 2 weeks until at 20 mg every other day, then taper by no more than 2.5 mg every 2 weeks.

In a retrospective study of 113 patients with idiopathic inflammatory myopathy, Joffe et al. *(6)* showed that after the first prednisone trial, 25% of patients had a complete remission, 61% of patients had a partial response, and 14% of patients had no response. Patients who either have known malabsorption or fail to show cushingoid features after many weeks of high-dose prednisone may benefit from a change to methylprednisone or dexamethasone. Patients who have a flare of disease during the steroid taper may respond to one of the following: (1) a small increase in the steroid dose (e.g., by 5–10 mg) to bring the flare back under control, followed by a slower rate of dose reduction; (2) a large increase in the steroid dose (up to 40–60 mg), followed by a rapid reduction (over 2–3 weeks), to a level just above that when the patient flared, then followed by a slower rate of dose reduction; (3) intravenous pulse methylprednisone (e.g., 0.5–1 g daily for 3 days). The severity of the flare and the patient's medical comorbidities are considerations in choosing a course of action.

In 1999, Nzeusseu et al. *(11)* published a retrospective study in which 15 patients treated with high doses of steroid (>0.5 mg/kg) were compared to 10 patients treated with steroids at less than 0.5 mg/kg; functional outcomes were similar for both groups. The conclusion was that patients who have milder disease may respond well to a lower initial starting dose of corticosteroids, although it is not clear if this requires early initiation of an immunosuppressive agent. It has also been suggested that patients with overlap of another systemic inflammatory illness may need less corticosteroid *(12)*. Several reports have suggested that patients who are treated earlier in their disease course tend to respond better to therapy *(6,13)*. This may be analogous to emerging paradigms in the treatment of RA, in which early aggressive therapy of the autoimmune condition leads to better long-term outcomes *(14)*.

While intravenous pulse methylprednisone is typically used as a second-line agent or in situations of severe, life-threatening disease, it has also been suggested as an initial therapy *(15,16)*. In a study by Matsubara et al. *(17)*, 11 patients with PM and DM were treated with three consecutive daily infusions of 500 mg methyl prednisone (average of 4.3 courses) in addition to oral daily prednisone. When compared with a group of 14 patients who received only daily oral prednisone, the intravenous pulse methylprednisone group had a higher rate of remission and a faster return to normal for serum level of creatine kinase.

Unfortunately, patients taking high doses of corticosteroids for a prolonged period suffer numerous side effects. Patients with diabetes will likely have a worsening of hyperglycemia and may even require insulin; others may develop steroid-induced diabetes, and this may or may not resolve as the dose is reduced. New hypertension or worsening of preexisting hypertension may require that antihypertensives are either initiated or adjusted. Other common side effects include weight gain, thinning of the skin, frequent bruising, cataracts, glaucoma, insomnia, labile mood, difficulty with concentration, and muscle cramps. A decrease in bone density as a result of steroids can begin within weeks of the first dose; therefore, patients should be started on calcium and vitamin D supplementation immediately, and the use of a bisphosphonate should be considered. While a patient is taking chronic steroids, bone density testing should be performed every year. Steroid myopathy may be seen with moderate-to-high doses of corticosteroids. This toxic myopathy does not usually cause the serum CK to be elevated but can nevertheless complicate the clinical picture. Muscle enzyme levels and MRI of involved muscles may help distinguish; for example, in the setting of worsening weakness during a reduction of steroid dose, rising serum CK and evidence of inflammation on MRI would suggest a flare of disease, while absence of these findings would be suggestive of steroid myopathy. Steroid myopathy usually resolves as the steroids are tapered.

## Immunosuppressive Agents and Other Treatments

Immunosuppressive drugs or intravenous immunoglobulin (IVIg) may often be added when adequate steroid therapy is not effective, if the patient flares frequently during steroid taper of appropriate rate, if the side effects of the steroids are not at all tolerable, if the patient responds but there is a need for a "steroid-sparing" agent, or if the disease is severe and rapidly progressive. In patients who have no response or a poor response to an adequate steroid trial, it is always important to reconsider the diagnosis, possibly repeating or performing new diagnostic tests. If the patient does not respond to an adequate trial of a second-line agent (at an appropriate dose for a reasonable duration) or is intolerant, then another second-line or third-line agent is added or substituted.

## Methotrexate and Azathioprine

Methotrexate and azathioprine are the most commonly used second-line agents. Methotrexate inhibits dihydrofolate reductase, an enzyme responsible for converting folic acid into a form required for synthesis of some nucleic and amino acids. Methotrexate also exerts a more direct anti-inflammatory effect by promoting the release of adenosine at sites of inflammation *(18)*. In general, the drug is prescribed at 15–25 mg weekly, taken orally, subcutaneously, or intramuscularly. For the treatment of inflammatory myopathy, several publications have described higher doses and have employed the intravenous route. Folic acid or folinic acid is given in addition to the methotrexate to help minimize the side effects. Azathioprine is a purine analog that inhibits the synthesis of purines, thus interfering with the proliferation and function of lymphocytes. Azathioprine is typically prescribed at 1.5–2.0 mg/kg/day orally. Patients who are homozygous, deficient in the enzyme thiopurine methyltransferase (TPMT) are more likely to suffer toxicity from this drug.

In 1973, Arnett et al. *(19)* treated five patients with steroid-resistant PM, using oral or intravenous methotrexate in doses up to 50 mg weekly. Four of five patients improved, but two developed pneumonitis, which contributed to the death of one patient. In 1974, Metzger et al. *(20)* treated 22 patients with steroid-resistant PM or DM using prednisone and methotrexate (average maintenance dose of 42 mg IV weekly). Patients were treated for an average of 15 months. Seventeen patients had improved muscle strength and a decrease in serum CK level, and steroid doses were significantly reduced. Toxicity was minimal and reversible on discontinuation of the drug. In a retrospective cohort study published in 1993, there were 55 patients with IIM (including IBM) previously treated with an adequate trial of steroids who were also treated with methotrexate (minimum of 5 mg/week for 8 weeks): 31 patients had a partial response, and 9 patients had a complete response *(6)*.

In 2000, Vencovsky et al. *(21)* published a randomized trial of methotrexate versus cyclosporine; 36 patients with DM and PM (either newly diagnosed or a relapse of previously quiescent myositis) were randomized to either 7.5–15 mg of weekly oral methotrexate or 3–3.5 mg/kg/day of cyclosporine. Both groups were also treated with prednisone at 0.5–1.0 mg/kg daily and were followed for 6 months. Both groups showed improvement as assessed by strength testing, serum muscle enzymes, and MRI. There was no significant difference in efficacy or toxicity.

In 1980, Bunch et al. *(22)* published an RCT in which 16 patients were treated with 60 mg of prednisone daily and either azathioprine (2 mg/kg/day) or placebo. After 3 months, there was no significant difference between the groups as measured by strength testing and histopathology on muscle biopsy. However, during the 3-year, uncontrolled follow-up, the group who received azathioprine had less functional disability and required a lower prednisone maintenance dose (1.6 mg/day vs. 8.7 mg/day) *(23)*.

In 2002, Miller et al. *(24)* published an abstract describing a randomized double-blind trial of methotrexate (15 mg weekly) plus steroids versus azathioprine (2.5 mg/kg/day) plus steroids in 28 patients with PM and DM. There was no significant difference in efficacy as measured by handheld myometry and change in timed walks, and there was no difference in the final steroid dose after 1 year.

In 1998, Villalba et al. *(25)* published a randomized crossover study of 30 patients with steroid-refractory PM and DM (most patients had also failed a trial of one immunosuppressive agent); patients were randomized to either escalating oral methotrexate (7.5 mg escalated to 22.5–25 mg/weekly) plus escalating azathioprine (50 mg escalating to 150 mg/day) versus intravenous methotrexate at 500 mg/m$^2$ followed by leucovorin rescue. Patients could cross over to the other arm at 3 or 6 months if they failed to improve. Eight of the 15 patients who received the oral combination therapy improved, while only 3 of the 15 who received intravenous methotrexate improved. After crossover, four people improved after receiving oral combination therapy, while one person improved after receiving intravenous methotrexate.

## Intravenous Immunoglobulin

IVIg preparations contain purified immunoglobulin (Ig) G from pooled human plasma. The dosage of IVIg is usually given at a total 2 g/kg, administered in monthly intervals. IVIg often contains a low level of IgA, which can cause an allergic reaction in patients who have IgA deficiency; therefore, it is important to check for IgA deficiency before initiating IVIg. Aseptic meningitis, a common side effect, appears to be related to the infusion rate; therefore, the dose is often split over 3–4 days at approximately 0.5 g/kg/day. There are many preparations of IVIg that are available, each with varied salt and sugar content; this may be a consideration in patients with medical comorbidities. The mechanism of action is unknown; however, many have been proposed: blockading of Fc receptors by the Fc portion of IgG; stimulation of inhibitory Fc receptors; binding to and occupying complement components; directly neutralizing autoantibodies by anti-idiotypes present in the IVIg; and reducing the half-life of autoantibodies by saturation of the IgG salvage receptor FcRn.

In 1993, Dalakas et al. *(26)* published a placebo-controlled trial in 15 patients with DM who were refractory to steroids or an immunosuppressive agent for at least 4 months. Patients continued to receive prednisone and either placebo or three monthly treatments of IVIg at 2 mg/kg. All patients in the IVIg group had improvement of strength; the placebo group did not. After a crossover phase, four patients who had previously received IVIg worsened or stayed the same after receiving placebo. Four patients who initially received placebo were crossed over to IVIg, and all patients improved. Biopsies taken after treatment with IVIg, compared with those taken before treatment, showed reduction of MHC class I, transforming growth factor beta (TGFβ), and adhesion molecules as well as a decrease in complement component deposition in muscle. Placebo-controlled studies performed in patients with IBM (also treated for 3 months at 2 mg/kg) failed to show statistically significant improvement of strength. However, in one trial there was a trend toward improvement with statistically significant benefit in muscles used for swallowing. In a second study, reduction in clinical progression was noted. For these reasons, many clinicians believe that some patients with IBM may benefit from a trial of IVIg *(27)*. In refractory PM, an uncontrolled study of IVIg (monthly doses at 2 g/kg for 4–5 months) in 35 patients showed significant improvement of strength in 71% of patients, with significant reductions in serum CK levels *(28)*. Steroid doses in these patients also were able to be reduced.

# Cyclosporine

Cyclosporine is an inhibitor of T-cell activation that has been used in transplant medicine (for the prevention of organ rejection) and as therapy for RA and psoriasis. Starting dose is usually 2.0–2.5 mg/kg/day and can be slowly increased to a maximum of 5.0 mg/kg/day.

In 1996, Zeller et al. *(29)* published a retrospective study of six patients with juvenile DM who had failed corticosteroids; four patients had also failed second-line agents. Patients were treated with 5–6 mg/kg/day of cyclosporine, were continued on corticosteroids, and were followed for a mean of 51.5 months. All patients exhibited improved control of disease and were able to taper their steroids. Three patients relapsed after discontinuation of cyclosporine, but their disease came under control once the drug was reintroduced.

In 1987, Jones and colleagues *(30)* published a letter describing two patients who failed treatment with cyclosporine and experienced significant side effects. In 2000, Qushmaq et al. *(31)* published their experience treating six patients (four with PM, two with DM) who had failed corticosteroids and at least one second-line agent. Doses used ranged from 2.4 to 4.2 mg/kg/day, and patients were followed for 3–44 months. All patients demonstrated a reduction in CK level and improvement in strength; all but one were able to taper their prednisone dose.

Also in 2000, Vencovsky et al. *(21)* published a randomized trial of methotrexate versus cyclosporine in patients with DM and PM (either newly diagnosed or a relapse of previously quiescent myositis). Thirty-six patients were randomized to either 7.5–15 mg of weekly oral methotrexate or 3–3.5 mg/kg/day of cyclosporine. Because in this study cyclosporine was not superior to methotrexate over 6 months, the authors concluded that methotrexate would be a better choice for a second-line therapy (due to cost and expectation of long-term toxicity).

# Mycophenolate Mofetil

Mycophenolate mofetil (MMF) has been commonly employed to suppress rejection of organ transplants. The drug inhibits inosine monophosphate dehydrogenase, an enzyme important for purine synthesis, and thereby impairs the proliferation of both

B and T lymphocytes. MMF is typically started orally at 250 or 500 mg twice per day and is escalated every few weeks up to 1,000 mg twice daily.

In 1999, Gelber et al. *(32)* treated four patients with classic skin manifestations of DM (two patients also had muscle involvement) with MMF. All patients had failed hydroxychloroquine, three of four failed corticosteroids and methotrexate. Patients were treated with 1,000–1,500 mg twice daily for 6–20 months. All patients saw improvement in the skin findings, one patient had an improvement in strength, and three patients were able to taper their steroid dose.

In 2005, Majithia et al. *(33)* published a case series of seven patients with biopsy-proven IIM who had an inadequate response to corticosteroids and other immunosuppressive agents. Patients were treated with MMF in doses up to 1,000 mg twice daily. Six of seven patients had improvement of weakness, and all patients had a decrease in the levels of their muscle enzymes.

In 2006, Edge et al. *(34)* published a retrospective chart review of 12 patients with DM who had failed conventional therapy; patients were treated with MMF in doses up to 1,000 mg twice daily. Ten of 12 patients had an improvement of skin findings and increased strength and were able to taper concomitant therapies. One patient developed B-cell lymphoma of the central nervous system.

## Tacrolimus

Tacrolimus is an inhibitor of T-cell activation that has been previously employed in transplant medicine. In 1999, Oddis et al. *(35)* published on the treatment of eight patients with IIM (six with anti-Jo-1 antibody) who had failed corticosteroids and at least one immunosuppressive agent. Patients were treated with oral tacrolimus at 0.075 mg/kg/day (target 12-h plasma trough of 5–20 ng/ml) for a mean of 4–6 months. All patients had improvement of strength, with five of the six anti-Jo-1 patients achieving normal strength (in three of these patients, CK levels became normal within 1 month of therapy). One patient developed hypertension and worsening renal function.

In 2005, Wilkes et al. *(36)* published a retrospective study of 13 patients with antisynthetase syndrome and interstitial lung disease. Patients were treated with the same dosing described above for an average of 51.2 months. A significant improvement was observed in all pulmonary function test (PFT) parameters. All patients had a decrease in their CK level; strength in most patients either was improved or was unchanged despite a significant reduction of steroid dose.

## Rituximab

CD20 is a transmembrane cell surface molecule found on all normal mature B cells thought to function as a calcium channel. Rituximab is a chimeric monoclonal antibody of human and murine origin that recognizes CD20 and binds to and causes the depletion of B cells in peripheral blood and lymph nodes. Recently, it has come to be used as first-line therapy in the treatment of some B-cell lymphomas. The therapeutic benefit of rutiximab in the treatment of autoimmune hemolytic anemia and immune thrombocytopenia purpura has led to its increased use in the treatment of other autoimmune diseases. Trials of rituximab in RA, and Wegner's granulomatosis have shown promising results.

Dermatomyositis displays several features that suggest that B cells may play an important role in pathogenesis. These include the presence of autoantibodies (which also may be present in the other inflammatory myopathies), the presence of immune complex deposits in the dermal-epidermal junction of skin lesions and capillaries in muscle, and the presence of B cells within the inflammatory muscle lesions. In 2005, a small open-label trial of rituximab in DM was reported (37). In addition to standard therapy, seven adults were treated with four weekly infusions of rituximab; B cells were depleted in all patients. All patients had improvement in muscle strength, between 36 and 113%. In four patients, return of symptoms correlated with return of B cells. Other symptoms, including rash, alopecia, and reduced forced vital capacity, also showed improvement.

Noss et al. (38) published three cases of patients with IIM (two with PM, one with DM) who had failed corticosteroids and either methotrexate or azathioprine; they were treated with intravenous rituximab at 1,000 mg on days 0 and 14. All three patients showed an improvement of strength, with two patients achieving normal strength. CK levels became normal in all patients (average time to normal CK was 4.6 months). The dose of corticosteroid was reduced in all. Two patients had disease flares manifested by weakness and increased CK at 6–10 months and were re-treated. After re-treatment, CK returned to normal, but changes in strength were not discussed.

Mok et al. (39) published a report of four patients with active PM who were refractory to conventional therapy. Patients were treated with four consecutive weekly doses of 375 mg/m$^2$ of intravenous rituximab. At 28 weeks, all patients had a reduction of CK level. Two patients returned to normal strength, while two patients had a mild improvement of strength.

Chung et al. (40) treated eight patients with refractory DM with two infusions of intravenous rituximab (1,000 mg for each infusion given 2 weeks apart). Three patients had an improvement in muscle strength, but muscle enzymes and skin scores were not significantly changed at 24 weeks.

## Tumor Necrosis Factor Alpha Blockade

The tumor necrosis factor alpha (TNFα) antagonists (infliximab, etanercept, adalimumab) have revolutionized the treatment of RA. In vitro, TNFα blockade was shown to significantly reduce production of other proinflammatory cytokines by leukocytes from patients with RA. In animal models of chronic arthritis, TNFα blockade has dramatically ameliorated disease. These observations placed TNFαat a critical point in a proinflammatory cytokine cascade. Currently, TNFα blockade is used for both acute and maintenance treatment of rheumatoid arthritis, the spondyloarthropathies, and Crohn's disease.

TNFα has been implicated in the pathogenesis of inflammatory myopathy. Utilizing immunohistochemistry and in situ hybridization, Kuru and colleagues *(41)* showed that muscle fibers from patients with DM and PM both expressed and synthesized TNFα. TNFα, messenger RNA (mRNA), and protein were also found in the muscle fibers taken from patients with Duchenne muscular dystrophy but not in muscle fibers taken from patients with neurogenic disorders or other comparison specimens, suggesting that TNFα expression is not disease specific but rather a common pathophysiologic factor in inflammation and cell damage. Observations such as these led investigators to employ TNFα blockade in both PM and DM.

Several reports, including either one or a few patients, have shown that treated patients have had improvement of strength and decrease of serum muscle enzymes activities *(42–44)*. Another report, however, described the development of myositis in a patient with RA who was treated with infliximab *(45)*. Efthimiou et al. *(46)* published a retrospective study of eight patients with DM and PM who had failed conventional therapy and were treated with etanercept (six patients), infliximab (one patient), or both (one patient). After follow-up for an average of 15.2 months, six patients had an improvement of strength (all treated with etanercept), and all of these patients saw a reduction in their CK. Hengstman et al. *(47)* published the results of an open-label trial of infliximab and methotrexate in drug-naïve patients with DM and PM. Six patients were treated, but the trial was terminated early because of a low inclusion rate and high dropout rate (a result of disease progression).

Dastmalchi et al. *(48)* published the results of an open-label pilot study of infliximab in 13 patients with PM (5 patients), DM (4 patients), and IBM (4 patients) who had failed conventional therapy. Three patients withdrew due to adverse events (weakness, severe erythema, and severe cough in one patient each). Of those who completed the study, three improved by 20% or more in three of the six IMACS (International Myositis Assessment and Clinical Studies Group) core variables for disease activity, four were unchanged, and two worsened.

## Plasma Exchange

Plasma exchange has been used to treat autoimmune conditions with the goal of reducing the levels of autoantibodies, cytokines, or circulating immune complexes. Miller et al. *(49)* published an RCT in which 39 patients with PM and DM were randomized to plasma exchange, leukopheresis, or sham apheresis. During the study period, the dose of corticosteroids was held constant, and no immunosuppressive drugs were used. Patients received three treatments per week for four consecutive weeks and were assessed at 1 month. At 1 month, there was no significant difference in strength between groups. Cherin et al. *(50)* reported the treatment of 57 patients with PM and DM (38 acute cases, 19 subacute or chronic cases). Patients were treated with three sessions weekly for 3 weeks, then two sessions bimonthly for a mean of 14.8 treatments. Thirty nine patients were continued on corticosteroids and an immunosuppressive agent. Clinical improvement was observed in 54% of patients; all of the patients who improved were treated early in the course of disease.

# References

1. Dalakas MC, Hohlfeld R. Polymyositis and dermatomyositis. Lancet 2003;362:971–82.
2. Askanas V, Engel WK. Inclusion-body myositis, a multifactorial muscle disease associated with aging: current concepts of pathogenesis. Curr Opin Rheumatol 2007;19:550–9.
3. Baer AN, Wortmann RL. Myotoxicity associated with lipid-lowering drugs. Curr Opin Rheumatol 2007;19:67–73.
4. Levine SM. Cancer and myositis: new insights into an old association. Curr Opin Rheumatol 2006;18:620–4.
5. Oddis CV, Medsger TA. Current management of polymyositis and dermatomyositis. Drugs 1989;37:382–90.
6. Joffe MM, Love LA, Leff RL, et al. Drug therapy of the idiopathic inflammatory myopathies: predictors of response to prednisone, azathioprine, and methotrexate and a comparison of their efficacy. Am J Med 1993;94:379–87.
7. Cohen MR, Sulaiman AR, Garancis JC, Wortmann RL. Clinical heterogeneity and treatment response in inclusion body myositis. Arthritis Rheum 1989;32:734–40.
8. Neeck G. Fifty years of experience with cortisone therapy in the study and treatment of rheumatoid arthritis. Ann N Y Acad Sci 2002;966:28–38.
9. Dalakas M. Treatment of polymyositis and dermatomyositis. Curr Opin Rheumatol 1989;1:443–9.
10. Amato AA, Griggs RC. Treatment of idiopathic inflammatory myopathies. Curr Opin Neurol 2003;16:569–75.
11. Nzeusseu A, Brion F, Lefebvre C, et al. Functional outcome of myositis patients: can a low-dose glucocorticoid regimen achieve good functional results? Clin Exp Rheumatol 1999;17:441–6.
12. Oddis CV. Idiopathic inflammatory myopathies: a treatment update. Curr Rheumatol Rep 2003;5:431–6.
13. Tymms KE, Webb J. Dermatopolymyositis and other connective tissue diseases: a review of 105 cases. J Rheumatol 1985;12:1140–8.
14. Quinn MA, Emery P. Window of opportunity in early rheumatoid arthritis: possibility of altering the disease process with early intervention. Clin Exp Rheumatol 2003;21(5)Suppl 31:S154–7.
15. Laxer RM., Stein LD, Petty RE. Intravenous pulse methylprednisolone treatment of juvenile dermatomyositis. Arthritis Rheum 1987;30:328–34.
16. Bolosiu HD, Man L, Rednic S. The effect of methylprednisone pulse therapy in polymyositis/dermatomyositis. Adv Exp Med Biol 1999;455:349–57.
17. Matsubara S, Sawa Y, Takamori M, Yokoyama H, Kida H. Pulsed intravenous methylprednisolone combined with oral steroids as the initial treatment of inflammatory myopathies. J Neurol Neurosurg Psychiatry 1994;57(8):1008.
18. Cronstein BN, Naime D, Ostad E. The anti-inflammatory effects of methotrexate are mediated by adenosine. Adv Exp Med Biol 1994;370:411–6.
19. Arnett FC, Whelton JC, Zizic TM, Stevens MB. Methotrexate therapy in polymyositis. Ann Rheum Dis 1973;32:536–46.

20. Metzger AL, Bohan A, Goldberg LS, Bluestone R, Pearson CM. Polymyositis and dermatomyositis: combined methotrexate and corticosteroid therapy. Ann Intern Med 1974;81:182–9.
21. Vencovsky J, Jarosova K, Machacek S, et al. Cyclosporine A versus methotrexate in the treatment of polymyositis and dermatomyositis. Scand J Rheumatol 2000;29:95–102.
22. Bunch TW, Worthington JW, Combs JJ, Ilstrup DM, Engel AG. Azathioprine with prednisone for polymyositis. A controlled, clinical trial. Ann Intern Med 1980;92:365–9.
23. Bunch TW. Prednisone and azathioprine for polymyositis: long-term followup. Arthritis Rheum 1981;24:45–8.
24. Miller J, Walsh Y, Saminaden S, Lecky BRF, Winer, JB. Randomized double blind trial of methotrexate and steroids compared with azathioprine and steroids in the treatment of idiopathic inflammatory myopathy. J Neurol Sci 2002;199(Suppl 1):S53.
25. Villalba L, Hicks JE, Adams EM, et al. Treatment of refractory myositis: a randomized crossover study of two new cytotoxic regimens. Arthritis Rheum 1998;41:392–9.
26. Dalakas MC, Illa I, Dambrosia JM, et al. A controlled trial of high-dose intravenous immune globulin infusions as treatment for dermatomyositis. N Engl J Med 1993;329:1993–2000.
27. Dalakas MC. Intravenous immunoglobulin in autoimmune neuromuscular diseases. JAMA 2004;291:2367–75.
28. Cherin P, Pelletier S, Teixeira A, et al. Results and long-term followup of intravenous immunoglobulin infusions in chronic, refractory polymyositis: an open study with thirty-five adult patients. Arthritis Rheum 2002;46:467–74.
29. Zeller V, Cohen P, Prieur AM, Guillevin L. Cyclosporin a therapy in refractory juvenile dermatomyositis. Experience and longterm followup of 6 cases. J Rheumatol 1996;23:1424–7.
30. Jones DW, Snaith ML, Isenberg DA. Cyclosporine treatment for intractable polymyositis. Arthritis Rheum 1987;30:959–60.
31. Qushmaq KA, Chalmers A, Esdaile JM. Cyclosporin A in the treatment of refractory adult polymyositis/dermatomyositis: population based experience in 6 patients and literature review. J Rheumatol 2000;27:2855–9.
32. Gelber AC, Nousari HC, Wigley, FM. Mycophenolate mofetil in the treatment of severe skin manifestations of dermatomyositis: a series of 4 cases. J Rheumatol 1999;27:1542–5.
33. Majithia V, Harisdangkul V. Mycophenolate mofetil (CellCept): an alternative therapy for autoimmune inflammatory myopathy [erratum appears in Rheumatology (Oxford) 2005;44(4):569]. Rheumatology 2005;44:386–9.
34. Edge JC, Outland JD, Dempsey JR, Callen JP. Mycophenolate mofetil as an effective corticosteroid-sparing therapy for recalcitrant dermatomyositis. Arch Dermatol 2006;142:65–9.
35. Oddis CV, Sciurba FC, Elmagd KA, Starzl TE. Tacrolimus in refractory polymyositis with interstitial lung disease. Lancet 1999;353:1762–3.
36. Wilkes MR, Sereika SM, Fertig N, Lucas MR, Oddis CV. Treatment of antisynthetase-associated interstitial lung disease with tacrolimus. Arthritis Rheum 2005;52:2439–46.
37. Levine TD. Rituximab in the treatment of dermatomyositis: an open-label pilot study. Arthritis Rheum 2005;52:601–7.
38. Noss EH, Hausner-Sypek DL, Weinblatt ME. Rituximab as therapy for refractory polymyositis and dermatomyositis. J Rheumatol 2006;33:1021–6.
39. Mok CC, Ho LY, To CH. Rituximab for refractory polymyositis: an open-label prospective study. J Rheumatol 2007;34:1864–8.
40. Chung L, Genovese MC, Fiorentino DF. A pilot trial of rituximab in the treatment of patients with dermatomyositis. Arch Dermatol 2007;143:763–7.
41. Kuru S, Inukai A, Kato T, et al. Expression of tumor necrosis factor-alpha in regenerating muscle fibers in inflammatory and non-inflammatory myopathies. Acta Neuropathol 2003;105:217–24.
42. Labioche I, Liozon E, Weschler B, et al. Refractory polymyositis responding to infliximab: extended follow-up. Rheumatology 2004;43:531–2.

43. Hengstman GJ, van den Hoogen FH, Barrera P, et al. Successful treatment of dermatomyositis and polymyositis with anti-tumor-necrosis-factor-alpha: preliminary observations. Eur Neurol 2003;50:10–5.
44. Sprott H, Glatzel M, Michel BA. Treatment of myositis with etanercept (Enbrel), a recombinant human soluble fusion protein of TNF-alpha type II receptor and IgG1. Rheumatology 2004;43:524–6.
45. Musial J, Undas A, Celinska-Lowenhoff M. Polymyositis associated with infliximab treatment for rheumatoid arthritis. Rheumatology 2003;42:1566–8.
46. Efthimiou P, Schwartzman S, Kagen LJ. Possible role for tumour necrosis factor inhibitors in the treatment of resistant dermatomyositis and polymyositis: a retrospective study of eight patients. Ann Rheum Dis 2006;65:1233–6.
47. Hengstman GJ, De Bleeker JL, Feist E, et al. Open-label trial of anti-TNF-a in dermato- and polymyositis treated concomitantly with methotrexate. Eur Neurol 2008;59:159–63.
49. Miller FW, Leitman SF, Cronin ME, et al. Controlled trial of plasma exchange and leukapheresis in polymyositis and dermatomyositis [see comment]. N Engl J Med 1992;326:1380–4.
50. Cherin P, Auperin I, Bussel A, Pourrat J, Herson S. Plasma exchange in polymyositis and dermatomyositis: a multicenter study of 57 cases. Clin Exp Rheumatol 1995;13:270–1.

# Index